The 5-Minute Patient Advisor

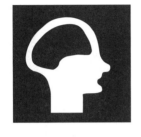

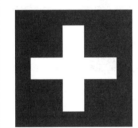

The 5-Minute Patient Advisor

MARK R. DAMBRO, MD, FAAFP

FORT WORTH, TEXAS

FORMERLY ASSISTANT PROFESSOR OF MEDICINE

AND

DIRECTOR OF MEDICAL COMPUTING

UNIVERSITY OF ARIZONA COLLEGE OF MEDICINE

TUCSON, ARIZONA

 LIPPINCOTT WILLIAMS & WILKINS
A **Wolters Kluwer** Company
Philadelphia · Baltimore · New York · London
Buenos Aires · Hong Kong · Sydney · Tokyo

Acquisitions Editor: Richard Winters
Developmental Editor: Delois Patterson
Production Editor: W. Christopher Granville
Manufacturing Manager: Tim Reynolds
Cover Designer: Christine Jenny
Compositor: TechBooks
Printer: RR Donnelley Willard

© 2001 by LIPPINCOTT WILLIAMS & WILKINS
530 Walnut Street
Philadelphia, PA 19106 USA
LWW.com

All rights reserved. This book is protected by copyright. No part of this book may be reproduced in any form or by any means, including photocopying, or utilized by any information storage and retrieval system without written permission from the copyright owner, except for brief quotations embodied in critical articles and reviews. Materials appearing in this book prepared by individuals as part of their official duties as U.S. government employees are not covered by the above-mentioned copyright.

Printed in the USA

Library of Congress Cataloging-in-Publication Data

Dambro, Mark R.
　The 5-minute patient advisor / Mark R. Dambro ; consulting author Bruce Goldfarb.
　　p. cm.
　Derived from Griffith's 5 minute clinical consult.
　Includes index.
　ISBN 0-7817-3067-8
　1. Family—Health and hygiene—Outlines, syllabi, etc.　2. Diseases—Outlines, syllabi, etc.　I. Title: Five minute patient advisor.　II. Goldfarb, Bruce.　III. Griffith's 5 minute clinical consult.　IV. Title.

RA777.7 .D364　2000
616'.002'02—dc21

00-049326

Care has been taken to confirm the accuracy of the information presented and to describe generally accepted practices. However, the author and publisher are not responsible for errors or omissions or for any consequences from application of the information in this book and make no warranty, expressed or implied, with respect to the currency, completeness, or accuracy of the contents of the publication. Application of this information in a particular situation remains the professional responsibility of the practitioner.

The author and publisher have exerted every effort to ensure that drug selection and dosage set forth in this text are in accordance with current recommendations and practice at the time of publication. However, in view of ongoing research, changes in government regulations, and the constant flow of information relating to drug therapy and drug reactions, the reader is urged to check the package insert for each drug for any change in indications and dosage and for added warnings and precautions. This is particularly important when the recommended agent is a new or infrequently employed drug.

Some drugs and medical devices presented in this publication have Food and Drug Administration (FDA) clearance for limited use in restricted research settings. It is the responsibility of the health care provider to ascertain the FDA status of each drug or device planned for use in their clinical practice.

10 9 8 7 6 5 4 3 2 1

Contents

Preface / ix

SECTION A

Acetaminophen Poisoning / 1
Acne / 5
Adenovirus Infections / 7
Alcoholism / 9
Alopecia / 13
Altitude Illness / 15
Alzheimer's Disease / 19
Amenorrhea / 23
Anaphylaxis / 25
Anemia, Pernicious / 27
Anemia, Sickle Cell / 29
Angina / 33
Animal Bites / 35
Anxiety / 37
Appendicitis, Acute / 41
Arteriosclerotic Heart Disease / 43
Arthritis, Osteo / 47
Arthritis, Rheumatoid (RA) / 49
Asthma / 51
Attention Deficit Hyperactivity Disorder / 55

SECTION B

Balanitis / 59
Basal Cell Carcinoma / 61
Bed Wetting / 63
Bell's Palsy / 65
Blepharitis / 67
Breast Cancer / 69
Breast Feeding / 73
Bronchitis, Acute / 77
Bulimia / 79
Burns / 83
Bursitis / 85

SECTION C

Candidiasis / 87
Carbon Monoxide Poisoning / 89
Carpal Tunnel Syndrome / 91
Cataract / 93
Cervical Dysplasia / 95
Chickenpox / 97
Child Abuse / 101
Chlamydial Sexually Transmitted Diseases / 103
Cholera / 105
Chronic Fatigue Syndrome / 107
Chronic Obstructive Pulmonary Disease and Emphysema / 109
Cirrhosis of the Liver / 113
Claudication / 115
Common Cold / 117
Congestive Heart Failure / 121
Constipation / 125
Contraception / 129
Crohn's Disease / 133
Croup / 137
Cutaneous (Skin) Drug Reactions / 139
Cystic Fibrosis / 141

SECTION D

Dehydration / 145
Dementia / 147
Depression / 149
Dermatitis, Contact / 153
Diabetes Mellitus, Insulin-Dependent (IDDM or Type I) / 155
Diabetes Mellitus, Non–Insulin-Dependent (NIDDM) / 159
Diaper Rash / 163
Diarrhea, Acute / 165
Dissociative Disorders / 167
Diverticular Disease / 171
Dysfunctional Uterine Bleeding / 173
Dysmenorrhea / 175

SECTION E

Eclampsia / 177
Endometriosis / 179
Epididymitis / 181
Epiglottitis / 183

SECTION F

Fatigue / 185
Fecal Incontinence / 187
Fertility Problems / 189
Fibrocystic Breast Disease / 191
Food Allergy / 193

Food Poisoning, Bacterial / 195
Frostbite / 197

SECTION G

Gallstones / 199
Gastritis / 201
Gastroesophageal Reflux Disease / 203
Genital Warts / 207
German Measles / 209
Gingivitis / 211
Glaucoma / 213
Glomerulonephritis, Acute / 215
Gonorrhea / 217
Gout / 219

SECTION H

Halitosis / 221
Headache, Cluster / 223
Headache, Tension / 225
Head Lice / 229
Heart Attack / 231
Heat Exhaustion and Heat Stroke / 235
Hemorrhoids / 237
Hepatitis, Viral / 239
Herpes Simplex / 241
Herpes, Genital / 243
Hirsutism / 245
HIV Infection and AIDS / 247
Hodgkin's Disease / 251
Huntington's Chorea / 253
Hypertension, Essential / 255
Hyperthyroidism / 259
Hypothermia / 261
Hypothyroidism, Adult / 265

SECTION I

Immunizations / 267
Impetigo / 269
Impotence / 271
Influenza / 273
Inner Ear Infection / 277
Insect Bites and Stings / 279
Insomnia / 283
Iron Deficiency Anemia / 287
Irritable Bowel Syndrome / 289

SECTION J

Jaundice / 291
Jet Lag / 293

SECTION K

Kaposi's Sarcoma / 295
Kidney Stones / 297

SECTION L

Laryngitis / 301
Lazy Eye / 303
Lead Poisoning / 305
Leukemia, Acute Lymphoblastic in Adults
   (ALL) / 309
Light Sensitivity / 311
Low Back Pain / 313
Lumbar Disk Disorders / 315
Lyme Disease / 317
Lymphoma, Burkitt's / 319
Lymphoma, Non-Hodgkin's / 321

SECTION M

Macular Degeneration, Age-Related
   (ARMD) / 323
Meniere's Disease / 325
Meningitis, Bacterial / 329
Meningitis, Viral / 331
Menopause / 333
Menorrhagia / 337
Middle Ear Infection / 339
Migraine / 341
Miscarriage / 345
Mitral Valve Prolapse / 347
Molluscum Contagiosum / 349
Mononucleosis / 351
Motion Sickness / 353
Multiple Sclerosis / 355
Mumps / 359

SECTION N

Nail Fungus / 361
Nosebleed / 363

SECTION O

Obesity / 365
Obsessive-Compulsive Disorder / 369
Osteoporosis / 371
Ovarian Cancer / 375

SECTION P

Painful Intercourse / 377
Pancreatitis / 379
Parkinson's Disease / 381
Parvovirus B19 Infection / 383
Pelvic Inflammatory Disease (PID) / 385
Peptic Ulcer Disease / 387
Pink Eye / 389
Pinworms / 391
Pneumonia, Bacterial / 393
Pneumonia, Viral / 395
Posttraumatic Stress Disorder (PTSD) / 397
Preeclampsia / 401
Premature Labor / 403
Premenstrual Syndrome (PMS) / 405
Prostate Cancer / 407
Prostatic Hyperplasia, Benign (BPH) / 409
Psoriasis / 411

SECTION R

Rabies / 413
Rape (Sexual Assault) / 415
Rash (Urticaria) / 419
Raynaud's Phenomenon / 423
Renal Failure, Acute (ARF) / 425
Retinal Detachment / 427
Rhinitis, Allergic / 429
Rocky Mountain Spotted Fever / 433
Rosacea / 435

SECTION S

Salmonella Infection / 437
Scabies / 441
Schizophrenia / 443
Scoliosis / 445
Seasonal Affective Disorder / 447
Seizure Disorders / 449
Seizures, Febrile / 451

Shingles / 453
Sinusitis / 455
Sleep Apnea, Obstructive / 457
Snakebite / 461
Sore Throat / 463
Sprains and Strains / 465
Stroke (Brain Attack) / 467
Stye / 471
Sudden Infant Death Syndrome (SIDS) / 473
Sunburn / 475
Swimmer's Ear / 477
Syphilis / 479
Systemic Lupus Erythematosus (SLE) / 481

SECTION T

Temporomandibular Joint (TMJ) Syndrome / 485
Tendinitis / 487
Tinea / 489
Toxic Shock Syndrome / 491
Toxoplasmosis / 493
Transient Ischemic Attack (TIA) / 497
Tuberculosis / 499

SECTION U

Ulcerative Colitis / 501
Urinary Incontinence / 505
Urinary Tract Infection in Men / 509
Urinary Tract Infection in Women / 511

SECTION V

Vaginal Bleeding During Pregnancy / 515
Vaginal Yeast Infection / 517
Varicose Veins / 519
Vitamin Deficiency / 521
Vulvovaginitis, Estrogen Deficient / 525

SECTION W

Warts / 527

Subject Index / 531

Preface

This *5 Minute Patient Advisor* will, I hope, provide both physician and patient a valuable reference. These pages, copied to be given to a patient with a specific condition, or kept at home as a reference, help patient's better understand their conditions. It is my firm belief that with better understanding comes better healthcare. While nothing can substitute for a clinician's experience, knowledge, understanding and sympathy, a quick reference sometimes can help us over a difficult issue or through a long night, as we struggle with questions and fears. If a few patient's fears are alleviated, or a few are motivated to follow treatment advice, or a few are empowered to not call after hours, then the *5 Minute Patient Advisor* will have succeeded.

The format of this edition encourages you to copy and distribute, as widely as possible, the information – please do so. I believe most patient's will appreciate the extra time spent in helping them achieve the goal of better understanding. And if you are a patient who has chosen to keep the entire set of topics for your personal library, I hope it helps you to understand these conditions just a bit better and helps you to be a better patient when you seek your physician's counsel.

This work is based on Griffith's 5 Minute Clinical Consult, a book covering over 1000 medical topics for the practicing clinician. I've tried in the *5 Minute Patient Advisor* to include the most common problems facing a patient-if I've missed a topic, let me know and I'll try to get it included in the next edition. Many thanks go to the authors of the parent book who have, every year, contributed their medical knowledge toward helping their peers, and now patients, better understand the conditions they write about. I'd like to also recognize the editorial staff at Lippincott Williams & Wilkins for their careful review of each page, Jo Griffith for her oversight of the initial review and update of this edition, and finally my family for their patience and support.

Your comments and suggestions help make this a better reference and I look forward to hearing from you.

Mark R. Dambro. M.D.
Fort Worth, Texas
e-mail: mrdambro@5mcc.com

The 5-Minute Patient Advisor

Acetaminophen Poisoning

 ## BASICS

DESCRIPTION

- Acetaminophen poisoning is a disorder marked by liver disease following ingestion of a large amount of acetaminophen (Tylenol). It is most often encountered following a large single ingestion of acetaminophen-containing medications. Usual toxic doses are >7.5 g in adults and 150 mg/kg in children. However, poisoning can occur after ingestion of lesser amounts in susceptible individuals, including those who regularly abuse alcohol, are chronically malnourished, or take medications that affect liver function. Therapeutic adults doses are 0.5 to 1.0 g every 4 to 6 hours up to a maximum of 4 g/day. Therapeutic pediatrics doses are 10 to 15 mg/kg every 4 to 6 hours, not to exceed 5 doses in any 24-hour period.

SIGNS AND SYMPTOMS

- Symptoms vary from nausea, vomiting, profuse sweating, and malaise to jaundice, confusion, sleepiness, coma, and death.
- Symptoms develop over the first 24 hours following a large ingestion and can last as long as 8 days.
- Severe symptoms indicate that a large amount of acetaminophen was consumed or that poisoning involves more than one substance.
- Serious liver disease occurs in less than 1% of adults and is very rare in children under 6 years of age.
- Symptoms can develop gradually in susceptible persons following long-term ingestion of smaller amounts of acetaminophen. Such individuals can develop liver disease without a history of excessive acetaminophen ingestion.

CAUSES

Accidental or intentional ingestion of acetaminophen or a combination of medications containing acetaminophen.

SCOPE

- More than 105,000 cases of ingestion of acetaminophen-containing medications were reported by poison control centers in 1995.
- A total of 103 deaths occurred in 1995, one involving a child less than 6 years of age.

MOST OFTEN AFFECTED

- Children and adults of any age
- About half of poisoning cases involve children under 6 years of age.

RISK FACTORS

- Age younger than 6 years
- Poisoning with other substances
- Psychiatric illness
- History of previous poisoning or suicide attempts
- Regular ingestion of large amounts of alcohol

 ## DIAGNOSIS

WHAT THE DOCTOR LOOKS FOR

- The doctor should consider the ingestion of other poisons, particularly those that affect liver function.
- The doctor will assess the degree of damage to the liver and other organs.

LABORATORY

- Blood tests to measure levels of acetaminophen and other possible poisons
- Blood tests to assess function of liver, heart, and pancreas

 ## TREATMENT

GENERAL MEASURES

- Contact a regional poison information center for first aid instructions.
- All persons suspected of acetaminophen poisoning should be evaluated at a healthcare facility.
- Nontoxic accidental ingestion can be managed on an outpatient basis.
- Toxic and intentional ingestion may require hospitalization.
- The person who has been poisoned may be treated by inducing vomiting with syrup of ipecac or having the stomach pumped, which must be performed within 4 hours of ingestion.
- Syrup of ipecac can be given at home if the victim is alert and unable to be seen at a hospital within 1 hour of ingestion.
- Activated charcoal should be given at a hospital.
- Antidote therapy may be effective 36 or more hours after ingestion.

ACTIVITY

Restricted if significant liver damage has occurred

DIET

No special diet except with severe liver damage

 ## MEDICATIONS

COMMONLY PRESCRIBED DRUGS

- Three classes of medicine:
  - Ipecac syrup: to induce vomiting
  - Activated charcoal: to absorb poisons
  - Acetylcysteine: antidote

CONTRAINDICATIONS

- Ipecac should not be given to persons with decreased responsiveness.
- Some people may have drug allergies.

PRECAUTIONS

- Ipecac therapy can result in severe vomiting.
- To reduce risks, activated charcoal should be given at least 30 minutes to 1 hour after ipecac and never before ipecac.

DRUG INTERACTIONS

Activated charcoal can interfere with antidote.

 ## FOLLOW-UP

PATIENT MONITORING

A person should have a psychiatric follow-up after intentional ingestion.

PREVENTION

- Homes with small children should be poison proofed.
- Keep syrup of ipecac in the home first aid kit.
- Keep a list of emergency telephone numbers in a convenient location.

Acetaminophen Poisoning

Doctor
Office
Phone
Pager

Special notes to patient:

Acetaminophen Poisoning

COMPLICATIONS

Complications are rare after recovery from acute poisoning.

WHAT TO EXPECT

- Complete recovery with early therapy
- Less than 1% of adult patients develop liver failure.
- Liver failure is rare in children younger than 6 years of age.

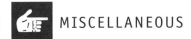

MISCELLANEOUS

OTHER FACTORS

PEDIATRIC

Risk of liver damage is decreased in children younger than 6 years of age.

GERIATRIC

Some medications increase risk of liver damage.

PREGNANCY

Increased incidence of miscarriage

FURTHER INFORMATION

Child Safety: How to keep your home safe for your baby. American Academy of Family Physicians, 8880 Ward Parkway, Kansas City, MO 64114-2797

Acetaminophen Poisoning

Doctor
Office
Phone
Pager

Special notes to patient:

Acne

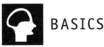
BASICS

DESCRIPTION
Acne, also called "acne vulgaris," is an inflammatory disorder of the sebaceous glands of the skin, resulting in pimples, boils, and occasionally scarring.

SIGNS AND SYMPTOMS
- Pimples (whiteheads or blackheads)
- Bumps or nodes of the skin
- Scars
- Pimples occur over the forehead, cheeks, and nose and may extend over the central chest and back.

CAUSES
Hormones stimulate the rate of skin growth in the sebaceous gland, blocking the pore. Bacteria stimulate an inflammatory response, resulting in a pimple.

SCOPE
Acne affects virtually 100% of adolescents to some degree. About 15% of people will seek medical advice for acne.

MOST OFTEN AFFECTED
Persons in early to late puberty, although some cases will persist into the 30s and 40s. Males and females are affected with equal frequency, although males tend to be affected more severely.

RISK FACTORS
- Adolescence
- Male gender
- Use of steroids or birth control pills
- Oily cosmetics, including cleansing creams, moisturizers, and oil-based foundations
- Rubbing or occluding the skin surface, as can occur with sports equipment (helmets and shoulder pads) or holding the telephone or hands against the skin
- Prescription drugs
- Hair growth disorders
- Hot, humid climate

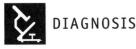
DIAGNOSIS

WHAT THE DOCTOR LOOKS FOR
- The doctor will evaluate the condition of the skin.
- Other causes of skin disorders will be considered, such as occupational exposure or drug side effects.

TESTS AND PROCEDURES
Levels of hormone in the blood may be measured in rare cases.

TREATMENT

GENERAL MEASURES
- Acne is managed on an outpatient basis.
- Pimples can be treated with surgery or injections.
- Gentle cleansing with a mild soap once or twice a day will control surface oiliness. More frequent washing will further irritate the skin and increase sebum (oil) production.
- Oil-free sunscreens: Ultraviolet (UV) light reacts adversely with the medications used to treat acne. Long-term UV exposure causes permanent skin damage. Oil-free sunscreens should be used to protect the skin.
- Stress management may be helpful if acne flares with stress.
- There is no cure for acne; treatment only controls the lesions.

ACTIVITY
Full activity; physical conditioning is important.

DIET
- Good nutrition is important to normal skin health.
- No special diet has been shown to diminish acne. Chocolate and fatty foods do not aggravate acne.

MEDICATIONS

COMMONLY PRESCRIBED DRUGS
- Topical medications
  - Benzoyl peroxide
  - Tretinoin (retinoic acid, Retin-A, Renova)
  - Topical erythromycin
  - Clindamycin (Dalacin T)
- Oral medications
  - Tetracycline
  - Erythromycin
- Oral contraceptives
  - Isotretinoin (Accutane)

CONTRAINDICATIONS
- Known allergies
- All oral medications could cause severe liver problems.
- Isotretinoin: causes birth defects; not for use in pregnancy or in women of reproductive age who are not using a reliable birth control method.
- Tetracycline: not for use in pregnancy or in children younger than 8 years of age.

PRECAUTIONS
- Tetracycline: can cause sensitivity to sunlight; sunscreen recommended.

DRUG INTERACTIONS
- Tetracycline: avoid antacids, dairy products, and iron.
- Erythromycin: Fexofenadine (Allegra) and astemizole
- Some antibiotics can reduce the effectiveness of oral contraceptives.

FOLLOW-UP

PATIENT MONITORING
- See the doctor monthly until adequate response is obtained.
- Blood tests should be done before treatment and monthly during treatment.
- Female patients taking isotretinoin should have pregnancy tests.

COMPLICATIONS
- Severe inflammatory acne with systemic symptoms
- Facial scarring
- Psychological scarring

WHAT TO EXPECT
- Acne gradually improves over time.
- Any treatment takes at least 4 weeks to show results.
- Topical agents cause redness and drying of the skin.

MISCELLANEOUS

PEDIATRIC
A mild form of acne, called "acne rosacea," can occur in the neonate.

PREGNANCY
- May result in an acute episode, or remission, of acne
- Isotretinoin causes severe birth defects; effective contraception should be ensured 1 month before and 1 month following isotretinoin therapy.
- Erythromycin can be used during pregnancy, but it is less preferable to topical agents.

FURTHER INFORMATION
American Academy of Dermatology, 930 N. Meacham Rd., P.O. Box 4014, Schaumberg, IL 60168-4014, (708) 330-0230

Acne

Doctor
Office
Phone
Pager

Special notes to patient:

Adenovirus Infections

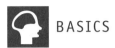 ## BASICS

DESCRIPTION
Adenovirus infections are usually self-limited illnesses characterized by fever and inflammation of eyes and the respiratory tract. Adenovirus infections occur in epidemics.

SIGNS AND SYMPTOMS
Vary depending on the type of virus; most respiratory adenovirus infections cause:

- Headache
- Malaise
- Sore throat
- Cough
- Fever (moderate to high)
- Vomiting
- Diarrhea

CAUSES
One of several types of adenovirus

SCOPE
Adenovirus infections are common in the United States. They are estimated to cause 2% to 5% of all respiratory infections.

MOST OFTEN AFFECTED
The disease can affect all ages—males and females equally—but it is more common in infants and children.

RISK FACTORS
- Large number of people gathered in a small area (e.g., military recruits, college students at the beginning of the school year, day-care centers, community swimming pools)
- Persons with immune system disorders are at risk for severe disease.

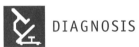 ## DIAGNOSIS

WHAT THE DOCTOR LOOKS FOR
- The doctor will perform a physical examination.
- Other similar conditions will be investigated (e.g., pneumonia, bronchitis, or other respiratory illnesses).

TESTS AND PROCEDURES
- Blood tests to evaluate for signs of infection or inflammation
- Sputum or other body fluids may be cultured for microbiological analysis.
- A chest x-ray study may be done to assess the respiratory system.
- Biopsy (lung or other) may be needed in severe or unusual cases.

 ## TREATMENT

GENERAL MEASURES
- Adenovirus is usually treated on an outpatient basis, except for severely ill infants.
- Treatment is supportive, aimed at relieving symptoms.
- Adenovirus infections are usually harmless and do not last long.
- Avoid giving aspirin to children.
- Nasal spray may help relieve nasal congestion.
- Wash hands frequently to avoid transmission of virus.

ACTIVITY
Rest during fever

DIET
No special diet

 ## MEDICATIONS

COMMONLY PRESCRIBED DRUGS
- Acetaminophen
- Topical corticosteroids for conjunctivitis (pink eye)
- Cough suppressants, expectorants, or both

CONTRAINDICATIONS
Read drug product information.

PRECAUTIONS
Read drug product information.

DRUG INTERACTIONS
Read drug product information.

 ## FOLLOW-UP

PATIENT MONITORING
Infants with severe pneumonia and conjunctivitis should be seen daily by the doctor until they are well.

PREVENTION
- Adenovirus vaccine reduces the incidence of acute respiratory disease.
- Frequent handwashing by office personnel and family members reduces the risk of virus transmission.

COMPLICATIONS
- Adenovirus infection causes few if any recognizable long-term problems.

WHAT TO EXPECT
- Adenovirus infection is self-limited, usually without lasting effects.
- Adenovirus can cause severe illness and death in very young persons and in those with immune system disorders.

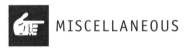 ## MISCELLANEOUS

PEDIATRIC
Viral pneumonia in infants may be fatal. Do not give aspirin to children.

GERIATRIC
Complications are more likely among elderly persons.

PREGNANCY
No special precautions

Adenovirus Infections

Doctor
Office
Phone
Pager

Special notes to patient:

Alcoholism

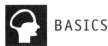
BASICS

DESCRIPTION
Alcoholism is an illness characterized by physiologic, psychological, or social problems associated with persistent and excessive use of alcohol.

SIGNS AND SYMPTOMS
- Behavioral psychological and social dysfunction
  - Marital problems (divorce or separation)
  - Anxiety, depression, insomnia
  - Social isolation, frequent moves
  - Child or spouse abuse
  - Alcohol-related arrests or legal problems (less likely in women)
  - Preoccupation with recreational drinking
  - Repeated attempts to stop or reduce drinking
  - Loss of interest in activities that do not involve drinking
  - Employment problems (tardiness, absenteeism, decreased productivity, interpersonal problems at work, frequent job changes)
  - Blackouts (not remembering what happened during drinking spells)
  - Complaints by family members or friends about alcohol-related behavior
- Physical
  - Gastrointestinal: anorexia, nausea, vomiting, abdominal pain, ulcer, pancreatitis, cancer
  - Cardiovascular: hypertension, irregular heart rhythms, heart disease
  - Respiratory: pneumonia, bronchitis, and chronic pulmonary disease
  - Genitourinary: impotence, menstrual irregularities, testicular atrophy
  - Dermatologic: signs of accidents and trauma, burns (especially cigarette burns), bruises in various stages of healing, poor hygiene
  - Musculoskeletal: old fractures and fractures in various stages of healing, myopathy
  - Neurologic: dementia, nerve disease

CAUSES
- Multiple factors, including biological, psychological, and sociocultural
- Evidence suggests a genetic link to alcoholism.

SCOPE
About 10% of men and 3.5% of women in the United States are alcoholics.

MOST OFTEN AFFECTED
- Alcoholism affects all ages.
- Highest prevalence of drinking problems is in the age group 18 to 29 years.
- Slightly more common in men than in women

RISK FACTORS
- Alcohol use
- Use of other psychoactive drugs, including nicotine
- Family history of alcohol abuse
- Young, single male
- Heavy drinking: five or more drinks in one sitting, getting drunk at least once per week
- Peer group pressure
- Family or sociocultural background promoting intoxication; accepting it as a norm
- Increased accessibility of alcohol
- Adolescence (alcohol and drug use by peers or parents, delinquency, sociopathy in the parents, poor self-esteem, social nonconformity, and stressful life changes)

DIAGNOSIS

WHAT THE DOCTOR LOOKS FOR
- The person with alcoholism can have a variety of medical and psychiatric disorders.
- The doctor will evaluate the person for depression, anxiety, or other mental health problems.
- The doctor will perform a physical examination to identify medical problems (e.g., hypertension, peptic ulcer, heart disease, liver disease, and diabetes).

TESTS AND PROCEDURES
- A variety of blood tests may be performed, including measuring the blood alcohol level.
- Psychological tests
- X-ray, computed tomography (CT) scan or magnetic resonance imaging (MRI) may be performed to assess structures of the head, chest, and abdomen.
- A sample of the liver may be obtained by biopsy for laboratory analysis.

TREATMENT

GENERAL MEASURES
- Treatment is inpatient or outpatient, depending on illness severity, the person's health, and other factors.
- In some cases, detoxification is done on an inpatient basis, with the remainder of treatment given on an outpatient basis.
- Primary care provider may want to consult an addiction specialist.

ACTIVITY
Fully active as tolerated

DIET
- Well-balanced diet (malnutrition from poor eating habits is common)
- Alcohol interferes with the metabolism of most vitamins.
- Person may require supplementation for specific vitamin or mineral deficiencies.

MEDICATIONS

COMMONLY PRESCRIBED DRUGS
- For detoxification and management of alcohol withdrawal:
  - Chlordiazepoxide (Librium)
  - Diazepam (Valium)
  - Lorazepam (Ativan)
  - Phenobarbital
- Detoxification adjuncts:
  - Beta-blockers (propranolol, atenolol)
  - Clonidine
- To promote sobriety:
  - Disulfirarn (Antabuse)
  - Naltrexone
- Thiamine

CONTRAINDICATIONS
Do not drink while taking detoxification medications.

PRECAUTIONS
- Medications should be used with caution in individuals with severe liver disease, organic pain, or other conditions.
- Watch for unsteadiness, excessive sleepiness, slurred speech, or other signs of intoxication.

SIGNIFICANT POSSIBLE INTERACTIONS
- Alcohol and benzodiazepines have additive effects.
- Do not mix medication with other sedatives.

Alcoholism

Doctor
Office
Phone
Pager

Special notes to patient:

___
___
___
___
___
___
___
___
___
___
___
___
___
___
___
___

Alcoholism

 FOLLOW-UP

PATIENT MONITORING
- Person should be seen daily during detoxification.
- Frequent visits (weekly) after patient completes treatment program
- Less frequent visits as patient becomes established in recovery

PREVENTION
People with a family history of alcoholism or other risk factors may benefit from preventive counseling.

POSSIBLE COMPLICATIONS
- Drinking relapse
- Nervous system disorders
- Alcoholic dementia
- Increased susceptibility to infection
- Cancer
- Cirrhosis (women sooner than men)

WHAT TO EXPECT
- Alcoholism is a chronic, relapsing disease.
- If untreated, alcoholism is progressive and fatal.

 MISCELLANEOUS

PEDIATRIC
- Substance abuse has a negative impact on normal maturation and development and on attainment of social, educational, and occupational skills.
- Signs and symptoms often include depression, suicidal thoughts or attempts, family disruption, disorderly behavior, violence or destruction of property, poor school or work performance, sexual promiscuity, social immaturity, lack of hobbies or interests, isolation, moodiness.

GERIATRIC
- Alcoholism is often missed in elderly individuals. The signs and symptoms of alcoholism may be different or attributed to a chronic medical problem or dementia.
- The elderly are more sensitive to alcohol effects.

PREGNANCY
- Alcohol causes birth defects. The greatest damage occurs during the early weeks of fetal development.
- Women should abstain from alcohol when planning conception and throughout pregnancy.

Alcoholism

Doctor
Office
Phone
Pager

Special notes to patient:

Alopecia

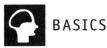
BASICS

DESCRIPTION
Alopecia is defined as the absence of hair from skin areas where it normally is present. Several forms of alopecia occur, depending on the type of hair loss.

SIGNS AND SYMPTOMS
- Hair loss
- Itching
- Scaling of the scalp
- Broken hairs
- Tapered hair
- Easily removable hairs
- Inflammation

CAUSES
Alopecia has many possible causes, including inherited disease, medication side effects, radiation therapy, infection, stress, malnutrition, and other conditions.

SCOPE
By 50 years of age, 50% of white men have noticeable male-pattern baldness. Nearly 40% of postmenopausal women show some evidence of hair loss.

MOST OFTEN AFFECTED
The incidence of androgenic alopecia (male-pattern baldness) increases with increasing age. Men are affected more often than women. A strong genetic tendency for baldness exists.

RISK FACTORS
- Family history of baldness
- Physical or psychological stress
- Pregnancy
- Poor nutrition

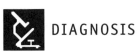
DIAGNOSIS

WHAT THE DOCTOR LOOKS FOR
The doctor will establish the type of alopecia and search for possible reversible causes.

TESTS AND PROCEDURES
- A variety of blood tests may be ordered, including hormone level. Hair may be studied microscopically.
- The scalp may be biopsied for microscopic evaluation and other special testing procedures may be performed.

TREATMENT

GENERAL MEASURES
- Alopecia is managed on an outpatient basis.
- Some forms of alopecia are permanent, whereas hair grows back in others.
- For male-pattern baldness, 39% of persons report moderate to marked hair growth after using minoxidil (Rogaine) after 12 months.

ACTIVITY
Fully active

DIET
No special diet

MEDICATIONS

COMMONLY PRESCRIBED DRUGS
- Male-pattern baldness: topical minoxidil (Rogaine); finasteride (Propecia)
- Alopecia areata: high-potency topical steroids, intralesional steroids
- Tinea capitis: griseofulvin or ketoconazole

CONTRAINDICATIONS
Drugs have many interactions; refer to product information.

PRECAUTIONS
- Topical minoxidil: burning and irritation of the eyes, salt and water retention, fast heart rate, chest pain
- Topical steroids: burning and stinging, itching, skin atrophy
- Griseofulvin: sensitivity to light
- Ketoconazole: allergic reactions, liver damage, lowering of sperm count, mental conditions

DRUG INTERACTIONS
Drugs have many interactions; read product information.

FOLLOW-UP

PATIENT MONITORING
Liver enzymes may be monitored if using ketoconazole.

WHAT TO EXPECT
- Recovery varies, depending on type of alopecia.
- Recovery from male-pattern baldness depends on treatments.
- Some forms of alopecia have complete recovery and hair regrowth.

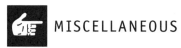

PEDIATRIC
Tinea capitis is the only common form of alopecia in children.

GERIATRIC
Male-pattern baldness is more common after 50 years of age.

PREGNANCY
Hair loss after giving birth is caused by altered physiology during pregnancy.

FURTHER INFORMATION
National Alopecia Areata Foundation, 714 C Street, San Rafael, CA 94901

Alopecia

Doctor
Office
Phone
Pager

Special notes to patient:

Altitude Illness

 ## BASICS

DESCRIPTION

Altitude illness is a medical problem ranging from mild discomfort to fatal illness that can occur on ascent to higher altitude. It can affect anyone, including those who are experienced and fit, who ascend to more than about 8,000 feet (2438 m). Several factors appear to be important in adaptation to altitude, including how long the ascent takes, how high, and length of stay. Much variation exists among people; in addition, an individual's response can vary from ascent to ascent.

SIGNS AND SYMPTOMS

- Mild to moderately severe symptoms:
  - Headache
  - Lack of energy and appetite
  - Mild nausea
  - Dizziness
  - Weakness
  - Insomnia
- Severe symptoms:
  - Increased headache
  - Irritability
  - Marked fatigue
  - Shortness of breath with exercise
  - Nausea and vomiting
  - Irregular or periodic breathing at night
  - Difficulty or cessation of breathing
- High altitude pulmonary edema (NAPE) symptoms:
  - Excessive shortness of breath on exertion
  - Severe respiratory distress
  - Shortness of breath at rest
  - Dry cough or wheezing
  - Increased heart rate and breathing rate
  - Marked irregular breathing at night
  - Gurgling breathing
  - Frothy cough
  - Wet crackling sounds in the lungs
  - Confusion
  - Coma
- High altitude cerebral edema (HACE) symptoms:
  - Progressive headache that is unrelieved by mild pain relievers
  - Lack of coordination
  - Confusion and bizarre behavior followed by unconsciousness
  - Other symptoms of moderate altitude sickness (e.g., dizziness, vomiting, irritability) are usually present.

CAUSES

The physiology of altitude illness is still not completely understood. The fundamental problem is a decrease in air pressure, resulting in less oxygen delivery to the body.

SCOPE

Unknown

MOST OFTEN AFFECTED

Altitude sickness can affect individuals of any age, men and women in equal proportion. Young, well-conditioned climbers have a higher incidence of altitude illness, probably because they push themselves more.

RISK FACTORS

- In general, the faster and higher the ascent, the more likely a person will experience symptoms of altitude illness.
- Chronic illness
- Lack of conditioning

 ## DIAGNOSIS

WHAT THE DOCTOR LOOKS FOR

The doctor will consider other respiratory problems (e.g, pneumonia, respiratory infection, or heart failure).

TESTS AND PROCEDURES

- A variety of blood tests may be performed.
- Arterial blood may be obtained to measure blood gasses.
- A chest x-ray study may be done to evaluate the respiratory system.
- An electrocardiogram (ECG) may be done to monitor heart function.

 ## TREATMENT

GENERAL MEASURES

- Severe cases of altitude sickness may require hospitalization.
- Treatment is tailored to fit the severity of disease and may be limited by the environment.
- Definitive treatment is to descend to a lower altitude. Dramatic improvement accompanies even modest reductions in altitude (as little as 1,000 feet).
- Giving oxygen helps relieve symptoms.
- Descent is rarely needed for mild cases. Drink fluids, eat a light diet, and curtail activity.
- For severe symptoms, the victim should be immediately evacuated to a lower altitude and given continuous oxygen.
- A portable hyperbaric chamber is another effective and practical alternative for severe symptoms when descent is not possible.

ACTIVITY

Rest until symptoms clear.

DIET

Increased intake of fluids, a light diet, and avoidance of alcohol

 ## MEDICATIONS

COMMONLY PRESCRIBED DRUGS

- Aspirin or codeine to relieve headache
- Antibiotics, if infection is present
- Dexamethasone or acetazolamide
- Corticosteroids

CONTRAINDICATIONS

Read drug product information.

PRECAUTIONS

Read drug product information.

DRUG INTERACTIONS

Read drug product information.

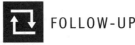 ## FOLLOW-UP

PATIENT MONITORING

- For mild cases, no follow-up is needed.
- For more severe cases, the patient should have follow-up by the doctor until symptoms subside.
- Person with underlying cardiopulmonary or cardiovascular disease should have follow-up by the doctor, as needed.

PREVENTION

- Staged ascent with appropriate acclimatization
- Sleeping elevation: "Climb high and sleep low" is a prudent practice for anyone going above 12,000 feet (3,656 m).
- Adequate hydration: Dehydration makes altitude sickness worse.
- Good physical conditioning
- Consider carrying a supply of oxygen.
- Some drugs can prevent or lessen the symptoms of altitude sickness.

COMPLICATIONS

- Without treatment, severe illness can cause motor and sensory problems, seizures, and coma.
- May progress to respiratory distress
- Patient may experience retinal hemorrhage–causing vision changes

Altitude Illness

	Doctor
	Office
	Phone
	Pager

Special notes to patient:

Altitude Illness

WHAT TO EXPECT

- Mild to moderate altitude sickness resolves over 1 to 3 days. Climbers can resume ascent once symptoms subside.
- People with severe symptoms but no underlying disease can expect complete recovery. They should not resume ascent.
- Problems are more likely among people who have had one or more attacks.

 MISCELLANEOUS

PEDIATRIC

Children younger than 6 years of age are more susceptible to altitude sickness than adults.

GERIATRIC

Elderly persons are more likely to have chronic conditions (e.g., coronary artery disease, congestive heart failure, chronic obstructive pulmonary disease) that may become worse at altitudes of 6,000 to 8,000 feet (1,829—2,438 m).

OTHERS

Women in premenstrual phase are more vulnerable to altitude sickness.

Altitude Illness

Doctor
Office
Phone
Pager

Special notes to patient:

Alzheimer's Disease

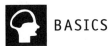 ## BASICS

DESCRIPTION

Alzheimer's disease is a degenerative mental disease characterized by progressive brain deterioration and dementia. It usually occurs after age 65 years. The diagnosis is made after ruling out treatable disorders with similar characteristics. The usual course of Alzheimer's disease is progressive and chronic.

SIGNS AND SYMPTOMS

- Anxiety
- Confusion
- Delusions
- Dementia
- Depression
- Impaired speech
- Intellectual decline
- Lack of concern or interest
- Occupational dysfunction
- Personality changes
- Recent memory loss
- Restlessness
- Sleep disturbances
- Social withdrawal
- Weight loss Late signs: seizures, muscle spasm, incontinence

CAUSES

Unknown

SCOPE

Nearly 4 million people in the United States have Alzheimer's disease, which strikes about 40% of individuals over 85 years of age.

MOST OFTEN AFFECTED

- Persons 50 to 90 years of age
- About half of individuals with Alzheimer's disease have a family history of the illness.
- Women are affected slightly more often than men.

RISK FACTORS

- Aging
- Head trauma
- Low education level
- Down syndrome
- Positive family history
- Smoking (two- to fourfold increase)

 ## DIAGNOSIS

WHAT THE DOCTOR LOOKS FOR

- The doctor will obtain a medical history and perform a thorough physical examination.
- Other conditions with similar symptoms should be investigated (e.g., Parkinson's disease and drug interactions).

TESTS AND PROCEDURES

- A number of blood tests may be performed to help rule out other causes of dementia.
- An electrocardiogram (ECG) may be done to assess heart function.
- An electroencephalogram (EEG) may be done to monitor brain activity.
- An x-ray study, computed tomography (CT) scan, or magnetic resonance imaging (MRI) may be done to evaluate internal structures.
- A sample of cerebrospinal fluid may be obtained for chemical and microscopic analysis.
- Psychological tests may be administered.

 ## TREATMENT

GENERAL MEASURES

- Management of the person with Alzheimer's disease is usually done on an outpatient basis, with adult daycare or nursing home care when needed.
- Management is primarily supportive.
- Other medical conditions should be identified and treated.
- Exercises to reduce restlessness
- The person may benefit from occupational therapy or music therapy.
- Challenging the mind slows the rate of deterioration.
- Make sure the person's home environment is safe and secure.
- Consider adult daycare, nursing home as needed.
- Plan advance directives (residential, medical preferences) as early as possible.
- Prepare a durable power of attorney.
- Person with Alzheimer's disease or family may benefit from referral to:
  ▸ Visiting nurse
  ▸ Social worker
  ▸ Physical therapist
  ▸ Occupational therapist
  ▸ Lawyer
  ▸ Support groups
  ▸ Alzheimer's special care group
- Assess driving safety

ACTIVITY

To whatever extent possible

DIET

No special diet

 ## MEDICATIONS

COMMONLY PRESCRIBED DRUGS

- No specific drug therapy is available for halting the disease.
- As few drugs as possible should be used; persons with Alzheimer's disease tolerate drugs poorly.
- No drugs are helpful for wandering, restlessness, fidgeting, uncooperativeness, hoarding, irritability.
- Depression: selective serotonin reuptake inhibitors or trazodone (Desyrel)
- Insomnia: trazodone, zolpidem (Ambien), zaleplon (Sonata), or temazepam (Restoril)
- Moderate anxiety or restlessness: benzodiazepines or buspirone
- Psychosis, severe aggressive agitation: butyrophenones or phenothiazine
- Severe aggressive agitation: carbamazepine (Tegretol) and propranolol (Inderal)
- Memory enhancement in mild to moderate disease: tacrine (Cognex), donepezil (Aricept)
- Nonsteroidal antiinflammatory drugs (NSAIDs) and estrogen replacement therapy (ERT) for women are related to lower incidence and slower progression of Alzheimer's disease.
- Selegiline, vitamin E, or both can be used to slow progression of disease.

CONTRAINDICATIONS

- Avoid tricyclic antidepressants and antihistamines
- Gingko biloba: avoid blood thinners and aspirin
- Read drug product information.

PRECAUTIONS

Read drug product information.

DRUGS INTERACTIONS

Drugs have many interactions; read drug product information.

Alzheimer's Disease

Doctor
Office
Phone
Pager

Special notes to patient:

Alzheimer's Disease

 ## FOLLOW-UP

PATIENT MONITORING

- The person with Alzheimer's disease should be seen by the doctor as often as necessary to manage nutrition, health, and drug therapy, and to support family caregivers.
- Periodic mental status testing may be helpful.
- Caregiver should be closely monitored to avoid burnout.

WHAT TO EXPECT

- Alzheimer's disease is a progressive disease with a poor outcome.
- A person with Alzheimer's disease has an average of 8 to 10 years survival.

PREVENTION

- None known for patient
- In near future, family members may seek genetic screening.

COMPLICATIONS

- Behavioral: hostility, agitation, wandering, uncooperative
- Medical: infection, dehydration, drug toxicity, malnutrition, falls
- Family or caregiver burnout
- Depression occurs in one third of patients.
- Suicide: in early stages, especially if patient is depressed

 ## MISCELLANEOUS

GERIATRIC

Alzheimer's disease is a frequent and serious problem in this age group.

FURTHER INFORMATION

Alzheimer's Association, 70 E. Lake Street, Suite 600, Chicago, IL, (312) 853-3060

Alzheimer's Disease

Doctor
Office
Phone
Pager

Special notes to patient:

Amenorrhea

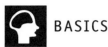 ## BASICS

DESCRIPTION
Amenorrhea is the absence of menstrual periods.

SIGNS AND SYMPTOMS
- The absence of menstrual periods
- Milky discharge from the nipple
- Temperature intolerance
- Symptoms of early pregnancy
- Signs of excess male hormone
- Signs of decreased female hormone

CAUSES
- Congenital disorders
- Pregnancy, breast feeding
- Hormone disorders
- Chemotherapy or hormone therapy
- Numerous other possible causes

SCOPE
About 3.3% of adult women have amenorrhea.

MOST OFTEN AFFECTED
Women between initial onset of menses and menopause

RISK FACTORS
- Overtraining (e.g., long-distance runner, ballet dancer)
- Eating disorders
- Psychosocial crisis

 ## DIAGNOSIS

WHAT THE DOCTOR LOOKS FOR
- The doctor will evaluate for possible causes of amenorrhea.
- One of the most common causes of amenorrhea is pregnancy.

TESTS AND PROCEDURES
- Several blood tests may be performed to assist with diagnosis.
- Pregnancy test should be performed.
- Internal structures may be assessed with ultrasound or x-ray imaging.
- The doctor may visually inspect internal organs by laparoscopy.

 ## TREATMENT

GENERAL MEASURES
- Amenorrhea is usually managed on an outpatient basis.
- Treatment depends on the cause of the amenorrhea.
- Not all cases require treatment, especially if amenorrhea is temporary.
- Surgery may be required if amenorrhea is the result of an intact hymen.
- Use appropriate contraceptive, as fertility returns before menses.

ACTIVITY
No restrictions

DIET
Correct overweight or underweight by dietary management.

 ## MEDICATIONS

COMMONLY PRESCRIBED DRUGS
- Progesterone replacement: medroxyprogesterone (Provera)
- Estrogen replacement: conjugated estrogen (Premarin)
- Hormonal therapies will not correct an underlying problem. Other drugs might be required to treat specific conditions.
- Hormonal replacement therapy is recommended after 6 months of amenorrhea, regardless of cause.
- Calcium supplementation if decreased estrogen is the cause

CONTRAINDICATIONS
- Pregnancy
- Blood clots
- Previous heart attack or stroke
- Estrogen-dependent malignancy
- Severe liver disease

PRECAUTIONS
- Diabetes
- Seizure disorder
- Migraine headache
- Smoker more than 35 years of age

DRUG INTERACTIONS
Barbiturates, phenytoin, rifampin, corticosteroids, theophyllines, tricyclics, oral anticoagulants

OTHER DRUGS
Oral contraceptives for hormonal replacement

 ## FOLLOW-UP

PATIENT MONITORING
- Follow-up depends on the cause and the treatment chosen.
- Hormonal replacement can be discontinued after 6 months to assess whether spontaneous menstruation resumes.

PREVENTION
Maintenance of proper body mass index (BMI)

COMPLICATIONS
- Estrogen deficiency symptoms (e.g., hot flushes, vaginal dryness)
- Osteoporosis
- Increase risk of endometrial cancer with production of excess estrogen

WHAT TO EXPECT
Depends on the underlying cause. In many cases, amenorrhea spontaneously resolves in time.

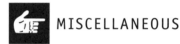 ## MISCELLANEOUS

PREGNANCY
One of the primary causes of amenorrhea

FURTHER INFORMATION
Society for Menstrual Cycle Research, 10559 N. 104th Place, Scottsdale, AZ 85258, (602) 451-9731

Amenorrhea

Doctor
Office
Phone
Pager

Special notes to patient:

Anaphylaxis

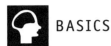 ## BASICS

DESCRIPTION

Anaphylaxis is an acute, systemic allergic reaction following exposure to an allergen in a sensitized person.

SIGNS AND SYMPTOMS

- Itching, flushing, rash, swelling
- Cough, difficult breathing
- Runny nose, congestion, noisy breathing
- Difficulty swallowing
- Nausea, vomiting, diarrhea, cramps, bloating
- Rapid heart rate, low blood pressure, shock, fainting
- Malaise, shivering
- Dilated pupils

CAUSES

- Allergic reaction following exposure to allergen
- Other anaphylaxis-like syndromes may have other causes. Some important causes of anaphylaxis are:
  - Antibiotics (e.g., penicillin)
  - Blood products
  - Diagnostic chemicals
  - Exercise
  - Foods (e.g., peanuts, nuts, fish, shellfish, cow's milk, eggs, soybean)
  - Insect stings (e.g., honeybees, wasps, kissing bugs, deer flies)
  - Latex rubber (condoms, gloves, catheters)
  - Vaccines

SCOPE

- The incidence of anaphylaxis is unknown.
- Between 20,000 and 50,000 cases of anaphylaxis occur annually in the United States.
- Anaphylaxis causes three to seven deaths per 10,000 people annually.

MOST OFTEN AFFECTED

Anaphylaxis affects all ages, males and females in equal proportion. Some allergies have a genetic predisposition.

RISK FACTORS

Previous anaphylaxis; history of allergies or asthma

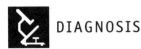 ## DIAGNOSIS

WHAT THE DOCTOR LOOKS FOR

- Signs and symptoms of allergic reactions
- Other conditions with similar signs should be investigated.

TESTS AND PROCEDURES

- Blood tests will be done to look for signs of inflammation or infection.
- Arterial blood may be obtained.

 ## TREATMENT

GENERAL MEASURES

- Treatment depends on the severity of the allergic reaction.
- Severe reaction requires first aid; seek hospital care as quickly as possible.
- Maintain airway, breathing, and circulation as needed.
- If sting or bite is on arm or leg, apply constrictive band between sting and body (do not apply too tightly and loosen if uncomfortable).
- Individuals with swelling, rash, or mild breathing problems may be released from the hospital when symptoms resolve; they are then managed on an outpatient basis.
- Moderate to severe anaphylaxis requires hospitalization, possibly mechanical breathing.
- An allergist can be consulted if the cause of anaphylaxis is unclear.
- Individuals with anaphylaxis from insect stings may benefit from desensitization immunotherapy.

ACTIVITY

Bed rest until anaphylaxis clears and patient is stable

DIET

Nothing by mouth until acute symptoms are controlled

 ## MEDICATIONS

COMMONLY PRESCRIBED DRUGS

- Epinephrine
- Antihistamine: diphenhydramine
- Cimetidine
- Corticosteroids
- Bronchodilators: inhaled beta-2 agonists, aminophylline

CONTRAINDICATIONS

Read drug product information.

PRECAUTIONS

Read drug product information.

 ## FOLLOW-UP

PATIENT MONITORING

The person with acute anaphylaxis should be followed closely during treatment and for several hours after symptoms resolve. Symptoms can recur for up to 72 hours.

PREVENTION

- Avoid drugs and foods that trigger allergic reaction.
- Carry a prefilled epinephrine syringe (bee sting kit); avoid areas where insect exposure is likely; and avoid wearing things that attract insects (e.g., perfumes, bright-colored clothing).
- Carry or wear medical alert identification about an anaphylaxis-causing substance or event.

WHAT TO EXPECT

- Anaphylaxis has a good outcome if treated immediately.
- The outcome is worse if medical care is delayed more than 30 minutes.
- Of individuals with anaphylaxis of unknown cause, 60% will not experience another episode after 2.5 years; most others have a decrease in the number of episodes.
- Allergy to one species of legume (e.g., peanuts) or one type of seafood (e.g., shrimp) does not mean that an allergy to all products in that category exists.

COMPLICATIONS

Inadequate oxygenation, cardiac arrest, death

 ## MISCELLANEOUS

GERIATRIC

Epinephrine can induce cardiac events in those with heart disease.

PREGNANCY

Epinephrine can induce blood flow to the placenta, but may save the life of mother and fetus.

FURTHER INFORMATION

- Asthma & Allergy Foundation of America, 1717 Massachusetts Avenue, Suite 305, Washington, DC 20036, (800) 7-Asthma
- American Allergy Association, P.O. Box 7273, Menlo Park, CA 94026, (415) 322-1663
- Medic-Alert Foundation, Turlock, CA 95381-1009

Anaphylaxis

_____ Doctor
_____ Office
_____ Phone
_____ Pager

Special notes to patient:

Anemia, Pernicious

 ## BASICS

DESCRIPTION
Pernicious anemia is a disorder caused by vitamin B_{12} deficiency. Usual course is slow but progressive.

SIGNS AND SYMPTOMS
- Abnormal reflexes
- Anorexia, weight loss
- Confusion
- Dementia
- Depression
- Dizziness
- Enlarged liver
- Heart failure
- Increased skin pigmentation
- Lack of coordination
- Numbness or tingling in extremities
- Pallor
- Prematurely gray-haired
- Rapid heartbeat, palpitations
- Ringing in ears (tinnitus)
- Shortness of breath on exertion
- Sore tongue
- Weakness

CAUSES
- Digestive disorder
- Metabolic disorder
- Immune system disorder

SCOPE
Unknown

MOST OFTEN AFFECTED
This disorder primarily affects adults 60 years of age or older. It occurs equally among males and females.

RISK FACTORS
- Vegetarian diet without B_{12} supplementation
- Digestive disease, surgery
- Drugs side effect
- Chronic pancreatitis
- Alcoholism

 ## DIAGNOSIS

WHAT THE DOCTOR LOOKS FOR
- The doctor will take a history and perform a thorough physical examination.
- Other causes of similar signs and symptoms should be investigated (e.g., neurologic disorder, liver disorders, hypothyroidism, bleeding, or alcoholism).
- The doctor will evaluate for the presence of other conditions associated with pernicious anemia.

TESTS AND PROCEDURES
- A number of blood tests may be done to assist in diagnosis.
- A sample of bone marrow may be obtained for analysis.
- Cerebrospinal fluid may be obtained for analysis.
- Cells from the digestive system may be microscopically analyzed.
- The digestive system may be visually inspected by endoscopy.

 ## TREATMENT

GENERAL MEASURES
- Pernicious anemia is managed on an outpatient basis.
- The underlying disorder leading to pernicious anemia must be identified and treated.
- Treatment must be continued for life.

ACTIVITY
No limitations

DIET
Emphasize meat, animal protein foods, and legumes, unless contraindicated.

 ## MEDICATIONS

COMMONLY PRESCRIBED DRUGS
Vitamin B_{12} (cyanocobalamin)

CONTRAINDICATIONS
None

PRECAUTIONS
Do not take folic acid supplements without vitamin B_{12}. Folic acid without vitamin B_{12} can cause neurologic problems.

OTHER DRUGS
None

 ## FOLLOW-UP

PATIENT MONITORING
- Monthly injections of vitamin B_{12}
- Endoscopy every 5 years to rule out gastric cancer

PREVENTION
Monitoring by primary care provider will help assure early detection and treatment of anemia.

WHAT TO EXPECT
- Pernicious anemia is reversible with vitamin B_{12} supplementation.
- Neurologic effects of pernicious anemia are not reversible with use of vitamin B_{12}.
- People with pernicious anemia have an increased risk of developing gastric cancer. Endoscopy should be done about every 5 years even if symptom-free.

COMPLICATIONS
- Neurologic problems may be permanent if pernicious anemia is not treated within 6 months of the onset of symptoms.
- Gastric polyps
- Stomach cancer

 ## MISCELLANEOUS

PEDIATRIC
- Juvenile pernicious anemia occurs in older children and is the same in most respects as in adults.
- Congenital pernicious anemia is usually evident before 3 years of age.

GERIATRIC
Pernicious anemia is more common among the elderly and is often associated with immune system disorders, depression, and dementia.

Anemia, Pernicious

Doctor
Office
Phone
Pager

Special notes to patient:

Anemia, Sickle Cell

 ## BASICS

DESCRIPTION
Sickle cell anemia is a chronic, inheritable blood disorder, marked by moderately severe chronic anemia, periodic acute episodes of painful "crises," and increased susceptibility to infections.

SIGNS AND SYMPTOMS
- Often no symptoms in the early months of life
- After 6 months of age, the earliest symptoms are pallor and symmetric, painful swelling of the hands and feet.
- Chronic anemia
- Painful "crises" in bones, joints, abdomen, back, and viscera
- Increased susceptibility to infections
- Delayed physical or sexual maturation, especially among boys
- Many multisystem complications, especially in later childhood and adolescence

CAUSES
- Genetic defect in hemoglobin
- Sickle red blood cells are inflexible and oddly shaped. They increase the thickness of blood and block smaller blood vessels.
- Chronic anemia

SCOPE
Sickle cell anemia affects about 1 in 500 black Americans; 8% to 10% black Americans carry the sickle trait.

MOST OFTEN AFFECTED
An inheritable disorder, primarily affecting blacks; males and females are affected equally.

RISK FACTORS
- Dehydration
- Infection
- Fever
- Cold
- Strenuous physical exercise
- Severe infections
- Folic acid deficiency
- Exposure to certain drugs
- Smoking

 ## DIAGNOSIS

WHAT THE DOCTOR LOOKS FOR
- Other types of anemia
- Other causes of acute pain in bones, joints, and abdomen

TESTS AND PROCEDURES
- Several blood tests may be performed to assist in diagnosis
- Radiologic imaging may be performed, including chest x-ray, computed tomography (CT) scan, magnetic resonance imaging (MRI), and bone scan.

 ## TREATMENT

GENERAL MEASURES
- Sickle cell anemia is usually managed on an outpatient basis.
- General healthcare maintenance should include assessment of growth/development, regular immunizations, vision/hearing screening, and regular dental care.
- Hospitalization is required for most crises and complications.
- Infections should be promptly treated with antibiotics.
- Transfusion may be required for severe crises.
- Maintaining good hydration is important to health.

ACTIVITY
- Bed rest with crises; otherwise, activity level as tolerated.
- Activity can be limited by chronic anemia and poor muscular development.

DIET
Well-balanced diet with folic acid supplementation. Avoid alcohol, which can lead to dehydration.

 ## MEDICATIONS

COMMONLY PRESCRIBED DRUGS
- Painful crises (mild, outpatient): non-narcotic analgesics (ibuprofen, acetaminophen)
- Painful crises (severe, hospitalized): morphine, meperidine (Demerol), acetaminophen-codeine, ibuprofen
- Corticosteroids
- Antibiotics
- Penicillin to prevent infection is controversial but often recommended.

CONTRAINDICATIONS
None

PRECAUTIONS
Avoid high-dose estrogen oral contraceptives.

DRUG INTERACTIONS
None

OTHER DRUGS
- Other nonsteroidal antiinflammatory drugs (NSAIDs)
- Folic acid supplements

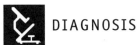 ## FOLLOW-UP

PATIENT MONITORING
- See the doctor as frequently as needed, depending on the crisis severity and complications.
- Temperature of 101°F (38.3°C) or above requires immediate medical attention.
- Counseling, tutoring, or vocational training may be needed.

PREVENTION
Avoid conditions that precipitate sickling (dehydration, cold, infection, fever).

COMPLICATIONS
- Bone disease
- Cardiovascular disease
- Liver disease
- Persistent erection (priapism)
- Hematuria or hyposthenuria
- Eye disease
- Respiratory disease
- Infections
- Decreased intellectual function–even without clinical stroke

Anemia, Sickle Cell

Doctor
Office
Phone
Pager

Special notes to patient:

Anemia, Sickle Cell

WHAT TO EXPECT
- Sickle cell anemia is a life-long condition.
- In the second decade of life, the number of crises diminish but complications become more frequent.
- Some patients die in childhood of stroke or infection.
- Most persons with sickle cell anemia live to early or mid adulthood; few live beyond 50 years of age.
- Common causes of death are infections, blood clots, or renal failure.

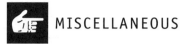

MISCELLANEOUS

PEDIATRIC
- Some signs and symptoms are seen only in infants and young children.
- The frequency of complications and tissue damage increases with age.
- Psychological complications of adolescents: body-image and sexual identity problems, interrupted schooling or career training, restriction of activities, stigma of chronic disease, low self-esteem, fear of future.

PREGNANCY
- Usually complicated and hazardous, especially in the third trimester and at delivery.
- Fetal death rate is 35% to 40%.
- Blood transfusion in third trimester reduces maternal morbidity and fetal death.

Anemia, Sickle Cell

	Doctor
	Office
	Phone
	Pager

Special notes to patient:

Angina

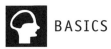 ## BASICS

DESCRIPTION

Angina is defined as chest pain and other symptoms that result when the oxygen demand of the heart exceeds the supply. Also called "angina pectoris."

SIGNS AND SYMPTOMS

- Pressure or heaviness in the center of the chest, brought on by exercise, emotional stress, meals, cold air, or smoking, and relieved by rest or nitroglycerine medication
- Pain can radiate to neck, lower jaw, teeth, shoulders, inner aspects of the arms, or back.
- Individuals with angina may describe their pain with a clenched fist over the sternum.
- Shortness of breath on exertion may be the only symptom.
- A choking sensation is a classic symptom

CAUSES

- Atherosclerosis of the coronary arteries (hardening of the arteries)
- Heart disease
- Disease of blood vessels

SCOPE

Angina is the presenting symptom of coronary artery disease (CAD) in 38% of men and 61% of women.

MOST OFTEN AFFECTED

It is most common in middle-aged and older men and postmenopausal women; males are affected more often than females.

RISK FACTORS

- Family history of premature CAD
- High cholesterol levels
- High blood pressure
- Smoking
- Diabetes mellitus
- Male gender
- Advanced age
- Morbid obesity

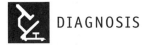 ## DIAGNOSIS

WHAT THE DOCTOR LOOKS FOR

- Other possible causes of chest pain should be investigated (e.g., digestive disorders, respiratory disease, anxiety).
- The doctor will evaluate for other conditions known to be associated with angina (e.g., high blood cholesterol level or high blood pressure).

TESTS AND PROCEDURES

- Blood tests, urinalysis
- An electrocardiogram (ECG) may show evidence of disease.
- Special imaging procedures can be done to assess heart function, including radionuclide scintigraphy, stress echocardiography, stress thallium, and coronary angiography.
- Exercise stress testing can be done to evaluate heart function.

 ## TREATMENT

GENERAL MEASURES

- The person's symptoms should be brought under control.
- The person with angina should be hospitalized if symptoms are unstable.
- The goal of treatment is to restore adequate levels of oxygen to the heart.
- Quit smoking.
- Minimize emotional stress.

ACTIVITY

- Physical activity, as tolerated, after consulting physician
- Exercise program after physician's approval

DIET

Low-fat, low-cholesterol diet

 ## MEDICATIONS

COMMONLY PRESCRIBED DRUGS

- Aspirin
- To slow heart rate, ease demand: beta-blockers (e.g., atenolol, metoprolol, propranolol)
- Acute anginal episodes: nitroglycerin. The dose can be repeated two to three times over a 10- to 15-minute; patients not experiencing relief, should seek medical attention immediately.
- Long-acting nitrates (e.g., skin patches)
- Calcium antagonists: verapamil, nifedipine, amlodipine
- Cholesterol-lowering drugs: pravastatin, lovastatin, and others
- Heparin: blood thinner; for those hospitalized with unstable angina

CONTRAINDICATIONS

Viagra plus nitrates should be avoided because of affects on blood pressure. Read drug product information.

PRECAUTIONS

Read drug product information.

SIGNIFICANT POSSIBLE INTERACTIONS

Read drug product information.

OTHER DRUGS

Cholesterol-lowering drugs are often given to individuals with an unfavorable lipid profile.

 ## FOLLOW-UP

PATIENT MONITORING

- The doctor should be seen with a frequency that depends on the severity of symptoms.
- Individuals with unstable angina should be hospitalized for observation and treatment.

PREVENTION

- Stop smoking.
- Adhere to a low-fat, low-cholesterol diet.
- Establish a regular aerobic exercise program.
- Cholesterol-lowering drugs

COMPLICATIONS

Heart conditions: heart muscle damage, irregular heartbeat, heart failure, cardiac arrest

WHAT TO EXPECT

- The outcome of angina is variable, depending on the extent of disease as well as heart function.
- The annual death rate is 3% to 4%.

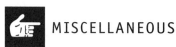 ## MISCELLANEOUS

GERIATRIC

The elderly can be sensitive to the side effects of medications (e.g., beta-blockers) and depression).

PREGNANCY

- Other causes of chest pain should be excluded.
- Requires close management by obstetrician and cardiologist as pregnancy worsens symptoms become worse and interferes with treatment.

FURTHER INFORMATION

American Heart Association, 7320 Greenville Avenue, Dallas, TX 75231, (214) 373-6300

Angina

Doctor
Office
Phone
Pager

Special notes to patient:

Animal Bites

 ## BASICS

DESCRIPTION
Animal bites include bite wounds from dogs, cats, and other animals (including humans).

SIGNS AND SYMPTOMS
- Bite wounds can be tears, punctures, scratches, avulsions, or crush injuries.
- Dog bites
  - Most commonly occur on the hands (up to 68% of bites)
  - Occur on the face in up to 29% of cases, the lower extremities in 10%
  - Do not commonly occur on the trunk
- Cat bites
  - Most commonly involve the hands, followed by lower extremities, face and trunk
  - Are more likely to become infected because of puncture wound

CAUSES
- Most bite wounds are from a domestic pet known to the victim, commonly a large dog.
- Human bites are often the result of one person striking another in the mouth with a clenched fist.

SCOPE
- Approximately 1,200 dog bites per 100,000 persons occur in the United States annually.
- About 160 cat bites per 100,000 persons
- Snake bites are relatively rare in the United States, with 15 nonvenomous bites per 100,000 persons and 3 venomous bites per 100,000 persons annually.
- About half of all people will experience an animal bite during a lifetime.

MOST OFTEN AFFECTED
Bites can occur in any age group, but are more likely to occur among children. They are more common among boys than girls.

RISK FACTORS
- Dog bites are more common in the early afternoon, especially during warm weather.
- Cat bites are more common in the morning.
- Clenched fist injuries are frequently associated with the use of alcohol.

 ## DIAGNOSIS

WHAT THE DOCTOR LOOKS FOR
The diagnosis of animal bite is straightforward. Of primary concern to the doctor is judging the risk from the injury and resulting infection.

TESTS AND PROCEDURES
- Routine blood tests
- Fluid from the wound may be cultured for microbiologic analysis.
- If bite wound is near a bone or joint, an x-ray study may be done.
- In human bite wounds from clenched fist injuries, x-rays may be taken of the hands.

 ## TREATMENT

GENERAL MEASURES
- Animal bites are managed in the outpatient setting unless the person has a serious infection that requires intravenous antibiotics, close observation, or surgery.
- Elevate the injured extremity to prevent swelling.
- The hand should be splinted if it is injured.

 ## MEDICATIONS

COMMONLY PRESCRIBED DRUGS
- Antibiotics
- Pain relievers: acetaminophen, ibuprofen

CONTRAINDICATIONS
Penicillin-derived antibiotics should not be used in people with penicillin allergy.

PRECAUTIONS
Read drug product information.

SIGNIFICANT POSSIBLE INTERACTIONS
Antibiotics may decrease effectiveness of oral contraceptives.

FOLLOW-UP

PATIENT MONITORING
- Bite victim should be rechecked within 24 to 48 hours.
- The doctor may be seen daily for treating active infections.

PREVENTION
Children should be instructed to use caution around animals.

COMPLICATIONS
Complications from bites can include arthritis, osteomyelitis, extensive soft tissue injuries with scarring, infection, bleeding, and death.

WHAT TO EXPECT
Wounds should steadily improve and close within 7 to 10 days.

 ## MISCELLANEOUS

PEDIATRIC
No special precautions

GERIATRIC
- Serious injury from any bite wound is more common among individuals older than 50 years of age, those with wounds in the upper extremities, or those with puncture wounds.
- The risk of infection is increased in individuals older than 50 years of age.

No special precautions

Animal Bites

Doctor
Office
Phone
Pager

Special notes to patient:

Anxiety

BASICS

DESCRIPTION

Anxiety is a common, acute or chronic, fearful emotion with associated physical symptoms. Types of anxiety disorders include:

- Acute situational anxiety: response to recent stressful event; usually transient
- Adjustment disorder with anxious mood: reaction following a psychosocial stressor that lasts up to 6 months
- Generalized anxiety disorder: persistent anxiety lasting more than 6 months
- Panic disorder: recurrent unexpected attacks of anxiety
- Posttraumatic stress disorder: recurrent flashbacks or nightmares of catastrophic event by a survivor, often associated with panic attacks and major depression
- Phobias: intense fear of an object or situation (simple phobia) or of public embarrassment (social phobia)
- Obsessive-compulsive disorder: persistent unwanted and disturbing thoughts and recurrent behavioral patterns (e.g., handwashing) that interfere with daily life

SIGNS AND SYMPTOMS

Patterns vary with the type of anxiety; not all signs and symptoms are present in each case.

- Unrealistic or excessive anxiety or worry
- Sense of impending doom
- Nervousness
- Rapid heart rate, palpitations
- Hyperventilation, choking sensation
- Sighing respiration
- Nausea or abdominal distress
- Tingling sensation in extremities
- Excessive sweating
- Dizziness or syncope
- Flushing
- Muscle tension
- Tremor
- Restlessness
- Chest tightness, pressure
- Headache, backaches, muscle spasm

CAUSES

- Panic disorder and obsessive compulsive disorder are associated with genetic factors.
- Psychosocial stressors commonly trigger anxiety disorders.

SCOPE

Anxiety, the most common psychiatric disorder in the United States, affects about 40 million persons.

MOST OFTEN AFFECTED

Mainly adults, highest among those aged 20 to 45 years; females are affected more often than males. Evidence is seen for a genetic cause of anxiety.

RISK FACTORS

- Social and financial problems
- Medical illness
- Family history
- Lack of social support

DIAGNOSIS

WHAT THE DOCTOR LOOKS FOR

The doctor will investigate the variety of medical conditions that can cause anxiety-like symptoms, including cardiovascular, respiratory, neurologic, hormonal, and nutritional disorders; alcohol or drug use; or other conditions.

TESTS AND PROCEDURES

- Blood tests, urinalysis, chest x-ray study, electrocardiogram (ECG)
- An electroencephalogram (EEG) may be done to assess brain activity.
- Psychological testing may be performed.

TREATMENT

GENERAL MEASURES

- Anxiety is managed on an outpatient basis.
- The doctor should do a thorough workup to identify the cause and type of anxiety disorder.
- Other substance abuse should be identified and treated.
- Counseling or psychotherapy along with medications
- Regular exercise program
- Biofeedback in selected cases

ACTIVITY

Fully active

DIET

No special diet

MEDICATIONS

COMMONLY PRESCRIBED DRUGS

- Acute situational anxiety:
  - Short-term (up to 1 month) treatment with benzodiazepines: alprazolam (Xanax), clonazepam (Klonopin), lorazepam (Ativan), diazepam (Valium)
- Adjustment disorder with anxiety mood:
  - Benzodiazepines
- Generalized anxiety disorder:
  - Azapirones: buspirone (BuSpar)
- Panic disorder:
  - Tricyclic antidepressants (TCAs): imipramine (Tofranil)
  - Serotonin reuptake inhibitors (SRIs): fluoxetine (Prozac), sertraline (Zoloft), paroxetine (Paxil)
- Obsessive-compulsive disorder:
  - Clomipramine (Anafranil)
  - SRIs: fluoxetine (Prozac), sertraline (Zoloft), paroxetine (Paxil)

CONTRAINDICATIONS

- Benzodiazepines: first-trimester pregnancy, acute alcohol intoxication with depressed vital signs, acute glaucoma, sleep apnea, history of personality disorder, or substance abuse. Long-term use should be avoided.
- Buspirone: concurrent monoamine oxidase (MAO) inhibitor use
- TCAs: acute myocardial infarction (heart attack)

PRECAUTIONS

Drugs used for anxiety have numerous precautions; read drug product information.

DRUG INTERACTIONS

- Benzodiazepines: cimetidine, disulfiram, oral contraceptives, ethanol, levodopa, rifampin
- Buspirone: MAO inhibitors
- TCAs: amphetamines, barbiturates, guanethidine, clonidine, epinephrine, ethanol, norepinephrine, MAO inhibitors, propoxyphene
- SRIs: MAO inhibitors

OTHER DRUGS

- Generalized anxiety disorder: short-term use of benzodiazepine or TCAs
- Panic disorder: TCAs, SRIs, benzodiazepines, MAO inhibitors
- Obsessive-compulsive disorder: fluoxetine (Prozac), sertraline (Zoloft), paroxetine (Paxil)

FOLLOW-UP

PATIENT MONITORING

- See the doctor on a regular basis.
- Development of associated depression should be noted and treated.
- Drug therapy should be evaluated.

Anxiety

Doctor
Office
Phone
Pager

Special notes to patient:

Anxiety

PREVENTION
- Manage stress to the extent possible.
- Learn relaxation techniques or meditation.

COMPLICATIONS
- Impaired social or occupational functioning
- Drug dependence (benzodiazepines)
- Cardiac rhythm disturbances (TCAs)

WHAT TO EXPECT
- With proper treatment, excellent results can be expected, especially with short-term anxiety disorders, including panic disorder.
- Obsessive-compulsive disorder and posttraumatic stress disorder are more difficult to treat, often requiring long-term psychotherapy and medication.

 MISCELLANEOUS

PEDIATRIC
Reduced dosage of medications

GERIATRIC
Reduced dosage of medications

PREGNANCY
- Benzodiazepines: These drugs are contraindicated in first-trimester pregnancy and should be used with caution later in pregnancy and during lactation. They can cause lethargy and weight loss in nursing infants; avoid breast-feeding if taking benzodiazepines.
- TCAs: Some evidence is seen of fetal risk, especially in the first trimester.
- SRIs: Taper and discontinue, if possible, in first trimester; they can be used later in pregnancy.

FURTHER INFORMATION
- American Academy of Family Physicians Foundation, P.O. Box 8418, Kansas City, MO 64114, (800) 274-2237, ext. 4400
- National Institute of Mental Health (NIMH), National Anxiety Awareness Program, 9000 Rockville Pike, Bethesda, MD 20892

Anxiety

_____ Doctor
_____ Office
_____ Phone
_____ Pager

Special notes to patient:

_____
_____
_____
_____
_____
_____
_____
_____
_____
_____
_____
_____
_____
_____
_____
_____
_____

Anxiety

Appendicitis, Acute

 ## BASICS

DESCRIPTION
Acute appendicitis is the acute inflammation of the vermiform appendix. It must be treated promptly by surgical removal to avoid rupture of the appendix, which can be life-threatening.

SIGNS AND SYMPTOMS
- Abdominal pain around the navel that later moves to the right lower quadrant of the abdomen. Pain lessens by flexing the thigh.
- Anorexia (almost 100%)
- Nausea (90%)
- Mild vomiting (75%)
- Severe constipation
- Mild diarrhea
- Sequence of symptom appearance in 95% of persons: anorexia, then abdominal pain, then vomiting
- Slight temperature elevation
- Slightly fast heartbeat

CAUSES
Obstruction of the appendix opening in the digestive tract

SCOPE
Acute appendicitis affects about 10 of 100,000 persons; 1 of 15 persons (7%) will have acute appendicitis at some point in their life. It is the most common acute surgical condition of the abdomen.

MOST OFTEN AFFECTED
- Between the ages of 10 and 30, appendicitis is more common in males than females.
- Among those over age 30, males and females are affected in equal numbers.

RISK FACTORS
- Adolescent males
- Family member with a history of appendicitis
- Abdominal tumors

 ## DIAGNOSIS

WHAT THE DOCTOR LOOKS FOR
- The doctor conducts a thorough physical examination, including checking for several classic signs of appendicitis.
- A rectal digital examination may be done to assess the appendix.
- Other conditions that can cause similar symptoms should be investigated (e.g., urologic causes, inflammatory bowel disease, colonic disorders, and gynecologic diseases).

TESTS AND PROCEDURES
- Blood tests, urinalysis
- Imaging may be done to assist in diagnosis, including ultrasound, x-ray study of the abdomen, barium enema, and computed tomography (CT) scan.
- Internal organs may be visually inspected by laparoscopy.

 ## TREATMENT

GENERAL MEASURES
Acute appendicitis is usually managed by inpatient surgery.

ACTIVITY
- Walking soon after surgery
- Return to full activity by 4 to 6 weeks

DIET
Regular diet with return of bowel function, usually within 24 to 48 hours after surgery

 ## MEDICATIONS

COMMONLY PRESCRIBED DRUGS
Antibiotics: cefoxitin (Mefoxin), cefotetan (Cefotan)

CONTRAINDICATIONS
Documented allergy to specific antibiotic

PRECAUTIONS
Read drug product information.

DRUG INTERACTIONS
Read drug product information.

OTHER DRUGS
- Metronidazole (Flagyl)
- Ampicillin-sulbactam (Unasyn)
- Ticarcillin-clavulanate (Timentin)

 ## FOLLOW-UP

PATIENT MONITORING
- See the doctor at 2 and 6 weeks after surgery.
- Contact the doctor if anorexia, nausea, vomiting, abdominal pain, fever, or chills develop after surgery.

COMPLICATIONS
- Wound infection
- Abdominal abscess
- Intestinal problems

WHAT TO EXPECT
- Young adults who have nonruptured appendicitis generally have a good course of recovery.
- Risks of complications increase with age and presence of ruptured appendix.

 ## MISCELLANEOUS

PEDIATRIC
- Rare in infancy
- Higher fever, more vomiting
- May return to full activities earlier

GERIATRIC
Patients over 60 years of age account for 50% of deaths from acute appendicitis.

Appendicitis, Acute

Doctor
Office
Phone
Pager

Special notes to patient:

Arteriosclerotic Heart Disease

BASICS

DESCRIPTION

Arteriosclerosis, also called "hardening of the arteries" or coronary artery disease, involves the thickening of the arterial wall, which, along with loss of elasticity of the artery, progressively blocks the coronary arteries supplying the heart. The process is chronic, developing over many years, and is the most common cause of cardiovascular disability and death. High levels of cholesterol and low-density lipoproteins in the bloodstream are involved in the development of arteriosclerosis.

SIGNS AND SYMPTOMS

- May not cause symptoms, even in advanced stages
- Chest pain
- Difficulty breathing
- Easier to breathe sitting up
- Shortness of breath during sleep
- Rapid or irregular heartbeat
- Ankle swelling

CAUSES

- Fat and cholesterol deposits within blood vessels (atherosclerosis)
- Narrowing of coronary arteries
- Blood clot formation
- Lesions within the blood vessels

SCOPE

Arteriosclerotic heart disease is common in the United States. It is responsible for 35% of deaths among men 35 to 50 years of age. The death rate among those 55 to 64 years of age is about 1%.

MOST OFTEN AFFECTED

Peak symptoms are seen in men aged 50 to 60 years, and in women aged 60 to 70 years; men are affected more often than women. The tendency to develop arteriosclerotic heart disease is inheritable.

RISK FACTORS

- High levels of cholesterol and fats in the bloodstream
- Smoking
- Family history of premature arteriosclerosis
- Obesity
- High blood pressure
- Stress
- Sedentary life style
- Increasing age
- Male gender
- Postmenopausal women
- Diabetes mellitus

DIAGNOSIS

WHAT THE DOCTOR LOOKS FOR

The doctor will take a history and perform a thorough physical examination, particularly listening to the heart and lungs.

TESTS AND PROCEDURES

- Blood tests
- Chest x-ray
- An electrocardiogram (ECG) can be done to assess the heart's electrical activity.
- An exercise stress test can be done to measure how the heart responds while working.
- Special imaging procedures (e.g., a stress thallium test, angiography, echocardiography) can be done to evaluate the heart and related structures.

➕ TREATMENT

GENERAL MEASURES

- Arteriosclerotic heart disease is managed on an outpatient basis, except for episodes of acute ischemia (decreased oxygen supply to the heart), which require hospitalization.
- Prevention of further progression of the disease:
  - Stop smoking
  - Treatment of high cholesterol (diet, drugs)
  - Blood pressure control
  - Diabetes mellitus treated early and adequately
  - Exercise
  - Aspirin to prevent blood clots
  - Stress reduction
  - Diet changes
  - Weight loss
  - Estrogen replacement therapy (ERT) in postmenopausal women
- Treatment of complications (e.g., angina, heart attack, heart failure, stroke).

ACTIVITY

Exercise may be helpful in preventing and treating heart disease.

DIET

- Low-fat (20–30 g/day total intake) diet
- Weight-loss diet, if obesity is a problem
- Increase soluble fiber

MEDICATIONS

COMMONLY PRESCRIBED DRUGS

- Aspirin: one 325 mg/day tablet, unless contraindicated, to prevent blood clots from forming in the coronary arteries. Do not take daily aspirin without a doctor's permission.
- Cholesterol-lowering agents: cholestyramine, colestipol, nicotinic acid, gemfibrozil, probucol, pravastatin (Pravachol), lovastatin (Mevacor), fluvastatin (Lescol), simvastatin (Zocor)

CONTRAINDICATIONS

Read drug product information.

PRECAUTIONS

Read drug product information.

DRUG INTERACTIONS

Read drug product information.

OTHER DRUGS

- Ticlopidine: prevents clots

🔁 FOLLOW-UP

PATIENT MONITORING

- Health status should be monitored regularly.
- Preventive programs (weight loss, smoking cessation)

PREVENTION

See *General Measures*.

COMPLICATIONS

- Heart attack (myocardial infarction)
- Irregular heartbeat
- Heart failure
- Angina pectoris
- Sudden death

WHAT TO EXPECT

The outcome of arteriosclerotic heart disease varies. In many cases, the outcome is favorable. Many risk factors can be changed and improved.

Arteriosclerotic Heart Disease

Doctor

Office

Phone

Pager

Special notes to patient:

Arteriosclerotic Heart Disease

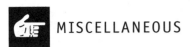 **MISCELLANEOUS**

PEDIATRIC

Preventive measures can begin early (e.g., proper nutrition, exercise, weight control).

GERIATRIC

The greatest incidence of arteriosclerotic heart disease is among the elderly.

PREGNANCY

Arteriosclerotic heart disease is practically nonexistent in pregnant women.

FURTHER INFORMATION

American Heart Association, 7320 Greenville Avenue, Dallas, TX 75231, (214) 373-6300

Arteriosclerotic Heart Disease

Doctor

Office

Phone

Pager

Special notes to patient:

Arthritis, Osteo

 ## BASICS

DESCRIPTION
Osteoarthritis (OA), the most common form of joint disease, involves progressive loss of cartilage and changes of the joint and bone.

SIGNS AND SYMPTOMS
- Joint pain that develops slowly
- Pain following use of a joint
- Stiffness, especially in the morning and after sitting
- Joint enlargement
- Decreased range of motion
- Crackling sensation in joint

CAUSES
Multiple factors are implicated.

SCOPE
- About 60 million Americans suffer from OA at any one time.
- OA affects 33% to almost 90% of individuals more than 65 years of age.

MOST OFTEN AFFECTED
- Persons over 40 years of age
- OA is the leading cause of disability in people older than 65 years of age.
- Male and females affected in equal proportions

RISK FACTORS
- Age more than 50 years
- Obesity
- Prolonged occupational or sports stress
- A joint injury

 ## DIAGNOSIS

WHAT THE DOCTOR LOOKS FOR
- The doctor will perform a thorough physical examination.
- Other causes of similar symptoms should be investigated (e.g., other forms of arthritis, cancer, or bone disorders).

TESTS AND PROCEDURES
- Blood tests
- A sample of joint fluid may be obtained for analysis.
- X-ray study may be done of the affected joint(s).

 ## TREATMENT

GENERAL MEASURES
- OA is managed in the outpatient setting.
- Weight reduction if obese
- General fitness program
- Heat (e.g., local, tub baths)
- Physical therapy to maintain or regain joint motion and muscle strength
- Protect joints from overuse (e.g., use of cane, crutches, walker, neck collar, elastic knee support).
- Surgery may be required for advanced disease.

ACTIVITY
As active as tolerated

DIET
No special diet

MEDICATIONS

COMMONLY PRESCRIBED DRUGS
- Pain relief: acetaminophen, ibuprofen, salsalate, choline-magnesium salicylate
- Other nonsteroidal antiinflammatory drugs (NSAIDs)
- Narcotic painkillers: codeine, oxycodone, propoxyphene

CONTRAINDICATIONS
NSAIDs are relatively contraindicated for individuals with kidney disease, heart failure, hypertension, peptic ulcer, or allergy to NSAIDs or aspirin.

PRECAUTIONS
Drugs used to treat OA have many precautions.
Read drug product information.

DRUG INTERACTIONS
- NSAIDs reduce effectiveness of angiotensin-converting enzyme (ACE) inhibitors and diuretics.
- Aspirin and NSAIDs may increase effects of anticoagulants.
- Aspirin may interfere with diabetes medication.
- Aspirin and other NSAIDs should not be taken together.

OTHER DRUGS
- Drug therapy should be tailored to symptoms and changed if not effective.
- Antiinflammatory drugs: magnesium salicylate, choline salicylate
- Capsaicin cream is a topical application that relieves pain. It is most effective in small joints of the hand, but can cause a local burning sensation.

 ## FOLLOW-UP

PATIENT MONITORING
- See the doctor regularly for monitoring of health status and drug therapy.
- Tests should be done periodically to detect gastrointestinal bleeding caused by NSAIDs.

COMPLICATIONS
- Side effects of medication
- Infection or accelerated cartilage loss

WHAT TO EXPECT
- OA tends to be progressive.
- Early in disease, rest relieves pain.
- As disease develops, pain may occur at rest and at night.
- Joint enlargement occurs later from bony enlargement.
- Spurs can form, especially at joint margins, as disease progresses.

 ## MISCELLANEOUS

GERIATRIC
- Becomes increasingly common with age
- Almost universal in persons over 65 years of age

PREGNANCY
NSAIDs pose some risk to the fetus during pregnancy; however, they can be taken while breast-feeding.

FURTHER INFORMATION
American Academy of Family Physicians Foundation, P.O. Box 8418, Kansas City, MO 64114, (800) 274-2237, ext. 4400

Arthritis, Osteo

Doctor
Office
Phone
Pager

Special notes to patient:

Arthritis, Rheumatoid (RA)

 ## BASICS

DESCRIPTION

Rheumatoid arthritis (RA) is a chronic, systemic, inflammatory disease of unknown cause that tends to involve the joints. The disease also causes effects throughout the body, including the nervous system, heart, and other internal organs.

SIGNS AND SYMPTOMS

- Joints
  - Most often involved are wrists, knees, elbows, shoulders, ankles, and feet
  - Swelling
  - Sensation of heat
  - Deformity
  - Morning stiffness
  - Pain
- Fatigue
- Depression
- Malaise
- Anorexia
- Anemia
- Swollen glands
- Eye disease

CAUSES

Immune disorder; cause unknown

SCOPE

- RA affects 0.3% to 1.5% of the population.
- Women are affected twice as often as men, although men tend to show more signs of systemic disease.
- Prevalence in Native Americans is 3.5% to 5.3%.

MOST OFTEN AFFECTED

Persons 30 to 60 years of age. RA tends to run in families.

RISK FACTORS

- Genetic factors
- Family history
- Native American ethnicity
- Female gender, 20 to 50 years of age

 ## DIAGNOSIS

WHAT THE DOCTOR LOOKS FOR

- The doctor will perform a thorough physical examination.
- Other possible causes of similar signs and symptoms (e.g., bone disorders, infection, or inflammatory diseases) will be investigated.

TESTS AND PROCEDURES

- Blood tests to look for signs of infection and inflammation
- A sample of joint fluid may be obtained for analysis
- X-ray study may be done to monitor progress of the disease
- Special imaging procedures may be done to assist in diagnosis, including arthrography, bone scan, computed tomography (CT) scan, and magnetic resonance imaging (MRI).

 ## TREATMENT

GENERAL MEASURES

- RA is managed on an outpatient basis, except for complicating emergencies or orthopedic procedures.
- Therapy emphasizes exercise and mobility and general healthcare.
- Special emphasis should be placed on reducing joint stress and on physical and occupational therapy.

ACTIVITY

- Full activity is encouraged, but heavy work and vigorous exercise during acute episodes should be avoided.
- Hydrotherapy or water exercise is effective.

DIET

No special diet

 ## MEDICATIONS

COMMONLY PRESCRIBED DRUGS

- Early disease or acute or chronic inflammation: aspirin or other nonsteroidal antiinflammatory drugs (NSAIDs)
- Severe disease: corticosteroids
- Persistent disease activity:
  - Steroid injections
  - Antimalarials: hydroxychloroquine (Plaquenil)
  - Gold: auranofin
  - Sulfasalazine
  - Penicillamine (d-penicillamine)
  - Methotrexate
  - Leflunomide (Arava)

CONTRAINDICATIONS

Depends on drugs used. Read drug product information.

PRECAUTIONS

Some drugs require careful monitoring of disease activity and signs of drug toxicity.

DRUG INTERACTIONS

- Numerous drugs interfere with NSAIDs, including antacids, anticoagulants, diabetes medication, blood pressure medication, and others.
- Read drug product information.

 ## FOLLOW-UP

PATIENT MONITORING

- See the doctor regularly for evaluation of RA and the effectiveness of therapy.
- Blood tests should be repeated periodically.

PREVENTION

- Oral contraceptive may decrease risk of RA.

COMPLICATIONS

- Joint destruction
- Skin disorders
- Heart disease
- Respiratory disease
- Other medical disorders
- Complications induced by treatment

WHAT TO EXPECT

The usual course of RA has been a progressive decline in function. Proper medical, surgical, and physiotherapeutic interventions can significantly improve the outcome.

 ## MISCELLANEOUS

GERIATRIC

- Onset in the geriatric population is less common.
- Elderly have less tolerance to medication and increased incidence of side effects.

PREGNANCY

- Labor and delivery pose no serious problems, unless the mother has severe joint disease (e.g., hips).
- More than 75% of patients with RA experience improvement during pregnancy. The cause of improvement is unclear. Relapse invariably occurs within 6 months after delivery.
- No increased number of birth defects have been reported from RA itself.

FURTHER INFORMATION

American Rheumatism Association, (800) 282-7023

Arthritis, Rheumatoid (RA)

Doctor
Office
Phone
Pager

Special notes to patient:

Asthma

BASICS

DESCRIPTION

Asthma, also called "reactive airway disease," is marked by mild to severe obstruction of airflow through the airway. Symptoms, which range from coughing to difficulty breathing, usually have a sudden onset.

- The clinical hallmark of asthma is wheezing, but some patients may complain primarily of only a cough.
- Acute symptoms are caused by the narrowing of large and small airways caused by bronchial smooth muscle spasm, swelling and inflammation of airway tissues, and mucus production.

SIGNS AND SYMPTOMS

- Chest pain or tightness with aerobic exercise
- Wheezing
- Cough
- Difficulty breathing
- Symptoms that become periodically acute
- Attacks during sleep
- A bluish discoloration of the skin around the eyes, lips, and nail beds.
- Increased heart rate

CAUSES

- Allergies to pollens, molds, house dust, mites, animal dander, feather pillows
- Other factors: smoke and other pollutants, infection, sinusitis, aspirin, exercise, gastroesophageal reflux, sleep

SCOPE

- Approximately 10 million new cases of asthma are seen each year. However, lack of a uniform definition of asthma leads to confusion about the diagnosis.
- Asthma affects 7% to 19% of children
- Asthma is a leading cause of missed school days, about 7.5 million days annually.

MOST OFTEN AFFECTED

- Asthma can occur at any age, but primarily affects young adults (16–30 years of age).
- Half of asthma cases occur in children younger than 10 years of age.
- Asthma is more common in males during childhood until puberty and is more common in females among adults.
- Asthma and allergies tend to run in families. Search for an asthma gene is presently underway.

RISK FACTORS

- Family history of asthma
- Viral infection of the lower respiratory tract during infancy

DIAGNOSIS

WHAT THE DOCTOR LOOKS FOR

- The doctor will evaluate breathing status and symptom severity.
- The doctor will rule out possible causes related to the heart (e.g., congestive heart failure or mitral valve prolapse).
- Other causes of breathing difficulty include infection, cystic fibrosis, or a foreign body in the airway.
- May be associated with sinusitis or irritation of the esophagus from reflux (heartburn)

TESTS AND PROCEDURES

- Blood tests may be done to determine the presence of inflammation or infection.
- The levels of salt in the sweat of a child with chronic asthma should be measured to rule out cystic fibrosis.
- In severe cases, arterial blood can be drawn to measure levels of oxygen and carbon dioxide.
- A chest x-ray study may be performed to assess the respiratory system.
- Pulmonary function tests can be done to evaluate breathing and detect reversible airway obstruction.
- Allergy testing may be done to identify causes of asthma.
- Exercise tolerance testing can be done to assess the impact of physical activity.
- Patients may be given peak flow meters for self-assessment of breathing status.

TREATMENT

GENERAL MEASURES

- Asthma is usually treated on an outpatient basis.
- A person may be hospitalized if asthma is not relieved by medication.
- Sources of irritants at the home and workplace should be eliminated.
- Antiinflammatory drugs (e.g., cromolyn sodium and inhaled steroids) are used to prevent the development of symptoms.
- Dosages of beta-agonist drugs are increased in response to symptoms.
- The person with asthma may be treated for allergies.
- Education about asthma and its management is essential for well-being.

ACTIVITY

A person with asthma should have no restrictions on activity if the asthma is diagnosed early and properly treated.

DIET

No special diet

MEDICATIONS

COMMONLY PRESCRIBED DRUGS

- Five major classes of drugs are used:
  - Cromoglycate and nedocromil
  - Steroids (budesonide, prednisone)
  - Beta-agonists (albuterol, bitolterol, salmeterol)
  - Methylxanthines (theophylline)
  - Anticholinergics (atropine, ipratropium bromide)
  - Leukotriene modifiers (montelukast, zafirlukast)
- Mild asthma (brief wheezing once or twice a week):
  - Intermittent use of beta-agonist by nebulizer or metered dose inhaler (MDI)
  - Oral beta-agonist or theophylline
- Moderate asthma: (weekly symptoms interfering with sleep or exercise, occasional visits to an emergency department, peak flow rate 60% to 80% of predicted)
  - Regular maintenance schedule
  - Inhaled steroids (beclomethasone dipropionate)
  - Cromolyn sodium four times a day or nedocromil twice a day
  - If asthma is not controlled with inhaled steroid, the doctor may prescribe slow-release xanthines by mouth or inhaled ipratropium bromide.
  - Acute episodes are treated with inhaled beta-agonists and steroids.
- Severe asthma: (frequent symptoms affecting activity, nocturnal symptoms, frequent hospital stays, peak flow rate less than 60% predicted)
  - Cromolyn sodium and ipratropium
  - Inhaled steroids; some patients may need oral steroids every other day.
  - Theophylline is often useful, particularly for nighttime symptoms.
- Acute episode-outpatient management
  - Inhaled beta-agonist (albuterol)
  - Short course of steroids
  - Observation for at least 1 hour
- Delivery systems
  - Children younger than 2 years of age: nebulizer or MDI with valved spacer and mask
  - Children 2 to 4 years of age: MDI and valved spacer
  - Over 5 years of age: MDI or powder inhaler

Asthma

Doctor
Office
Phone
Pager

Special notes to patient:

Asthma

- Hospital management
  - Intravenous (IV) steroids
  - Other medications may be given by inhalation or IV if symptoms do not improve.
  - In rare cases, mechanical ventilation may be needed to support breathing.

CONTRAINDICATIONS

- Sedatives
- Beta-adrenergic blocking drugs should be avoided.

PRECAUTIONS

Chronic use of beta-agonists can result in harmful effects. Use only when experiencing symptoms of asthma. Chronic asthma may require chronic use of beta-agonists.

DRUG INTERACTIONS

Some antibiotics increase levels of theophylline.

OTHER DRUGS

- Ketotifen
- H_1-antagonists
- Troleandomycin (TAO)
- Methotrexate
- Immune globulin, intravenous (IVIG)
- Furosemide (Lasix)

FOLLOW-UP

PATIENT MONITORING

- The person with asthma may be given a device to monitor peak flow rates while at home. The patient should keep a record to track trends and report if flow drops below 70% of baseline.
- The patient should have blood drawn periodically for testing, including arterial blood for blood gases and pH.
- The doctor may order a test called oximetry that measures the oxygen-carrying ability of blood.
- The patient should be tested for tuberculosis annually.

PREVENTION

- Management of asthma by the patient is essential. A person with asthma should:
  - Understand medication, inhalers, nebulizers, peak flow meters
  - Monitor symptoms and peak flows
  - Have written guidelines prepared by a doctor
  - Have prearranged action plan for an acute episode
- If symptoms are severe, control triggering factors: pollutants, exercise, mites, molds, animal dander.
- Have flu shots every year.
- Avoid the use of aspirin.
- Avoid sulfites and tartrazine (food additives).

COMPLICATIONS

- Collapsed lung, pneumothorax, or other lung conditions.
- Respiratory failure; mechanical ventilation may be needed to support breathing.
- Muscle conditions caused by steroids
- Death

WHAT TO EXPECT

- In most cases, the outcome is excellent with attention to general health and use of medications to control symptoms.
- Less than 50% of children with asthma "outgrow it."
- If the response to treatment is poor, the doctor should review the diagnosis and compliance with therapy before prescribing stronger drugs.

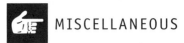

MISCELLANEOUS

PEDIATRIC

Half of new cases of asthma occur in children younger than 10 years of age.

GERIATRIC

It is unusual for an initial episode of asthma to occur in an elderly person.

PREGNANCY

- About 50% of asthma patients have no change in symptoms during pregnancy, 25% seem to improve, and 25% have worse symptoms.
- It is important to prevent stress during pregnancy.
- Avoid medications that are contraindicated during pregnancy.

FURTHER INFORMATION

- American Lung Association, 1740 Broadway, New York, NY 10019, (212) 315-8700
- Asthma and Allergy Foundation of America, 1125 15th St., NW, Washington, DC 20005, (800) 7-ASTHMA, (800) 727-8462

Asthma

Doctor
Office
Phone
Pager

Special notes to patient:

Attention Deficit Hyperactivity Disorder

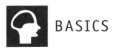 BASICS

DESCRIPTION

Attention deficit hyperactivity disorder (ADHD), also called "hyperactivity," is a behavior problem marked by a short attention span, low frustration tolerance, impulsivity, distractibility, and usually, hyperactivity. ADHD can result in poor school performance, difficulty in peer relationships, and parent-child conflict.

SIGNS AND SYMPTOMS

- Fidgets
- Difficulty remaining seated
- Easily distracted
- Cannot wait turn
- Blurts out answers before question is complete
- Difficulty following instructions
- Difficulty sustaining attention
- Shifts from one uncompleted task to another
- Difficulty playing quietly
- Talks excessively
- Interrupts others
- Does not seem to be listening
- Loses things
- Engages in physically dangerous activities without considering consequences

CAUSES

Multiple factors

SCOPE

ADHD affects about 5% of school-aged children.

MOST OFTEN AFFECTED

- Onset before 7 years of age
- Lasts into adolescence and adulthood
- By age 4, 50% of cases can be diagnosed
- May affect more than one family member
- Males affected four to six times more often than females

RISK FACTORS

- Poor prenatal health (preeclampsia, drug and alcohol use, smoking)
- Associated with, but not caused by, other conditions:
  - Learning disabilities
  - Tourette's syndrome
  - Mood disorders
  - Conduct disorder

 DIAGNOSIS

WHAT THE DOCTOR LOOKS FOR

- The doctor will obtain a history and perform a thorough physical examination.
- Other possible causes of the behavior will be investigated (e.g., learning disability, or hearing or vision disorder).

TESTS AND PROCEDURES

- Laboratory testing rarely needed
- Lead level in the blood may be measured.
- Behavioral or psychological testing may be done.

 TREATMENT

GENERAL MEASURES

- ADHD is managed in the outpatient setting.
- Doctor and parents must work closely with teachers and other school officials.
- Avoid unproved therapies.
- Reinforce good behavior with rewards and attention.
- Make eye contact with each request.
- Keep child on one task at a time.
- Administer time-out (brief) for problems.
- Stop behavior before it escalates.
- Find things the child is good at and emphasize these tasks.
- Some families benefit from anger training, social training, and family therapy.
- Keep realistic expectations during growth stages (newborn to adulthood).
- Discuss pros and cons of drug therapy with doctor.
- Parents may need help dealing with feelings (guilt, shame, anxiety, exhaustion, and blame).
- At school:
  - Keep work sessions short.
  - Make sure rules are clear.
  - Consequences for unacceptable behavior must be immediate.
  - Reinforce good behavior.
  - Teachers should coordinate homework with parent (child may not bring home messages).

ACTIVITY

- Allow for increased activity in a safe environment.
- Children with ADHD often respond well to water play or bathtubs.

DIET

- No dietary changes have been proven to help ADHD.
- Parents can experiment with nonharmful diets by eliminating sugar, dyes, additives.

COMMONLY PRESCRIBED DRUGS

- Methylphenidate (Ritalin)
- Pemoline (Cylert)
- Dosage should start low and be increased as needed.
- Some physicians give "holidays" off drugs in the summer, and a few patients can have weekend "holidays."
- Some children experience withdrawal (tearfulness, agitation) after a missed dose.

PRECAUTIONS

Do not crush sustained-release tablets.

OTHER DRUGS

- Dextroamphetamine (Dexedrine)
- Clonidine
- Tricyclics

Attention Deficit Hyperactivity Disorder

Doctor
Office
Phone
Pager

Special notes to patient:

Attention Deficit Hyperactivity Disorder

 FOLLOW-UP

PATIENT MONITORING
- Person with ADHD and family should be tested regularly.
- See the doctor at least every 3 months to have medication monitored.

PREVENTION
- Children are at risk for abuse, depression, and social isolation.
- Parents need regular support and advice.
- Establish contact with teacher each school year.

COMPLICATIONS
- Medications can cause headaches, abdominal pain, growth delay.
- Untreated ADHD can lead to failing in school, parental abuse, social isolation, poor self-esteem.

WHAT TO EXPECT
- ADHD lasts through school years and into adulthood.
- The condition becomes easier to control with increasing age.
- Encourage career choices that allow autonomy and mobility.
- Delinquency is not increased unless other conditions exist (e.g., conduct disorder).

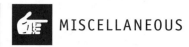 **MISCELLANEOUS**

PREGNANCY
Avoid stimulants in pregnancy.

Attention Deficit Hyperactivity Disorder

Doctor
Office
Phone
Pager

Special notes to patient:

Balanitis

 ## BASICS

DESCRIPTION
Balanitis is the inflammation of the glans penis.

SIGNS AND SYMPTOMS
- Penile pain
- Difficult or painful urination
- Infection
- Reddening
- Swelling of the prepuce (foreskin)
- Ulcers or plaques

CAUSES
- Allergic reaction (condom latex, contraceptive jelly)
- Fungal and bacterial infections
- Drug side effects
- Other medical problems

MOST OFTEN AFFECTED
Adult males

RISK FACTORS
- Presence of foreskin (uncircumcised)
- Oral antibiotics in male infants can predispose to infection.

 ## DIAGNOSIS

WHAT THE DOCTOR LOOKS FOR
- The doctor will perform a physical examination and consider other possible causes of similar signs and symptoms.
- The doctor will check for known associated conditions (e.g., diabetes mellitus).

TESTS AND PROCEDURES
- Blood tests
- Cells or fluid may be analyzed in the laboratory.

 ## TREATMENT

GENERAL MEASURES
- Balanitis is managed in the outpatient setting.
- Warm compresses or sitz baths may relieve symptoms.
- Practice good hygiene.
- Circumcision can be considered as preventive measure.
- Avoid substances that trigger an allergic reaction.

ACTIVITY
No Limitations

DIET
No special diet

 ## MEDICATIONS

COMMONLY PRESCRIBED DRUGS
- Antifungal drugs: clotrimazole (Lotrimin), nystatin (Mycostatin)
- Antibacterial drug: bacitracin or neomycin-polymyxin B-bacitracin (Neosporin), cephalosporin, sulfa drugs
- Topical steroids

CONTRAINDICATIONS
Read drug product information.

PRECAUTIONS
Read drug product information.

DRUG INTERACTIONS
Read drug product information.

 ## FOLLOW-UP

PATIENT MONITORING
- See the doctor every 1 to 2 weeks until the cause of balanitis has been identified.
- Persistent inflammation may require biopsy to rule out cancer.

PREVENTION
- Proper hygiene
- Avoid allergy-triggering substances.
- Circumcision

COMPLICATIONS
- Narrowing or scarring of the urinary opening
- Cancerous changes from chronic irritations
- Urinary tract infections

WHAT TO EXPECT
Balanitis should resolve once the cause has been identified and appropriate treatment instituted.

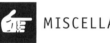 ## MISCELLANEOUS

PEDIATRIC
Oral antibiotics predispose infants to infection.

GERIATRIC
Condom-type urinary catheters can lead to balanitis.

Balanitis

_____ Doctor
_____ Office
_____ Phone
_____ Pager

Special notes to patient:

Basal Cell Carcinoma

 ## BASICS

DESCRIPTION
Basal cell carcinoma is a slow-growing malignant cancer of the skin. Tumors rarely spread but are capable of local tissue destruction.

SIGNS AND SYMPTOMS
- Basal cell carcinoma begins as a small, smooth-surfaced, well-defined lump on the skin.
- The affected area is pink to red in color, with a pearly translucent border.
- Area may be covered with blood vessels.
- May be pigmented to varying degrees
- A crusting ulcer develops as the lesion grows.

CAUSES
Sun exposure

SCOPE
Approximately 400,000 cases occur each year in the United States.

MOST OFTEN AFFECTED
More common in fair-skin blondes and redheads. Generally affects individuals over 40 years of age, but the incidence of basal cell carcinoma is increasing in younger populations. It is more common in males than females, although the incidence is increasing in females.

RISK FACTORS
- Chronic sun exposure
- Light complexion
- Tendency to sunburn
- Male gender, although risk is increasing in women because of lifestyle changes (e.g., use of tanning salons)

 ## DIAGNOSIS

WHAT THE DOCTOR LOOKS FOR
The diagnosis is confirmed by biopsy, in which a small sample of tissue is obtained by needle or surgical procedure. The tissue sample is then examined microscopically for the presence of cancer cells.

TESTS AND PROCEDURES
A sample of tissue will be examined microscopically.

 ## TREATMENT

GENERAL MEASURES
- Basal cell carcinoma is treated on an outpatient basis unless the lesion is extensive.
- Lesions can be surgically removed or treated with freezing or electrical devices.
- Treatment selected depends on the location, extent, and nature of the lesion.
- Radiation therapy can be used for patients unable to tolerate minor surgery (e.g., the elderly). It can also be used to preserve tissue, such as that near lips and eyelids.

ACTIVITY
No restrictions on physical activity except to avoid overexposure to sun

DIET
No special diet

 ## MEDICATIONS

COMMONLY PRESCRIBED DRUGS
Topical antibiotic medication may be prescribed for the first 24 to 48 hours after skin cancer is removed by surgery.

FOLLOW-UP

PATIENT MONITORING
The patient is usually seen in the doctor's office or clinic every month for the first 3 months after treatment, then twice a year for 5 years, and once a year thereafter.

PREVENTION
- Reduce the risk of skin cancer with the use of sunscreen lotion.
- Wear a hat and a long-sleeve shirt when outdoors in bright sunlight.
- Avoid excessive tanning.
- Examine the skin regularly to detect changes in moles, freckles, and other spots.

COMPLICATIONS
- The lesion could recur, usually within 5 years, if at all.
- The lesion could spread, which rarely occurs.

WHAT TO EXPECT
- Between 90% and 95% of people who receive proper treatment are cured.
- Most recurrences happen within 5 years.
- About 36% of patients will develop a new basal cell carcinoma lesion within 5 years.

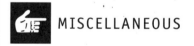 ## MISCELLANEOUS

PEDIATRIC
Rare in children

ELDERLY
More common among the elderly

Basal Cell Carcinoma

Doctor
Office
Phone
Pager

Special notes to patient:

Bed Wetting

 ## BASICS

DESCRIPTION

Enuresis is involuntary urination. Nocturnal enuresis, or bed-wetting, is involuntary urination during sleep more than once a month in girls older than 5 years and in boys older than 6 years.

SIGNS AND SYMPTOMS

- Inability to keep from urinating while asleep at least once per month.
- Some children may be withdrawn and shy; some may show aggressive behaviors.
- Stress factors (e.g., family discord, significant life events, and psychosocial or emotional problems) may be present.

CAUSES

- Hormone disorder
- Reduced bladder capacity
- Food allergies can influence bladder capacity.
- Infection
- Other urinary tract disorders

SCOPE

Enuresis affects about 10% of children.

MOST OFTEN AFFECTED

Enuresis affects 40% of 3-year-olds, 10% of 6-year-olds, 3% of 12-year-olds, and 1% of 18-year-olds. It is more common in males than females. It may be an inheritable trait.

RISK FACTORS

- History of enuresis in one or both parents
- First-born child

 ## DIAGNOSIS

WHAT THE DOCTOR LOOKS FOR

- The doctor will perform a physical examination to rule out causes of enuresis (e.g., infection, diabetes, or other disorders).

TESTS AND PROCEDURES

- Urinalysis and culture
- Pregnancy test, if indicated
- The volume of the bladder can be measured by urinating into a measuring cup.
- Imaging that may be performed includes ultrasound, intravenous pyelogram, and voiding cystourethrogram.
- X-ray study of the spine may be obtained.

 ## TREATMENT

GENERAL MEASURES

- Enuresis is managed in the outpatient setting.
- Counseling and behavior modification
- Encourage daytime fluids and less frequent urination to help increase bladder size.
- Discourage any fluids during the 2 hours before bedtime.
- Protect the bed from urine by covering the mattress with plastic, have the child wear extra thick underwear (not diapers), and put a towel on the bed in the area of the child's bottom.
- Encourage the child to take responsibility for the problem.
- Encourage the child to get up to urinate during the night, but parents should not awaken the child to urinate.
- When enuresis occurs, the child should rinse pajamas and underwear and the towel.
- Do not punish the child for wet nights, but act sympathetically.
- Heap praise on the child for dry nights: A possible incentive is a calendar for gold stars or happy faces.
- Bladder stretching exercises may be helpful.
- Self-awakening or hypnotherapy programs may be helpful.
- Bed-wetting alarms have the greatest rate of success (70%) and the lowest rate of relapse (30%).

ACTIVITY

No restrictions

DIET

No fluids for 2 hours before bedtime

 ## MEDICATIONS

COMMONLY PRESCRIBED DRUGS

Tricyclic antidepressants: imipramine, desipramine

CONTRAINDICATIONS

Read drug product information.

PRECAUTIONS

Imipramine is one of the leading causes of childhood drug-related deaths in the United States, usually from unintentional overdose; read drug product information.

DRUG INTERACTIONS

Read drug product information.

OTHER DRUGS

Desmopressin (DDAVP)

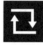 ## FOLLOW-UP

PATIENT MONITORING

See the doctor as often as necessary.

PREVENTION

No preventive measures are known.

COMPLICATIONS

Urinary tract infection

WHAT TO EXPECT

- Enuresis is a self-limited problem.
- Most children overcome the problem between 6 and 10 years of age; in a very few cases, the problem persists beyond 16 years of age.
- By age 4.5 years, 12% of children will not have complete urinary control. These 12% convert to complete control at a rate of 15% per year. By puberty, only 2% to 3% have not achieved complete control.

Bed Wetting

Doctor
Office
Phone
Pager

Special notes to patient:

Bell's Palsy

 ## BASICS

DESCRIPTION

Bell's palsy is paralysis or weakness of facial muscles, usually only on one side, resulting from the inflammation of the facial nerve.

- May be a complication of zoster (shingles)
- The development of Bell's palsy on both sides of the face is highly unusual. Other possible explanations should be considered (e.g., Guillain-Barré syndrome, chronic meningitis).

SIGNS AND SYMPTOMS

- Total or partial paralysis of the muscles on one side of the face
- Mild numbness on the affected side
- One-sided ear ache
- Loss of flavor perception
- Excessive production of tears, or dry eye, on one side
- Develops suddenly, within hours or days

CAUSES

- Inflammation of the facial nerve
- Infection, usually viral
- Exposure to cold
- Cause may be unknown

SCOPE

Bell's palsy affects about 25 of 100,000 persons.

MOST OFTEN AFFECTED

Affects all ages, but it is most common among individuals more than 30 years of age. Males and females are affected equally often. Bell's palsy tends to run in families.

RISK FACTORS

- Age more than 30 years
- Exposure to a cold environment

 ## DIAGNOSIS

WHAT THE DOCTOR LOOKS FOR

- The doctor will evaluate the extent of facial paralysis and related signs and symptoms.
- Other causes of signs and symptoms, including infection, cancer, and nerve conditions, should be considered as possible explanations for the symptoms.
- The patient should be observed for corneal abrasions caused by dry eye.

TESTS AND PROCEDURES

- A sample of cerebrospinal fluid (CSF) may be obtained by spinal tap. Analysis of CFS may reveal signs of inflammation or infection.
- Magnetic resonance imaging (MRI) can be done to make sure a lesion or tumor is not affecting the nerves or bone.
- A test known as electromyography can be performed to measure and record the electrical activity of facial muscles.
- Tests can be done to evaluate the conduction of impulses along the nerve.
- The doctor can test the blink reflex by tickling or stimulating the eyelashes.

 ## TREATMENT

GENERAL MEASURES

- Typically managed on an outpatient basis
- Surgery is rarely performed.
- Cover the eye on the affected side with a patch.
- Lubricating drops may be prescribed if the eye is dry.

ACTIVITY

No limitations on physical activity. Caution should be used when performing activities that require keen depth perception.

DIET

No special diet

 ## MEDICATIONS

COMMONLY PRESCRIBED DRUGS

A course of steroids should begin immediately after onset of Bell's palsy. Little benefit is seen in starting steroids after 4 days.

CONTRAINDICATIONS

Preexisting infections (e.g., tuberculosis)

PRECAUTIONS

Steroids should be used with caution in pregnancy, peptic ulcer disease, and diabetes.

DRUG INTERACTIONS

May interact with vaccines

 ## FOLLOW-UP

PATIENT MONITORING

- The patient should be evaluated once a month for 6 to 12 months.
- The eye should be examined for signs of corneal abrasion.

COMPLICATIONS

- Steroids may unmask infection (e.g., tuberculosis).
- Steroids can cause psychological disturbances.
- Corneal abrasion and ulceration

WHAT TO EXPECT

Recovery of function may be partial or complete, and in some cases does not occur at all. Patients with partial nerve loss typically fully recover. Patients with total nerve loss usually have partial recovery, but may have long-term complications (e.g., tearing or spasm of facial muscles).

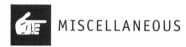 ## MISCELLANEOUS

PREGNANCY

Steroids should be used cautiously if the patient is pregnant. The primary care provider should consult with the patient's obstetrician.

Bell's Palsy

Doctor
Office
Phone
Pager

Special notes to patient:

Blepharitis

 ## BASICS

DESCRIPTION
Blepharitis, an inflammation of the edge of the eyelid, can occur as either an ulcerous or nonulcerous form. It commonly occurs as a combination of both forms.

SIGNS AND SYMPTOMS
- Ulcerous (staphylococcus) blepharitis
  - Itching
  - Excessive tearing
  - Burning sensation
  - Light sensitivity
  - Usually worse in morning
  - Recurring stye
  - Ulcerations at the base of eyelashes
  - Broken, sparse, misdirected eyelashes
- Nonulcerous (seborrheic) blepharitis
  - Reddening at the edge of the eyelid
  - Dry flakes, oily skin on lid edge, lashes, or both
  - Dandruff of scalp, eyebrows
  - Sometimes reddening or flaking of skin on the nose and lips
- Mixed blepharitis (seborrheic with associated staphylococcus)
  - Most common type of blepharitis
  - Symptoms and signs of both staphylococcus and seborrheic present

SCOPE
Common: blepharitis is the most common eye disease in the United States.

MOST OFTEN AFFECTED
Adults: males and females in equal proportion

CAUSES
- Sebaceous gland dysfunction
- Bacterial (*Staphylococcus*) infection
- Dermatitis

RISK FACTORS
- Infection
- Dermatitis
- Rosacea
- Diabetes mellitus
- Immune system disorders

 ## DIAGNOSIS

WHAT THE DOCTOR LOOKS FOR
- The doctor will assess the eye and consider other similar conditions.

TESTS AND PROCEDURES
- Blood tests can be done to assist in diagnosis.
- Fluid or cells from the affected area can be analyzed in the laboratory.

 ## TREATMENT

GENERAL MEASURES
- Blepharitis is managed in an outpatient setting.
- Wash affected area with cleanser at least once daily.
- If infection is suspected, topical antibiotic should be applied with cotton-tipped swab.
- Clean lids and apply ointment nightly in mild cases, up to four times daily in severe cases.
- Discontinue soft contact lens wear until condition clears.
- Chronic blepharitis requires referral to ophthalmologist for evaluation.

ACTIVITY
No restrictions

DIET
No restrictions

 ## MEDICATIONS

COMMONLY PRESCRIBED DRUGS
- Topical antibiotic: bacitracin, erythromycin ointment
- In some cases, oral antibiotics: tetracycline

CONTRAINDICATIONS
- Allergy to medication
- Tetracycline: not for use in pregnancy or in children younger than 8 years of age

PRECAUTIONS
- Avoid medication containing neomycin as it is sensitizing.
- Tetracycline can cause photosensitivity; sunscreen is recommended.

DRUG INTERACTIONS
- Tetracycline: avoid antacids, dairy products, and iron.
- Antibiotics can reduce the effectiveness of oral contraceptives.

OTHER DRUGS
Quinolones may be helpful for persistent or recurrent blepharitis.

 ## FOLLOW-UP

PATIENT MONITORING
See the doctor every 2 months.

PREVENTION
Follow treatment guidelines.

COMPLICATIONS
- Stye
- Eyelid scarring
- Eyelash misdirection
- Corneal infection

WHAT TO EXPECT
- Blepharitis is a chronic condition, likely to recur if hygiene is not maintained after antibiotic treatment is discontinued.
- Long-term eyelid hygiene is required to control blepharitis.

Blepharitis

Doctor
Office
Phone
Pager

Special notes to patient:

Breast Cancer

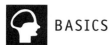 ## BASICS

DESCRIPTION

Breast cancer is malignant neoplasm of the breast. Breast cancers are classified as noninvasive (in situ) or invasive (infiltrating). Approximately 70% of all breast cancers have a component of invasion.

SIGNS AND SYMPTOMS

- Palpable lump (55%)
- Abnormal mammogram without a palpable mass (35%)
- Change in the color or texture of breast skin
- Dimpling of breast skin
- Nipple retraction
- Breast enlargement
- Lump in the armpit
- Bone pain (rare)
- Discharge

CAUSES

Unknown

SCOPE

- One of eight women in the United States will develop breast cancer within a lifetime.
- 150,000 new cases are diagnosed annually, and 50,000 women die.

MOST OFTEN AFFECTED

Women 30 to 80 years of age, with a peak at ages 45 to 65. More common in females, although 1% occurs in males. About 20% of women have a family history of breast cancer. A breast cancer gene has been identified that affects about 1 of 400 women.

RISK FACTORS

- Family history of breast cancer
- Early menarche, late menopause, no births, or first full-term pregnancy after age 30
- Women with a history of breast cancer or previous breast biopsies revealing atypical changes
- Other risk factors include estrogen use, high dietary fat, high alcohol use

 ## DIAGNOSIS

WHAT THE DOCTOR LOOKS FOR

- The doctor will perform a thorough physical examination.
- Other diseases with similar signs and symptoms will be investigated (e.g., abscess and other benign breast conditions).
- If cancer is identified, the doctor will "stage" the disease (i.e., determine the extent of involvement).

TESTS AND PROCEDURES

- Several blood tests can be done to assist in diagnosis, particularly those to assess liver function and hormone activity.
- Chest x-ray study
- Specialized radiologic imaging that may be done includes mammography, ultrasound, bone scan, liver imaging, computed tomography (CT) scan.
- Tissue can be obtained by biopsy for analysis in the laboratory.

 ## TREATMENT

GENERAL MEASURES

- Persons with breast cancer are usually treated by a team consisting of a medical oncologist, a surgeon, and a radiation oncologist.
- Treatment of breast cancer involves period of hospitalization for surgery and other treatment.
- The decision to treat with hormone therapy or chemotherapy is complex. Premenopausal women tend to respond more to cytotoxic (cell-killing) chemotherapy, and postmenopausal women tend to obtain greater benefit from hormone therapy.
- Treatment of early disease:
  - Local control measures
  - Modified radical mastectomy or lumpectomy followed by radiation
  - The optimal treatment is unclear.
- Treatment of locally advanced breast cancer:
  - Combination chemotherapy and radiation therapy before mastectomy
- Treatment of metastatic cancer (cancer that has spread to adjacent lymph nodes)
  - Measures to provide symptom improvement
  - Combinations of chemotherapy, hormone therapy, or radiation therapy

ACTIVITY

Minimal activity restrictions during treatment

DIET

No proven relationship exists between breast cancer and diet.

 ## MEDICATIONS

COMMONLY PRESCRIBED DRUGS

- Chemotherapy
- Hormone therapy: tamoxifen
- Combination chemotherapy

PRECAUTIONS

Monitoring for infection is important for patients receiving chemotherapy.

SIGNIFICANT POSSIBLE INTERACTIONS

Drug interactions are common and depend on the combinations used. The oncologist will provide information about drug interactions.

OTHER DRUGS

- Ondansetron (Zofran), dronabinol (Marinol), metoclopramide (Reglan), and others to control nausea.

Breast Cancer

Doctor
Office
Phone
Pager

Special notes to patient:

Breast Cancer

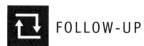 **FOLLOW-UP**

PATIENT MONITORING

- Regular follow-up physical examinations by the doctor are important to detect relapses.
- Up to 60% of patients with invasive disease will have a relapse within 5 years despite initial therapy.

PREVENTION

- Decreasing dietary fat or alcohol has not been shown to alter breast cancer risk.
- The synthetic antiestrogen drug tamoxifen may be a useful preventive agent in women at high risk (e.g., those with a family history).
- The estrogen receptor modulator drug raloxifene (Evista) may reduce the risk of breast cancer and play a role in prevention in the future
- Perform a monthly breast self-examination to detect lumps, skin, or nipple changes.
- Clinical breast examination (breast examination by a doctor) should be part of the gynecologic examination.

- Mammography:
  - In women more than 50 years of age, mammography screening can reduce breast cancer deaths by 30%.
  - All women more than 35 years of age should have baseline screening mammogram.
  - Mammography should be repeated every 1 to 2 years between the ages of 40 and 49 and annually after age 50.

COMPLICATIONS

- Postoperative: lymphedema, wound infection, limited shoulder motion
- Chemotherapy: nausea, vomiting, hair loss, bladder irritation, inflamed mouth, fatigue, and menstrual abnormalities
- Tamoxifen: hot flashes, menstrual irregularities including menopause, vaginal discharge, skin rashes, possibly uterine cancer
- Irradiation: skin reaction, rib fracture, swelling of the arm, pulmonary disease, and rarely second breast cancer

WHAT TO EXPECT

- 10-year survival rates:
  - Noninvasive: 95%
  - Stage I occult: 90%
  - Stage II: 40%
  - Stage III: 15%
  - Stage IV (metastatic): 0%

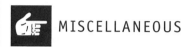 **MISCELLANEOUS**

PEDIATRIC

Breast cancer rarely occurs in children.

GERIATRIC

A higher percentage of hormone-positive tumors is found among the elderly. These cancers are responsive to hormone therapy and, thus, disease-free survival may be improved.

Breast Cancer

	Doctor
	Office
	Phone
	Pager

Special notes to patient:

Breast Feeding

 ## BASICS

DESCRIPTION

- Advantages
  - Babies who are breast-fed have fewer respiratory, gastrointestinal, and ear infections.
  - Breast milk is an ideal food. It is easily digestible, nutrients are well-absorbed, and breast-fed babies have less constipation.
  - Increased contact between mother and baby
  - Economical, portable, easy and easily meets needs
  - Breast feeding may decrease incidence of allergies in childhood.
  - More rapid and complete recovery from pregnancy
- Contraindications
  - Human immunodeficiency virus (HIV) infection; active tuberculosis
  - Drugs of abuse will pass into human milk.
- Technique
  - Mother should get in comfortable position, usually sitting or reclining with baby's head in crook of mother's arm (side-lying position is often useful following cesarian section delivery).
  - Mother should bring baby to her, not lean toward baby, to avoid stress on back.
  - Baby's belly and mother's belly should face each other or touch (belly-to-belly).
  - Mother initiates the rooting reflex by tickling baby's lips with nipple or finger. As baby's mouth opens wide, mother guides her nipple to back of her baby's mouth while pulling the baby closer. This will ensure that the baby's gums are sucking on the areola, not the nipple.

SCOPE

About 56% of new mothers breast feed in the early postpartum period and 21% were breast feeding at 5 to 6 months.

MOST OFTEN AFFECTED

Females 16 to 45 years of age

 ## TREATMENT

GENERAL MEASURES

See *Patient Education*

ACTIVITY

No restrictions

DIET

- Adequate calorie and protein intake while nursing
- Drink plenty of fluids.
- Continue prenatal vitamins.
- Fluoride supplement unnecessary

PATIENT EDUCATION

- Consider plans after birth (e.g., if returning to work). It is possible to nurse parttime after returning to work. Some mothers wean (stop breast-feeding) the week before returning to work.
- For some mothers, an occasional supplemental bottle can be used.
- Colostrum (a fluid that appears before milk that is rich in antibodies) is present in the breast at birth but may not be seen.
- Milk will not come in before the third day after birth.
- Frequent nursing (at least nine or more times in 24 hours) will lead to milk coming in sooner and in greater quantities.
- Allow baby to determine duration of each feeding; baby will lose weight the first few days and may not get back to birth weight until day 10.
- Immediately after birth, baby should stay in mother's room, as much as possible, to encourage on-demand feeding.
- Signs of adequate nursing:
  - Breasts become hard before and soft after feeding
  - Six or more wet diapers in 24 hours
  - Baby satisfied; appropriate weight gain (average 1 oz/day in first few months)
  - Anticipate growth spurts around 10 days, 6 weeks, 3 months, and 4 to 6 months. Baby will nurse more often at these times for several days. More frequent feedings will increase milk production to allow for further adequate growth.
  - Supplemental baby vitamins are unnecessary unless the baby has very limited exposure to sun. (If this is so, then the baby needs vitamin D.)
- Weaning
  - Breast milk alone is adequate food for the first 6 months.
  - Solids may be introduced at 4 to 6 months.
  - For mothers going to work, start switching the baby to bottle-feeding during the hours mother will be gone about a week ahead of time. Do this by eliminating a breast-feeding every few days and substituting pumped breast milk or formula, preferably given by another caregiver.
  - To increase the likelihood that baby will take a bottle occasionally, introduce it at 3 to 4 weeks and give once or twice a week.

 ## FOLLOW-UP

PATIENT MONITORING

Mother and baby should be seen by the doctor within a few days of hospital discharge if mother is breast-feeding for the first time.

COMPLICATIONS

- Clogged ducts
  - Sore lump in one or both breasts without fever
  - Use moist hot packs on lump before and during nursing.
  - More frequent nursing on affected side
  - Use good technique.

Breast Feeding

Doctor
Office
Phone
Pager

Special notes to patient:

Breast Feeding

- Mastitis (infection of the breast duct)
  - Sore lump in one or both breasts plus fever or redness on skin overlying lump
  - Use moist hot packs on lump before and during nursing.
  - More frequent nursing on affected side
  - Antibiotics
  - Mastitis can make a person ill.
  - Other possible sources of fever should be ruled out (e.g., uterine or kidney disorders). Get increased rest, use acetaminophen (Tylenol) as necessary.
  - Fever should resolve within 48 hours; if it does not, type of antibiotic may be changed. Lump should also resolve. If it continues, minor surgery may be required to drain abscess.
- Milk supply inadequate
  - Check baby's weight gain.
  - Review technique, frequency, and duration of nursing.
  - Supplementing with formula decreases breast milk production.
- Sore nipples
  - Check technique.
  - Take baby off the breast by breaking the suction with a finger in the mouth.
  - Air-dry nipples after each nursing.
  - Do not use breast creams
  - Do not wash nipples with soap and water.
- Engorgement
  - Usually develops after milk first comes in (day 3 or 4).
  - Signs are warm, hard, sore breasts.
  - To resolve, offer baby more frequent nursing.
  - May have to hand-express a little milk to soften areola enough to let baby latch on.
  - Nurse long enough to empty breasts.
  - Generally resolves within a day or two.
- Flat or inverted nipples
  - When stimulated, inverted nipples will retract inward, flat nipples remain flat.
  - Nipple shells, a doughnut-shaped insert, can be worn inside the bra during the last month of pregnancy to gently force the nipple through the center opening of the shell.
  - Babies can nurse successfully even if the shell does not correct the problem before birth. A lactation consultant or La Leche League member may be a good resource in this situation.

WHAT TO EXPECT

A healthy baby

Breast Feeding

	Doctor
	Office
	Phone
	Pager

Special notes to patient:

Bronchitis, Acute

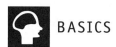 ## BASICS

DESCRIPTION
Acute bronchitis is an inflammation of the airway resulting from a respiratory tract infection. It is generally self-limited with complete healing and full return of function.

SIGNS AND SYMPTOMS
- Follows respiratory tract infection (e.g., a common cold—runny nose, malaise, chills, slight fever, sore throat, back and muscle pain)
- Cough: initially dry and unproductive, then productive
- Fever
- Fatigue, aching muscles
- Spitting up blood
- Burning sensation in chest
- Difficulty breathing (sometimes)
- Wheezing or noisy breathing

CAUSES
- Viral or bacterial infection
- Less often, infection by fungi or other microbe

SCOPE
Acute bronchitis is common in the United States.

MOST OFTEN AFFECTED
All ages are affected by acute bronchitis, males and females equally.

RISK FACTORS
- Chronic lung diseases
- Chronic sinusitis
- Allergies
- Enlarged tonsils and adenoids in children
- Immune system disorders
- Air pollutants
- Elderly
- Infants
- Smoking
- Second-hand smoke
- Alcoholism
- Reflux esophagitis
- Tracheostomy
- Environmental changes
- Immunologic deficiency

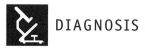 ## DIAGNOSIS

WHAT THE DOCTOR LOOKS FOR
- The doctor will take a history and perform a thorough physical examination.
- Other conditions with similar signs and symptoms will be investigated (e.g., influenza [flu], pneumonia, or asthma).

TESTS AND PROCEDURES
- A number of blood tests may be performed to assist in diagnosis.
- Arterial blood may be obtained.
- Complete blood count (CBC) may be obtained.
- Fluids may be cultured for microbiologic analysis.
- Chest x-ray study
- Pulmonary function tests may be done to assess the respiratory system.

 ## TREATMENT

GENERAL MEASURES
- Acute bronchitis is usually managed on an outpatient basis unless the person is elderly or the bronchitis is complicated by severe underlying disease.
- Rest
- Steam inhalations
- Vaporizers
- Antibiotics, if bacterial infection is suspected
- Maintain adequate hydration.
- Stop smoking.

ACTIVITY
Rest until fever subsides.

DIET
Increased fluids (up to 3 to 4 L/day) if fever present

 ## MEDICATIONS

COMMONLY PRESCRIBED DRUGS
- Amantadine if influenza A is suspected; most effective if started within 24 to 48 hours of development of symptoms.
- Decongestants if accompanied by sinus condition
- Fever-reducing pain reliever (e.g., aspirin [do not give to children] or acetaminophen).
- Antibiotics: amoxicillin, trimethoprim-sulfamethoxazole (TMP-SMX), cephalosporin, doxycycline, clarithromycin
- Cough suppressant for troublesome cough
- Bronchodilators (aerosols or steroids)

CONTRAINDICATIONS
- Doxycycline should not be used during pregnancy.

PRECAUTIONS
Read drug product information.

SIGNIFICANT POSSIBLE INTERACTIONS
Read drug product information.

OTHER DRUGS
- Other antibiotics
- Antiviral drugs

 ## FOLLOW-UP

PATIENT MONITORING
- See the doctor as necessary, depending on the nature of the disease and the person's health status.

PREVENTION
- Avoid smoking.
- Control underlying risk factors (asthma, sinusitis, reflux).
- Avoid exposure.
- Vaccinations

COMPLICATIONS
- Pneumonia
- Acute respiratory failure

WHAT TO EXPECT
- Usually, complete healing occurs with good return of function.
- Bronchitis can be serious in elderly or debilitated patients.
- Cough can persist for several weeks after initial improvement.
- Can result in reactive airway disease or other serious conditions (rare)

 ## MISCELLANEOUS

PEDIATRIC
- Bronchitis among children usually occurs in association with other upper and lower respiratory tract conditions.
- Some children seem to be more susceptible than others. If attacks of bronchitis recur, child should be further evaluated.
- If acute bronchitis is caused by respiratory syncytial virus, it may be fatal.

GERIATRIC
Bronchitis can be a serious illness among the elderly, particularly if part of influenza.

FURTHER INFORMATION
American Lung Association, 1740 Broadway, New York, NY 10019, (212) 315-8700

Bronchitis, Acute

Doctor
Office
Phone
Pager

Special notes to patient:

Bulimia

 ## BASICS

DESCRIPTION

Bulimia nervosa is defined as body dissatisfaction. Persons with bulimia nervosa engage in repeated binge eating, with or without purging by self-induced vomiting, laxatives, or diuretics. An alternative pattern is bingeing followed by sharply restricted diet, vigorous exercise, or both.

SIGNS AND SYMPTOMS

- Person may switch back and forth between bingeing and purging.
- Onset may be related to stress.
- Affected person may be average weight or even somewhat obese; most are slightly below average weight but have frequent fluctuations in weight.
- Denial of problem
- Eating high-calorie foods during binge
- Claim to feel fat even when thin
- Preoccupation with weight control
- Food collection and hoarding
- Drug or alcohol abuse
- Diet pill, diuretic, laxative, ipecac, and thyroid medication abuse
- Calories used up through vigorous exercise, especially running, aerobics
- Diabetic patients often withhold insulin.
- Depressed mood and self-depreciation following binges
- Relief and increased ability to concentrate following binges
- Vomiting (may be effortless)
- Abdominal pain
- Salivary gland swelling
- Eroded teeth
- Scarred hands

CAUSES

Unknown; thought to be largely emotional

SCOPE

About 2% of females suffer from bulimia nervosa. True incidence is unknown because it is a secretive disease. It is more common among university women.

MOST OFTEN AFFECTED

Bulimia nervosa is most common among adolescents and young adults, more often seen in females than males.

RISK FACTORS

- Depression
- Impulsiveness
- Low self-esteem
- Pressure to achieve; high self-expectations
- Acceptance of the culturally condoned ideal of slimness
- Ambivalence about dependence or independence
- Stress caused by multiple responsibilities, tight schedules, competition
- Unstable body image, perceptual distortions
- High risk: ballet dancers, models, cheerleaders, athletes

 ## DIAGNOSIS

WHAT THE DOCTOR LOOKS FOR

- The doctor will take a history and perform a thorough physical examination.
- Other medical problems should be identified (e.g., gastrointestinal disorders).
- Any mental health issues should be identified and addressed.

TESTS AND PROCEDURES

- A number of blood tests can be done to assist in diagnosis.
- The function of the gastrointestinal system may be evaluated.
- An electrocardiogram (ECG) can be done to assess heart activity.
- Psychological testing may be performed.

 ## TREATMENT

GENERAL MEASURES

- Most patients can be treated as outpatients.
- A person may require hospitalization if suicidal; with evidence of marked electrolyte imbalance or marked dehydration; or unresponsive to outpatient therapy.

ACTIVITY

- Monitor excess activity.
- Playful, pleasurable activities are important.

DIET

- Goal is a balanced diet with adequate calories and a normal eating pattern. Affected person needs support in eliminating preoccupation with calories, weight, purging.
- Feared foods should be gradually introduced.

 ## MEDICATIONS

COMMONLY PRESCRIBED DRUGS

- Medication is indicated for patients who are severely depressed or who have not responded to an adequate trial of therapy.
- Tricyclic antidepressants (TCAs), monoamine oxidase inhibitors (MAOs), serotonin reuptake inhibitors (SRIs).

CONTRAINDICATIONS

Read drug product information.

PRECAUTIONS

Read drug product information.

DRUG INTERACTIONS

Read drug product information.

OTHER DRUGS

- Patients with an underlying bipolar disorder may benefit from lithium (Eskalith).
- Opiate antagonist (e.g., naltrexone [Trexan]) to suppress consumption of sweet and high fat foods.
- Metoclopramide (Reglan) or cisapride before each meal and at bedtime for after-meal abdominal discomfort.

Bulimia

	Doctor
	Office
	Phone
	Pager

Special notes to patient:

Bulimia

 ## FOLLOW-UP

PATIENT MONITORING

The person with bulimia nervosa should see the doctor as often as necessary to monitor health status and disease activity.

PREVENTION

- Maintain rational attitude about weight.
- Moderate overly high self-expectations.
- Enhance self-esteem.
- Diminish stress.

COMPLICATIONS

- Suicide
- Drug and alcohol abuse
- Potassium depletion, irregular heart rhythm, cardiac arrest

WHAT TO EXPECT

- The outcome of treatment is highly variable; bulimia nervosa tends to wax and wane.
- The illness may spontaneously remit.
- People who stay in therapy tend to improve.

 ## MISCELLANEOUS

OTHERS

Infrequently diagnosed in men or in older women

PREGNANCY

- Poor nutritional status can affect fetus.
- Bingeing and purging may increase or decrease during pregnancy.

Bulimia

	Doctor
	Office
	Phone
	Pager

Special notes to patient:

Burns

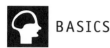 ## BASICS

DESCRIPTION

Burns are tissue injuries caused by heat, chemicals, electricity, or irradiation. The extent of injury (depth of burn) reflects the intensity of heat and the duration of exposure.

SIGNS AND SYMPTOMS

- First-degree burn (superficial layers of the skin)
  - Reddening of affected tissue
  - Skin blanches with pressure.
  - Skin may be tender.
- Second-degree burn (varying degrees of skin, with blister formation)
  - Skin is red and blistered.
  - Skin is very tender.
- Third-degree burn (destruction of the full thickness of skin and underlying tissues)
  - Burned skin is tough and leathery.
  - Skin is not tender.

CAUSES

- Open flame and hot liquid (most common)
- Caustic chemicals or acids
- Electricity
- Excess sun exposure

SCOPE

- Between 2 and 5 million Americans annually receive burns requiring treatment. One million people require hospitalization for burn injuries each year, and 12,000 people die.
- Burns are the leading cause of accidental death in children.

MOST OFTEN AFFECTED

Burns affect all age groups and both genders in equal proportions.

RISK FACTORS

- Hot water heaters set too high.
- Work place exposure to chemicals, electricity, or radiation
- Young children and elderly adults with thin skin are more susceptible to injury.
- Carelessness with burning cigarettes
- Inadequate or faulty electrical wiring

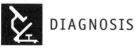 ## DIAGNOSIS

WHAT THE DOCTOR LOOKS FOR

- The doctor will perform a physical examination, measuring the depth of the burn and percentage of body surface area affected.
- The doctor will diagnose and treat other associated conditions (e.g., smoke inhalation).

TESTS AND PROCEDURES

- A number of blood tests can be done to assist in diagnosis and treatment.
- Chest x-ray study
- Arterial blood can be obtained to measure blood gasses.
- An electrocardiogram (ECG) may be done to evaluate the heart's activity.
- Urinalysis
- Bronchoscopy may be necessary to evaluate the respiratory tract.

 ## TREATMENT

GENERAL MEASURES

- Initiate first aid.
- Remove all objects (e.g., rings, watches) from injured extremities to avoid tourniquet effect.
- Remove clothing and cover all burned areas with dry sheet.
- Cool burned skin with water.
- Do not apply ice to burn site.
- Flush area of chemical burn (for approximately 2 hours).
- Serious burns require hospitalization.
- Surgery may be required.

ACTIVITY

Early mobilization is the goal of treatment.

DIET

High-protein, high-calorie diet when bowel function resumes; nasogastric tube feedings may be required in early postburn period.

 ## MEDICATIONS

COMMONLY PRESCRIBED DRUGS

- Morphine
- Silver sulfadiazine (Silvadene) topically to burn site
- Cimetidine, ranitidine, famotidine, or nizatidine for stress ulcer prevention in severely burned patients

CONTRAINDICATIONS

Specific drug allergies

DRUG INTERACTIONS

Read drug product information.

OTHER DRUGS

- Third-degree burn: mafenide (Sulfamylon)
- Silver nitrate (0.5%)
- Povidone-iodine (Betadine)

 ## FOLLOW-UP

PATIENT MONITORING

See the doctor as often as necessary, according to the extent of burn and treatment.

PREVENTION

- Use sunscreen when out of doors.
- Keep electrical cords and outlets in the home safe.
- Isolate household chemicals.
- Use low-temperature setting for hot water heater.
- Household smoke detectors with special emphasis on maintenance
- Prepare household evacuation plan.
- Store and use flammable substances properly.
- Skin grafts and healing skin are highly sensitive to sun exposure and heat.

COMPLICATIONS

- Gastroduodenal ulcer
- Skin cancer developing in old burn site
- Burn wound sepsis
- Pneumonia
- Decreased mobility with possibility of future flexion contractures

WHAT TO EXPECT

- First-degree burn: complete resolution
- Second-degree burn: healing in 10 to 14 days (deep second-degree burns will probably require skin graft)
- Third-degree burn: skin graft required
- Length of hospitalization and need for intensive care depend on extent of burn, smoke inhalation, and age.
- 50% survival rates: with 62% of body burned in ages 0 to 14 years, with 63% burn in ages 15 to 40 years, with 38% burn in ages 40 to 65 years, and with 25% burn in patients more than 65 years of age.
- 90% of survivors can be expected to return to work.

 ## MISCELLANEOUS

PEDIATRIC

Child abuse should be considered with hot water burns in children.

GERIATRIC

The outcome is poorer for elderly persons with severe burns.

Burns

Doctor
Office
Phone
Pager

Special notes to patient:

Bursitis

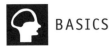 BASICS

DESCRIPTION

Bursitis is inflammation of a bursa, a fluid-filled sac that serves as a cushion between tendons and bones. Bursae are located in areas subject to friction (e.g., where tendons pass over bone). Bursae essentially lubricate the area with fluid. Common sites of bursae are the shoulder, elbow, and knee.

SIGNS AND SYMPTOMS

- Pain and tenderness of the affected area
- Decreased range of motion
- Redness of the skin (if infected)
- Swelling
- Crackling or popping noise when moving

CAUSES

- The cause of bursitis is often unknown.
- Bursitis can be acute or chronic.
- Many types of bursitis are seen, including inflammatory, infectious, traumatic, and gouty.

SCOPE

Bursitis is common in the United States.

MOST OFTEN AFFECTED

Individuals 15 to 50 years of age; males more often than females. Traumatic bursitis is more common in patients younger than 35 years of age.

RISK FACTORS

Repeated vigorous physical training or a sudden increase in level of activity (e.g., "weekend warriors"). Improper or overzealous stretching can cause injury.

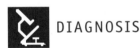 DIAGNOSIS

WHAT THE DOCTOR LOOKS FOR

- The doctor evaluates the patient to determine the presence, type, and severity of bursitis.
- Conditions with signs and symptoms similar to bursitis include tendinitis, strains and sprains, gout, rheumatoid arthritis, osteoarthritis.
- Bursitis can be associated with tendinitis, sprains and strains, stress fractures.

TESTS AND PROCEDURES

- Blood tests will help discriminate bursitis from other conditions.
- X-ray film may show deposits of calcium within the affected bursa.
- Computed tomography (CT) scan or magnetic resonance imaging (MRI) can be performed to evaluate the affected area.
- Fluid from the affected bursa can be withdrawn by needle to look for signs of inflammation or infection.
- If the pain is located in the chest or left arm, the doctor may order an electrocardiogram (ECG) to make sure the pain is not being caused by a cardiac condition.

 TREATMENT

GENERAL MEASURES

- Usually treated on an outpatient basis, with only difficult cases referred to a specialist
- Conservative therapy includes rest, ice, gentle compression, and elevation of the affected area.
- Invasive therapy includes the withdrawal of fluid from the bursa, injection of steroids.
- Treatment can include physical therapy and the application of moist heat.
- A splint or sling can be used to protect and support the affected arm or leg.
- Antibiotic is prescribed if bursitis is caused by infection.
- In severe cases, the bursa can be removed by surgery.

ACTIVITY

Rest and elevation of affected arm or leg

DIET

Changes to the diet may be recommended if bursitis is related to obesity or the formation of mineral deposits.

 MEDICATIONS

COMMONLY PRESCRIBED DRUGS

- Nonsteroidal antiinflammatory drugs (NSAIDs) or aspirin
- Steroids or stronger pain-killing drugs can be injected if needed.
- Antibiotic can be prescribed if bursitis is caused by infection.

CONTRAINDICATIONS

Read drug product information.

PRECAUTIONS

Read drug product information.

DRUG INTERACTIONS

Read drug product information.

OTHER DRUGS

- Topical analgesic or capsaicin creams can be used for symptomatic relief of bursitis.
- Oral steroids may be prescribed.

 FOLLOW-UP

PATIENT MONITORING

- The patient should stop taking NSAIDs as soon as possible to avoid side effects (e.g., ulcers).
- Some patients require repeated injections of steroid and analgesic, although usually no more than three.

PREVENTION

- Appropriate warm-up and cool-down routines can help prevent the symptoms of bursitis.
- Do not overdo physical activity.
- Get adequate rest between work-outs.
- Perform exercises to increase range of motion.
- Maintain high level of fitness and general good health.

COMPLICATIONS

- Acute bursitis can lead to chronic bursitis.
- Long-lasting limitation of range of motion

WHAT TO EXPECT

- Most bouts of acute bursitis heal without long-term effects.
- Repeated bouts of acute bursitis can lead to chronic bursitis.
- The affected bursae may need to be repeatedly drained of fluid or ultimately surgically removed.

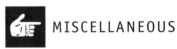 MISCELLANEOUS

PEDIATRIC

Other causes of signs and symptoms of bursitis should be investigated.

ELDERLY

Bursitis is more common among the elderly.

Bursitis

	Doctor
	Office
	Phone
	Pager

Special notes to patient:

Candidiasis

 ## BASICS

DESCRIPTION

Candidiasis is an infection with *Candida albicans* (a fungus) or a related species. Candidiasis affecting the skin causes lesions or a rash between the fingers or toes, ingrown or inflamed hair follicles, inflammation of the penis, a rash at the armpits or other folds of skin, inflammation or infection of the nails, or diaper rash. Infections can also affect mucous membranes, such as the mouth or vagina. The most serious form of the illness is acute systemic candidiasis.

SIGNS AND SYMPTOMS

- Fever
- Malaise
- Rapid heart rate
- Low blood pressure
- Altered mental status
- Skin rash

CAUSES

- Most Candida infections are caused by *Candida albicans*. Other species of Candida are important causes of disease.
- Candida species grow on mucous membranes, and most infections are acquired from the *Candida* organisms growing on these membranes.
- Human-to-human transmission of these organisms can occur (e.g., through sexual contact).

SCOPE

Candidiasis affects at least 120,000 persons annually in the United States.

MOST OFTEN AFFECTED

Persons of all ages are susceptible to candidiasis. Premature infants are at particularly high risk. Males and females are affected equally often.

RISK FACTORS

- White blood cell disorders
- Antibiotic therapy
- Indwelling intravenous access devices
- Dialysis

 ## DIAGNOSIS

WHAT THE DOCTOR LOOKS FOR

- The doctor will evaluate for other causes of similar signs and symptoms (e.g., bacterial infection or immune system disorder).

TESTS AND PROCEDURES

- Blood or cells from a lesion can be analyzed microscopically.
- Imaging of internal organs may be done by liver scan, ultrasound, or computed tomography (CT) scan to assist in diagnosis.

 ## TREATMENT

GENERAL MEASURES

- Candidiasis is usually managed on an inpatient basis.
- Fluids and electrolytes may be needed.
- Medication and mechanical breathing support may be required in seriously ill patients.

ACTIVITY

As tolerated

DIET

No special diet

 ## MEDICATIONS

COMMONLY PRESCRIBED DRUGS

Antifungal drugs: fluconazole, amphotericin B

CONTRAINDICATIONS

The safety of amphotericin B during pregnancy has not been established.

PRECAUTIONS

Amphotericin B is highly toxic. Acute reactions commonly occur at the beginning of therapy.

DRUG INTERACTIONS

- Fluconazole: Potentially important drug interactions can occur in patients receiving oral diabetes medication, anticoagulants, phenytoin, cyclosporine, rifampin, theophylline, terfenadine, or astemizole.
- Read drug product information for other interactions.

OTHER DRUGS

Other antifungal drugs

 ## FOLLOW-UP

PATIENT MONITORING

- Blood tests may be required as often as twice weekly.
- See the doctor as often as necessary, depending on the patient's health status.

COMPLICATIONS

- Kidney disease
- Eye disease
- Heart disease
- Arthritis or other joint or bone disease
- Respiratory disease
- Central nervous system infection

WHAT TO EXPECT

The overall mortality rate for patients with serious candidiasis infection is 40% to 75%.

Candidiasis

Doctor
Office
Phone
Pager

Special notes to patient:

Carbon Monoxide Poisoning

 ## BASICS

DESCRIPTION
Carbon monoxide poisoning results from the inhalation of carbon monoxide (co). co is produced by incomplete combustion of wood, gas, or other material. Inhalation of co prevents hemoglobin in red blood cells from carrying oxygen.

SIGNS AND SYMPTOMS
- Headaches
- Ringing or buzzing in the ear (tinnitus)
- Nausea
- Dizziness
- Weakness
- Confusion
- Lethargy or sleepiness
- Fainting
- Chest pain
- Fast or irregular heart rate
- Cardiac dysrhythmias
- Uncoordination
- Seizures
- Coma
- Cardiopulmonary arrest

CAUSES
co inhalation

SCOPE
co poisoning is responsible for about 3,800 deaths and 10,000 injuries annually.

MOST OFTEN AFFECTED
co affects all age groups and both genders.

RISK FACTORS
- Cigarette smoke
- Smoke inhalation
- Closed space with faulty furnaces or stoves
- Coal mining
- Inhalation of car exhaust
- Use of paint strippers
- Solvent manufacturing

 ## DIAGNOSIS

WHAT THE DOCTOR LOOKS FOR
- The doctor will perform a complete physical examination.
- Other possible toxic exposure will be considered (e.g., cyanide poisoning).
- The doctor will look for other associated injuries (e.g., burns).

TESTS AND PROCEDURES
Blood tests to measure the level of co

 ## TREATMENT

GENERAL MEASURES
- Provide emergency care as needed.
- Remove the person from the source of co.
- Provide rescue breathing and cardiopulmonary resuscitation (CPR) if needed.
- People with mild co poisoning can be treated in the emergency room.
- People with moderate or severe co poisoning require hospitalization.

ACTIVITY
Rest until co levels are reduced and symptoms ease.

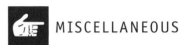 ## MEDICATIONS

COMMONLY PRESCRIBED DRUGS
Oxygen: a hyperbaric chamber may be used for severe cases.

 ## FOLLOW-UP

PATIENT MONITORING
- co levels and blood gases may be measured.
- See the doctor as often as needed based on symptoms.
- Psychiatric evaluation and follow-up for intentional exposure

PREVENTION
- Make sure furnaces, stoves, and fireplaces are properly maintained.
- People who work in high-risk occupations should have adequate ventilation.

COMPLICATIONS
- Heart attack
- Brain damage
- Personality changes

WHAT TO EXPECT
Most survivors recover completely.

MISCELLANEOUS

GERIATRIC
Complications are more common among the elderly.

PREGNANCY
co poisoning affects the fetus. co poisoning can cause significant birth defects, depending on the developmental stage.

Carbon Monoxide Poisoning

Doctor
Office
Phone
Pager

Special notes to patient:

Carpal Tunnel Syndrome

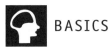 **BASICS**

DESCRIPTION
Carpal tunnel syndrome is the compression of the median nerve as it passes through the carpal tunnel in the wrist and hand. The tunnel contains flexor tendons and the median nerve. Symptoms tend to affect the dominant hand, but more than one half of people with carpal tunnel syndrome have symptoms in both hands.

SIGNS AND SYMPTOMS
- Tingling or prickling sensations in the fingers
- Burning pain in the fingers, particularly at night
- Loss of sensation in the fingers
- Symptoms usually relieved by shaking or rubbing the hands
- Arm pain
- During waking hours, symptoms occur when driving the car, reading the newspaper, and occasionally when using the hands repetitively.
- Symptoms usually affect the thumb, and index and middle fingers, although the entire hand can be affected.
- Weakness of the hand while performing tasks (e.g., opening a jar)

CAUSES
- Disorders affecting the musculoskeletal system in the area of the wrist (e.g., injury or arthritis)
- Often associated with hypothyroidism and diabetes, which also occur more often during pregnancy
- Other diseases

SCOPE
Carpal tunnel syndrome is a common nerve disorder.

MOST OFTEN AFFECTED
Carpal tunnel syndrome primarily affects individuals between 40 and 60 years of age; it affects women three to six times more often than it does men. It can affect more than one member of a family.

RISK FACTORS
Jobs that involve repetitive motion of the wrist can influence the development of carpal tunnel syndrome. However, no universal agreement is found that carpal tunnel syndrome is job related.

 DIAGNOSIS

WHAT THE DOCTOR LOOKS FOR
- The doctor will look for signs that are diagnostic of carpal tunnel syndrome.
- Other conditions that can cause similar conditions should be identified and treated.

TESTS AND PROCEDURES
- Blood tests
- Studies of muscle and nerve (electromyography) may be performed.
- X-ray study may be done of the wrist and arm.

 TREATMENT

GENERAL MEASURES
- Carpal tunnel syndrome is usually managed in the outpatient setting.
- Splinting the wrist may provide significant relief of symptoms.
- Surgery may be necessary, usually as an outpatient under local anesthesia.

ACTIVITY
As tolerated

DIET
No special diet

 MEDICATIONS

COMMONLY PRESCRIBED DRUGS
- Nonsteroidal antiinflammatory agents: ibuprofen, naproxen
- Steroids

CONTRAINDICATIONS
Gastrointestinal intolerance

DRUG INTERACTIONS
Read drug product information.

 FOLLOW-UP

PATIENT MONITORING
- Patients treated with wrist splints and other symptomatic measures should see the doctor for a follow-up within 4 to 12 weeks to assess treatment.
- Patients who receive surgery rarely experience recurrence of the disorder.
- Routine follow-up once the incision has healed is not necessary.

PREVENTION
Take a break once an hour when doing repetitive work involving the hands.

COMPLICATIONS
- Infection after surgery (rare)
- Nerve injury

WHAT TO EXPECT
- Untreated, the condition can lead to numbness and weakness in the hand, atrophy of hand muscles, and permanent loss of function of the extremity.
- Surgery is effective in about 95% of cases.

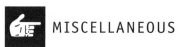 **MISCELLANEOUS**

PREGNANCY
May occur in pregnancy

FURTHER INFORMATION
American Academy of Family Physicians Foundation, P.O. Box 8418, Kansas City, MO 64114, (800) 274-2237, ext. 4400

Carpal Tunnel Syndrome

Doctor
Office
Phone
Pager

Special notes to patient:

Cataract

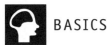 ## BASICS

DESCRIPTION
A cataract is a clouding of the lens of the eye. It is the single greatest cause of blindness in the world, blinding an estimated 17 million people at any point in time.

SIGNS AND SYMPTOMS
- Blurred vision and distortion or "ghosting" of images
- Visual problems in bright light or night driving (glare)
- Falls or accidents
- Injuries (e.g., hip fracture)

CAUSES
- Age
- Numerous other causes

SCOPE
Cataracts affect 5% of people 52 to 62 years of age and 46% of people 75 to 85 years of age. Of people 75 to 85 years of age, 92% have some degree of visual impairment.

MOST OFTEN AFFECTED
Cataracts affect males and females with equal frequency. Some forms of cataract may be inherited.

RISK FACTORS
- Aging
- Predisposing diseases

 ## DIAGNOSIS

WHAT THE DOCTOR LOOKS FOR
- The doctor will thoroughly examine the eyes, looking for clouding of the lens as well as other eye conditions.
- Special visual tests may be performed.
- Because cataracts develop gradually, the person may not be aware of how it has changed his or her lifestyle. The doctor may note cataracts when the patient is unaware of problems.
- The doctor will also look for other diseases known to be associated with cataract (e.g., diabetes).

 ## TREATMENT

GENERAL MEASURES
- Cataracts are surgically removed and the affected lens replaced.
- Cataract surgery can be done in an outpatient setting, or hospitalization may be required.
- An evaluation will be performed before surgery, including blood tests and an electrocardiogram (ECG).
- A second opinion by another ophthalmologist (eye specialist) may be indicated before surgery.

 ## MEDICATIONS

COMMONLY PRESCRIBED DRUGS
No medication is currently available to prevent or slow the progression of cataracts.

 ## FOLLOW-UP

PATIENT MONITORING
- As cataract develops, an ophthalmologist may change a patient's eyeglass prescription to maintain vision. When these changes are no longer practical or successful, surgery is recommended.
- Following surgery, eyeglasses may be required to maximize vision. Eyes are tested several weeks after surgery.

PREVENTION
- Sunglasses that filter ultraviolet rays may slow the development of cataract, although scientific studies have not proved this.
- Antioxidants (e.g., vitamins C, E) may be helpful, but benefit from their use has not been proved.

COMPLICATIONS
Blindness

WHAT TO EXPECT
The outcome is good after cataract surgery if the patient has no other eye disease.

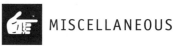 ## MISCELLANEOUS

PEDIATRIC
Congenital cataracts can occur in newborns; outcome is poor.

GERIATRIC
Of people more than 75 years of age, 92% have cataracts.

Cataract

Doctor
Office
Phone
Pager

Special notes to patient:

Cervical Dysplasia

 ## BASICS

DESCRIPTION

Cervical dysplasia is defined as precancerous changes in the tissue of the cervix, often associated with infection by human papilloma virus (warts). The changes may involve partial or full thickness of the tissue.

SIGNS AND SYMPTOMS

- Often no symptoms
- Occasionally associated with genital warts
- Occasionally occurs with sexually transmitted diseases (e.g., chlamydia, gonorrhea)

CAUSES

Cervical dysplasia is strongly linked to infection by human papilloma viruses, the virus that causes genital warts.

SCOPE

The scope has been difficult to assess. Cervical dysplasia has been found in 3,600 of 100,000 women 27 to 28 years of age.

MOST OFTEN AFFECTED

The average age for noninvasive cancer of the cervix is 28 years. Cervical dysplasia probably can be expected to occur at younger ages.

RISK FACTORS

- Multiple pregnancies and births before 20 years of age
- Multiple sexual partners
- Early age of first sexual intercourse
- Warts elsewhere in the body
- Cigarette smoking
- Prostitution
- Lower socioeconomic status

 ## DIAGNOSIS

WHAT THE DOCTOR LOOKS FOR

- The doctor will perform a physical examination of the lower reproductive tract.
- Other diseases of the cervix will be investigated (e.g., cancer and genital warts).

TESTS AND PROCEDURES

- A sample of cervical tissue (a Pap smear) can be examined microscopically.
- The lower reproductive tract can be visually examined by colposcopy.
- Other special tests can be performed (e.g., cervicography and speculoscopy).
- A sample of cervical tissue can be obtained by biopsy.

 ## TREATMENT

GENERAL MEASURES

- Cervical dysplasia is managed in an outpatient setting.
- Outpatient surgery may be performed.

ACTIVITY

Pelvic rest (4 weeks) after biopsy

DIET

No restrictions

 ## MEDICATIONS

COMMONLY PRESCRIBED DRUGS

- Treatment is primarily surgical and aimed at removing the abnormal tissue.
- Fluorouracil (Efudex) vaginal cream is used as supplemental therapy.

CONTRAINDICATIONS

Allergy to 5-fluorouracil

PRECAUTIONS

- If the hand is used to apply 5-fluorouracil, wash hand immediately afterward.
- Avoid getting 5-fluorouracil in the eyes, nose, or mouth.

 ## FOLLOW-UP

PATIENT MONITORING

- See the doctor every 4 months during the first year after treatment for repeat Pap smears, then every 6 months thereafter.
- For less serious cases, the doctor may repeat Pap smear annually.

PREVENTION

- Monogamy of both sexual partners
- Use of condom during intercourse, if unable to practice monogamy
- Abstain from smoking
- Annual Pap smear to detect changes early

COMPLICATIONS

- Some cases of severe dysplasia will develop into cancer.
- Possible complications of biopsy include:
  - Bleeding
  - Infection
  - Infertility
  - Incomplete removal of affected tissue
  - Recurrence of dysplasia
  - Other cervical disorders

WHAT TO EXPECT

- The outcome of cervical dysplasia is generally excellent.
- The condition can persist if it is not completely removed.
- The condition can return.

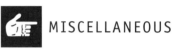 ## MISCELLANEOUS

PEDIATRIC

Very rare among children

GERIATRIC

Less frequent among the elderly

OTHERS

Cervical dysplasia is usually a problem for women in the reproductive age group. The median age is 28 years for severe dysplasia. For less severe cervical dysplasia, the median ages tend to be much lower.

PREGNANCY

- Dysplasia can get worse during pregnancy.
- Dysplasia does not require definitive treatment during pregnancy.
- Dysplasia by itself is not an indication for cesarean section.

Cervical Dysplasia

Doctor
Office
Phone
Pager

Special notes to patient:

Chickenpox

 ## BASICS

DESCRIPTION

Chickenpox, also called "varicella," is a common, highly contagious disease marked by the development of blisters on the skin and mucous membranes.

- The virus that causes chickenpox (varicella zoster virus) is spread directly by breathing air or contact with blisters, or indirectly through contact with freshly soiled articles.
- Outbreaks of chickenpox tend to occur from January to May.
- Incubation period is 14 to 16 days (range is 11-21 days).
- Patients are infectious from approximately 48 hours before onset of the rash until the final lesions have crusted.
- Most people acquire chickenpox during childhood and develop long immunity.
- A vaccination can prevent chickenpox.

SIGNS AND SYMPTOMS

- Symptoms that develop before appearance of the rash include fever, malaise, lack of appetite, and mild headache.
- The chickenpox rash is characterized by crops of "teardrop" blisters on reddened bases.
- Blisters erupt in successive crops.
- The individual blisters form from a pimple-like lesion.
- Eventually, the blisters begin to crust over.
- The rash causes intense itching.
- Rash usually begins on trunk, then spreads to face and scalp.
- Rash does not usually affect the arms or legs.
- Blisters may be present on mucous membranes (e.g., the mouth and vagina).

CAUSES

Infection by the varicella zoster virus

SCOPE

Chickenpox is common in the United States.

MOST OFTEN AFFECTED

- Chickenpox has a peak incidence among children 5 to 9 years of age, but it can occur at any age.
- Males and females are affected equally as often.

RISK FACTORS

- No prior history of chickenpox
- Lack of vaccination
- Immune system disorders

 ## DIAGNOSIS

WHAT THE DOCTOR LOOKS FOR

The doctor will perform a physical examination to rule out other similar-appearing conditions (e.g., herpes, impetigo, or scabies).

TESTS AND PROCEDURES

- Blood tests to look for signs of infection
- Virus can be isolated from tissue culture and examined by electron microscopy.
- Specialized tests can be done to analyze the genetic material of a virus.

 ## TREATMENT

GENERAL MEASURES

- Chickenpox is managed in the outpatient setting, except when complicating emergencies occur.
- Treatment involves providing support and relief of symptoms.
- Good hygiene is important to prevent infection of blisters.

ACTIVITY

As tolerated. Children can return to school when lesions have scabbed over, temperature is normal, and sense of well-being has returned.

DIET

No special diet

 ## MEDICATIONS

COMMONLY PRESCRIBED DRUGS

- Fever-reducing drugs (e.g., acetaminophen)
- Aspirin should be avoided because of its link to Reye's syndrome.
- Local and/or systemic antiitching agents
- Acyclovir: This antiviral drug decreases duration of fever and shortens time of viral shedding. It is recommended for adolescents, adults, and patients at high risk. It is most helpful if given early in the disease.

CONTRAINDICATIONS

Drug allergies

PRECAUTIONS

Possible kidney disease with acyclovir

OTHER DRUGS

Other antiviral drugs

 ## FOLLOW-UP

PATIENT MONITORING

- Usually no follow-up is needed for mild cases.
- If complications occur, intensive supportive care may be required.

PREVENTION

- People who have been exposed to chickenpox and who are susceptible to it (i.e., have not been vaccinated or have never had it) are considered infectious for 21 days.
- Varicella zoster virus vaccine (Varivax) is a vaccine against chickenpox. It is made from live, attenuated (changed in the laboratory to be non–disease-causing) varicella zoster virus.
- Vaccine recipients should avoid contact with individuals with immune system disorders and pregnant women who have never had chickenpox and their newborns for up to 6 weeks after vaccination.
- Varicella zoster immune globulin (VZIG) can also protect against chickenpox, but it is not as effective as Varivax. VZIG is given to individuals who should not receive Varivax (e.g., people with immune system disorders).

COMPLICATIONS

- Secondary bacterial infection
- Pneumonia
- Encephalitis
- Reye's syndrome
- Skin bruising
- Inflammation of the lymph nodes
- Inflammation of the kidney

Chickenpox

Doctor
Office
Phone
Pager

Special notes to patient:

Chickenpox

WHAT TO EXPECT

- In the healthy child, chickenpox is rarely a serious disease and recovery is complete.
- The illness provides long immunity.
- A second illness is rare.
- The virus can remain latent in the body and be reactivated later, causing herpes zoster (shingles).
- Deaths rarely occur from complications.

 MISCELLANEOUS

PEDIATRIC

Neonates born to mothers who develop chickenpox 5 days before or 2 days after delivery are at risk for serious disease.

GERIATRIC

- Infection is more severe than in children.
- Latent virus can reactivate and cause shingles.

PREGNANCY

- The risk of infection across the placenta following maternal infection is 25%.
- Birth defects are seen in 5% of newborns infected during the first or second trimester of pregnancy.
- An increased risk exists of pneumonia or other complications in women infected during pregnancy

Chickenpox

Doctor
Office
Phone
Pager

Special notes to patient:

Child Abuse

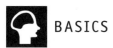 ## BASICS

DESCRIPTION

- Abuse can be emotional, psychological, or physical.
- Sexual abuse is any contact or interaction between a child and another person in which the child is sexually exploited for the gratification or profit of the perpetrator. Offenders can be juveniles.
- Neglect occurs when those responsible for meeting the basic needs of a child fail to do so.

SIGNS AND SYMPTOMS

- Nonspecific symptoms of abuse include:
  - Behavior regression
  - Anxiety, depression
  - Sleep disturbances, night terrors
  - Increased sex play
  - School problems
  - Self-destructive behaviors
- Physical abuse:
  - May be no physical signs
  - Skin markings (lacerations, burns, bruises)
  - Bruises with definite shapes (coat hangers, belt buckles)
  - Circular bruises on trunks or limbs (finger pressure points)
  - Bites
  - Cigarette burns on palms, arms, or legs
  - Immersion injuries
  - Oral injury
  - Ear injury
  - Eye injury
  - Abdominal injury
  - Fractures
  - Head injury
- Sexual abuse:
  - Unequivocal signs are found in only a small number of children (2% to 8%).
  - Abuse often consists of fondling, rubbing, and other contacts that are not likely to produce injuries.
  - Unexplained vaginal injuries or bleeding
  - Pregnancy
  - Sexually transmitted diseases
  - Reddening of tissues
  - Anal injury
  - May be no physical signs
- Neglect:
  - Child may be small, scrawny, dirty, with rashes
  - Fearful or too trusting
  - Clinging to or avoiding mother
  - Flat or balding area on the back of the head
  - Abnormal development or growth

SCOPE

More than 1 million cases of child abuse are seen annually in the United States.

MOST OFTEN AFFECTED

The most common age of abused children is 7 years; boys and girls are affected in equal proportion.

CAUSES

Not well-defined

RISK FACTORS

- May be many risk factors for child abuse
- Poverty (fivefold greater risk)
- Parental substance abuse
- Lower educational status
- Maternal history of abuse
- Unwanted pregnancy

 ## DIAGNOSIS

WHAT THE DOCTOR LOOKS FOR

The doctor will perform a thorough physical examination, paying particular attention to other possible causes of signs (e.g., accidental injury, bleeding disorders, or medical diseases).

TESTS AND PROCEDURES

- Urinalysis, culture
- Blood tests
- X-ray study
- In cases of suspected sexual abuse, special tests may be done to detect semen or sexually transmitted disease.
- Photographs

 ## TREATMENT

GENERAL MEASURES

- Acute episodes, especially of sexual abuse, are often best managed in an emergency room equipped for collecting forensic specimens and maintaining "chain of evidence."
- Children with moderate to severe injuries, unstable physical condition, or acute psychological trauma may be hospitalized.
- If not hospitalized, a child should be sent to another relative or placed in foster care should the suspected abuser live with the child.
- Counseling is imperative.
- Reporting to child protective authorities is mandatory.
- After initial evaluation, child victim of sexual abuse should be referred to a sexual assault center.
- Do not use negative terms such as "ruined," "violated," or "dirty" in reference to the child. The child's emotional reaction to abuse will be profoundly influenced by the responses of adult caretakers.

ACTIVITY

As allowed by doctor

DIET

As allowed by doctor

 ## MEDICATIONS

COMMONLY PRESCRIBED DRUGS

Antibiotics for sexually transmitted diseases

CONTRAINDICATIONS

Read drug product information.

PRECAUTIONS

Read drug product information.

DRUG INTERACTIONS

Read drug product information.

OTHER DRUGS

"Morning-after" contraceptive drugs

 ## FOLLOW-UP

PATIENT MONITORING

The child must be referred to the appropriate state protective services and followed as closely as necessary.

PREVENTION

Early detection and intervention whenever possible

COMPLICATIONS

Long-term physical and psychological damage

WHAT TO EXPECT

Without intervention, child abuse is a recurrent and escalating phenomenon.

Child Abuse

Doctor
Office
Phone
Pager

Special notes to patient:

Chlamydial Sexually Transmitted Diseases

 ## BASICS

DESCRIPTION

The most common sexually transmitted disease (STD) in the United States is infection by the bacteria *Chlamydia trachomatis*. Chlamydial STD often has no symptoms and is difficult to diagnose. The infection has serious consequences, and its transmission is difficult to control.

SIGNS AND SYMPTOMS

- In both genders: inflammation of the urinary or reproductive tract
- Most women infected with *Chlamydia trachomatis* have no symptoms.
- In women: inflammation of the cervix with production of mucus, pelvic inflammatory disease (PID)
- In infants: conjunctivitis (pink eye), airway or gastrointestinal disorders

CAUSES

Infection by *Chlamydia trachomatis*

SCOPE

Chlamydial infection affects 3% to 5% of the general population and up to 20% of individuals who seek treatment at STD clinics.

MOST OFTEN AFFECTED

Males and females 15 to 25 years of age

RISK FACTORS

- Sexual promiscuity
- Lower socioeconomic groups
- Youth

 ## DIAGNOSIS

WHAT THE DOCTOR LOOKS FOR

The doctor will examine the urinary and reproductive organs and will look for signs of other STDs (e.g., syphilis, gonorrhea).

TESTS AND PROCEDURES

Cells from the urinary or reproductive tract can be cultured and analyzed in the laboratory.

 ## TREATMENT

GENERAL MEASURES

- Chlamydial infection is managed in the outpatient setting.
- Human immunodeficiency virus (HIV) counseling and testing should be offered.
- Sex partners should be evaluated and treated.

ACTIVITY

Abstain from sexual activity until the infection is treated.

 ## MEDICATIONS

COMMONLY PRESCRIBED DRUGS

Antibiotics: doxycycline, azithromycin, erythromycin, tetracycline, ceftriaxone, cefoxitin, quinolone

CONTRAINDICATIONS

Tetracycline should not be used during pregnancy or by children younger than 8 years of age.

PRECAUTIONS

Tetracycline can cause light sensitivity; sunscreen recommended.

DRUG INTERACTIONS

- Tetracycline: avoid antacids, dairy products, and iron.
- Antibiotics can reduce the effectiveness of oral contraceptives; barrier method is recommended.
- Erythromycin plus fexofenadine (Allegra) can cause heart rhythm disturbances.

OTHER DRUGS

Other antibiotics

 ## FOLLOW-UP

PATIENT MONITORING

- See the doctor for retesting weeks to months after treatment.
- Sexual partners need to be evaluated and treated to prevent passage of the disease back and forth between partners.
- Contact the doctor if symptoms persist or return.

PREVENTION

- Practice safe sex, such as barrier protection (condoms).
- It is important to finish the entire course of antibiotics to insure care.

COMPLICATIONS

- Males
  - Temporary infertility
  - Scarring of urethra
- Females
  - Tubal infertility
  - Tubal pregnancy
  - Chronic pelvic pain

WHAT TO EXPECT

The outcome of chlamydial infection is good with early and complete therapy.

 ## MISCELLANEOUS

OTHERS

After the onset of sexual activity, incidence drops off with age.

PREGNANCY

Infection during pregnancy can affect the fetus.

FURTHER INFORMATION

American Academy of Family Physicians Foundation, P.O. Box 8418, Kansas City, MO 64114, (800) 274-2237, ext. 4400

Chlamydial Sexually Transmitted Diseases

Doctor
Office
Phone
Pager

Special notes to patient:

_____
_____
_____
_____
_____
_____
_____
_____
_____
_____
_____
_____
_____
_____
_____
_____

Cholera

 ## BASICS

DESCRIPTION
Cholera is an acute infectious disease caused by the bacteria *Vibrio choleroe*. Characteristics include severe diarrhea with extreme fluid and electrolyte depletion, vomiting, muscle cramps, and prostration.

SCOPE
Cholera is rare in the United States. It is endemic in India, Southeast Asia, Africa, the Middle East, southern Europe, Oceania, and South and Central America. The few cases of cholera in the United States have occurred in returning travelers or have been associated with food brought into the country illicitly.

MOST OFTEN AFFECTED
Affects all ages, males and females equally

SIGNS AND SYMPTOMS
- Abdominal discomfort, lack of appetite
- Apathy, lethargy, malaise, listlessness
- Cyanosis
- Dehydration
- Vomiting
- Severe diarrhea, which eventually turns gray in color with flecks of mucus; it is called "rice-water diarrhea" because the mucus flecks resemble grains of rice.
- Profuse sweating
- Rapid or irregular heart rate
- Fever
- Shock
- Weakness

CAUSES
Infection by *Vibrio choleroe*

RISK FACTORS
- Traveling or living in areas where cholera is endemic
- Exposure to contaminated food or water
- Person-to-person transmission (rare)

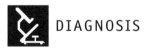 ## DIAGNOSIS

WHAT THE DOCTOR LOOKS FOR
The doctor will investigate other possible causes of severe diarrhea and dehydration.

TESTS AND PROCEDURES
- Blood tests
- A sample of stool may be cultured for laboratory analysis.
- X-ray study of the chest and abdomen

 ## TREATMENT

GENERAL MEASURES
- Mild cases of cholera are managed in the outpatient setting.
- Moderate or severe cases of cholera may require hospitalization.
- Rehydration therapy: oral fluids for mild to moderate cases, intravenous (IV) fluids for severe dehydration

ACTIVITY
Bed rest until symptoms resolve and strength returns

DIET
Small, frequent meals when vomiting stops and appetite returns

 ## MEDICATIONS

COMMONLY PRESCRIBED DRUGS
- Oral fluids: Pedialyte, Rehydralyte, Resol, Rice-Lyte
- IV fluids
- Antibiotics: doxycycline (Vibramycin), tetracycline, trimethoprim, sulfamethoxazole (SMX-TMP, Bactrim, Septra), furazolidone (Furoxone)

CONTRAINDICATIONS
- Tetracycline should not be used during pregnancy or by children younger than 8 years of age.
- Do not drink alcohol when taking furazolidone.

PRECAUTIONS
Tetracycline can cause sensitivity to sunlight; sunscreen recommended.

SIGNIFICANT POSSIBLE INTERACTIONS
Tetracycline: avoid antacids, dairy products, and iron

 ## FOLLOW-UP

PATIENT MONITORING
See the doctor regularly until symptoms resolve.

PREVENTION
- Use precautions in endemic areas: purify water, select food carefully (i.e., do not eat raw shellfish)
- Vaccination

POSSIBLE COMPLICATIONS
- Hypovolemic (low fluid volume) shock
- Chronic gallbladder infection
- Up to 50% death rate with untreated shock

WHAT TO EXPECT
- Clinical course is 3 to 5 days.
- Prompt oral or IV treatment can be lifesaving.
- Antibiotic treatment reduces duration and infectivity of disease.
- Mortality rate is less than 1% with appropriate supportive care.
- The risk of death increases with untreated shock.

 ## MISCELLANEOUS

PEDIATRIC
- Breast-feeding protects against cholera.
- Vaccine is not recommended for children younger than 6 months of age.

FURTHER INFORMATION
- Centers for Disease Control. Travelers Information Hotline: (404) 332-4559 (available 24 hours via a touch-tone telephone)
- International Association for Medical Assistance to Travelers, 417 Center St., Lewiston, NY 14092, (716) 754-4883

Cholera

Doctor
Office
Phone
Pager

Special notes to patient:

Chronic Fatigue Syndrome

 ## BASICS

DESCRIPTION
Chronic fatigue syndrome (CFS) is characterized by profound fatigue and multiple physical and emotional symptoms, lasting at least 6 months, and which are severe enough to reduce or impair daily activity.

SIGNS AND SYMPTOMS
- Fatigue
- Unexplained general muscle weakness
- Pain or ache of muscles or joints
- Forgetfulness, inability to concentrate
- Confusion
- Mood swings, irritability, depression
- Low-grade fever (99.5°F to 101.5°F; 37.5° to 38.6°C)
- Prolonged fatigue lasting 24 hours after exercise
- Headaches
- Sensitivity to light
- Difficulty sleeping, night sweats
- Allergies
- Vertigo
- Swollen or painful glands
- Shortness of breath
- Chest pain
- Nausea
- Weight loss or gain
- Hot flushes
- Palpitations
- Gastrointestinal complaints
- Rash

CAUSES
Unknown

SCOPE
Chronic fatigue syndrome affects about 10 of 100,000 persons in the United States.

MOST OFTEN AFFECTED
Young adults; females slightly more often than males

RISK FACTORS
Unknown

 ## DIAGNOSIS

WHAT THE DOCTOR LOOKS FOR
The doctor will conduct a history and perform a thorough physical examination to identify and treat other potential causes of fatigue (e.g., infection, chronic inflammation, immune system disorders, or cancer).

TESTS AND PROCEDURES
- A number of blood tests may be ordered.
- Urinalysis, chest x-ray study

 ## TREATMENT

GENERAL MEASURES
- Chronic fatigue syndrome is managed in the outpatient setting.
- As the cause of CFS is unknown and no specific therapy has shown consistent results, mainstay of therapy is supportive care.
- Although not a cure, a program consisting of moderate exercise (with rest periods during acute episodes), a healthy diet, stress reduction, and support groups or counseling is likely to be helpful.
- Alternative therapies (chiropractic, homeopathy, acupuncture, enforced rest) are helpful for some, but have not been proven to work. However, they may be worth trying.

ACTIVITY
As tolerated, but strenuous exercise tends to make symptoms worse in most persons with CFS.

DIET
No restrictions. Rich in vitamins and minerals.

 ## MEDICATIONS

COMMONLY PRESCRIBED DRUGS
- None
- Ampligen, essential fatty acid therapy, intravenous (IV) immune globulin, vitamin B_{12}, and bovine liver extract (LEFAC) have been used experimentally.
- Relief of symptoms with nonsteroidal antiinflammatory drugs (NSAIDs) and antidepressants

CONTRAINDICATIONS
Read drug product information.

PRECAUTIONS
Read drug product information.

DRUG INTERACTIONS
Read drug product information.

 ## FOLLOW-UP

PATIENT MONITORING
See the doctor as often as necessary.

PREVENTION
Unknown

COMPLICATIONS
- Depression
- Socioeconomic problems (e.g., inability to work)

WHAT TO EXPECT
- CFS is indolent; it waxes and wanes over time.
- Generally very slow improvement over months or years

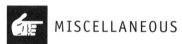 ## MISCELLANEOUS

PEDIATRIC
CFS has been reported in children.

GERIATRIC
CFS has been reported in elderly persons.

FURTHER INFORMATION
- CFS Association, 3521 Broadway, Suite 222, Kansas City, MO 64111, (816) 931-4777
- CFIDS Association. P.O. Box 220398, Charlotte, NC 28222-0398.
- International Chronic Fatigue Syndrome Society. P.O. Box 230108, Portland, OR 97223

Chronic Fatigue Syndrome

	Doctor
	Office
	Phone
	Pager

Special notes to patient:

Chronic Obstructive Pulmonary Disease and Emphysema

 ## BASICS

DESCRIPTION

- The term "chronic obstructive pulmonary disease" (COPD) encompasses several pulmonary diseases, including chronic bronchitis, asthma, cystic fibrosis, and emphysema. COPD usually refers to a mixture of chronic bronchitis and emphysema.
- Symptoms of chronic bronchitis include increased mucus production and recurrent cough.
- Emphysema involves the destruction of deep airway tissue.

SIGNS AND SYMPTOMS

- Chronic bronchitis
  - Cough
  - Sputum production
  - Frequent infections
  - Difficulty breathing
  - Swelling around the feet and ankles
  - A bluish discoloration around the lips, eyes, and nail beds
  - Wheezing
  - Weight gain
- Emphysema
  - Minimal cough
  - Scant sputum
  - Difficulty breathing
  - Often significant weight loss
  - Occasional infections
  - Barrel chest
  - Less wheezing
  - Use of accessory muscles of respiration
  - Pursed-lip breathing
  - Slight bluish discoloration around lips, eyes, and nail beds

SCOPE

- COPD affects 20% to 30% of the adult population in the United States and is responsible for more than 60,000 deaths annually.
- Of Americans, 8 million have chronic bronchitis; 2 million people have emphysema.

MOST OFTEN AFFECTED

- Persons older than 40 years of age; males are affected more frequently than females.
- Although not a genetic disease, a predisposition to developing COPD may be inheritable. A rare form of emphysema is inherited.

CAUSES

- Cigarette smoking
- Air pollution
- Genetic defect (rare)
- Occupational exposure (e.g., firefighters)
- Viral infection (possibly)

RISK FACTORS

- Passive smoking (especially adults whose parents smoked)
- Severe viral pneumonia early in life
- Aging
- Alcohol consumption
- Asthma or allergies

 ## DIAGNOSIS

WHAT THE DOCTOR LOOKS FOR

- The doctor will conduct a physical examination and investigate other possible respiratory diseases (e.g., acute bronchitis, asthma, cancer, or acute viral infection).
- The doctor will look for other conditions known to be associated with COPD, including coronary artery disease and peptic ulcer disease.

TESTS AND PROCEDURES

- Blood tests
- Arterial blood may be obtained.
- Pulmonary function may be tested to assist with diagnosis.
- Chest x-ray study

 ## TREATMENT

GENERAL MEASURES

- COPD is usually managed adequately in the outpatient setting. Hospitalization may be needed for complications or diagnostic procedures.
- Respiratory failure may require intensive care and possibly mechanical breathing assistance.
- Smoking cessation
- Infections should be aggressively treated.
- Respiratory therapy
- Pulmonary rehabilitation
- Home oxygen may be required.
- Surgery may be indicated in selected cases.

ACTIVITY

As tolerated. Full activity should be encouraged.

DIET

A well-balanced, high-protein diet is suggested. Low carbohydrate intake may be helpful.

 ## MEDICATIONS

COMMONLY PRESCRIBED DRUGS

- Theophylline: Theo-Dur, Slo-bid, Uni-Dur, Uniphyl
- Metaproterenol (Alupent), albuterol, levalbuterol (Proventil, Ventolin), pirbuterol (Maxair), terbutaline (Brethaire), salmeterol (Serevent)
- Ipratropium: Atrovent
- Prednisone: Deltasone

CONTRAINDICATIONS

Read drug product information.

PRECAUTIONS

Read drug product information.

DRUG INTERACTIONS

Read drug product information.

OTHER DRUGS

Home oxygen

 ## FOLLOW-UP

PATIENT MONITORING

- Individuals with severe disease or who are unstable should see the doctor monthly.
- When condition is stable, the doctor may be seen twice a year.
- Theophylline level may be checked every 6 to 12 months.
- If home oxygen is required, blood gasses should be checked annually or with any change in condition.
- Avoid travel at high altitude. Air travel with oxygen requires prearrangement.

PREVENTION

Smoking avoidance is the most important way to prevent COPD. Passive smoke also has been shown to be harmful.

Chronic Obstructive Pulmonary Disease and Emphysema

Doctor
Office
Phone
Pager

Special notes to patient:

Chronic Obstructive Pulmonary Disease and Emphysema

COMPLICATIONS

- Infection is common.
- Other complications include circulatory and respiratory disease, respiratory failure, pulmonary hypertension, and malnutrition.

WHAT TO EXPECT

- Younger patients with mild disease have a fairly good prognosis. Older patients with more severe lung disease do worse.
- Supplemental oxygen, when indicated, has been shown to increase survival.
- Smoking cessation is also important for an improved prognosis.

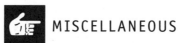 MISCELLANEOUS

PEDIATRIC

Repeated childhood respiratory illnesses increase the risk of COPD later in life.

GERIATRIC

The elderly have up to twice the risk as younger persons.

OTHERS

COPD is unusual among individuals younger than 25 years of age unless a genetic defect is present. The incidence of COPD increases as age approaches 60.

Chronic Obstructive Pulmonary Disease and Emphysema

Doctor
Office
Phone
Pager

Special notes to patient:

_____

_____

_____

_____

_____

_____

_____

_____

_____

_____

_____

_____

_____

_____

Cirrhosis of the Liver

 ## BASICS

DESCRIPTION
Cirrhosis is a degenerative disease of the liver.

SIGNS AND SYMPTOMS
- Fatigue
- Loss of appetite
- Nausea
- Discomfort or a feeling of fullness in the abdomen
- Weakness and malaise
- Vomiting of blood
- Encephalopathy
- Yellowish discoloration of the skin and eyes (jaundice)
- Enlarged liver
- Enlargement of the breasts in men
- Testicular atrophy
- "Spider veins"

CAUSES
- Alcohol abuse
- Viral infection
- Genetic defect
- Other medical conditions

SCOPE
Cirrhosis of the liver accounts for more than 30,000 deaths annually in the United States.

MOST OFTEN AFFECTED
Depends on cause

RISK FACTORS
See *Causes*

 ## DIAGNOSIS

WHAT THE DOCTOR LOOKS FOR
- The doctor will perform a physical examination to evaluate liver function.
- The doctor will investigate conditions known to be associated with cirrhosis of the liver (e.g., hepatitis, gallbladder disease, cystic fibrosis, and heart failure).
- Possible sources of gastrointestinal bleeding will be investigated.

TESTS AND PROCEDURES
- A number of blood tests may be performed.
- The liver can be visually examined by laparoscopy.
- A sample of liver tissue can be obtained by biopsy for laboratory analysis.
- An imaging procedure called cholangiography can be done to evaluate the liver and gallbladder.
- Ultrasound, computed tomography (CT) scan, or other specialized procedures can be performed to assist in diagnosis.
- The upper digestive system may be evaluated by endoscopy.

GENERAL MEASURES
- Cirrhosis of the liver is usually managed on an outpatient basis, except for complicating emergencies such as gastrointestinal bleeding or kidney failure.
- Treatment is aimed at the underlying cause of cirrhosis, preventing further liver damage, and preventing complications.
- Therapies involve drug treatment, dietary restrictions, rest, and other supportive measures. Adequate protein intake is necessary for liver healing.
- Surgery or transplantation may be necessary.

ACTIVITY
Patients should be as active as possible. Leg elevation may be necessary for swelling of the feet and ankles.

DIET
- Adequate protein and generous calories to help the liver heal
- In some cases, protein restriction is necessary.
- In some cases, salt restriction is necessary.
- In some cases, fluid restriction is necessary.
- No alcohol

 ## MEDICATIONS

COMMONLY PRESCRIBED DRUGS
- Propranolol
- Spironolactone, furosemide
- Lactulose (Cholac)
- Ampicillin plus aminoglycoside, cefotaxime, norfloxacin, penicillamine
- Corticosteroids, azathioprine
- Interferon
- Ursodeoxycholic acid (Ursodiol)

CONTRAINDICATIONS
Read drug product information.

PRECAUTIONS
Read drug product information.

SIGNIFICANT POSSIBLE INTERACTIONS
Read drug product information.

 ## FOLLOW-UP

PATIENT MONITORING
- Stable patients need a yearly battery of liver tests.
- Unstable patients may need weekly tests.
- Patients should monitor weight and record in a daily diary.

PREVENTION
- Limit use of alcohol and other substances that are toxic to the liver.
- Do not share syringes.
- Practice safe sex.

COMPLICATIONS
- Jaundice
- Bleeding disorders
- Brain damage
- Gastrointestinal bleeding
- Liver failure
- Liver cancer (uncommon)
- Infection
- Kidney failure

WHAT TO EXPECT
The course of cirrhosis depends on liver function. If a cause is identified and treated, the outcome may be good.

GERIATRIC
Cirrhosis is one of the leading causes of death in people more than 65 years of age.

PREGNANCY
Cirrhosis may become worse during pregnancy. Higher rates of miscarriage, premature birth, and infant death occur in women with cirrhosis.

FURTHER INFORMATION
- American Liver Foundation, (800) 223-0179
- National Digestive Diseases Information Clearinghouse, Box NDDIC, Bethesda, MD 20892, (301) 468-6344

Cirrhosis of the Liver

Doctor
Office
Phone
Pager

Special notes to patient:

Claudication

 BASICS

DESCRIPTION

Claudication is a feeling of muscle fatigue that occurs after a period of minimal exercise. The feeling may progress to a cramp-like pain, usually in the calf muscles. The pain is relieved by rest. Claudication can occur in the arms but is more common in the legs; calf more frequently than the thigh.

SIGNS AND SYMPTOMS

- May start gradually or suddenly
- Unable to walk distances
- Pain varies from muscle tiredness to a cramp
- May be a loss of hair on toes

CAUSES

Blockage of an artery, usually because of arteriosclerosis

SCOPE

Claudication is common in the United States.

MOST OFTEN AFFECTED

Claudication is common in men more than 55 years of age, women more than 60 years of age. Males are affected four times as often as females.

RISK FACTORS

- Smoking
- Diabetes
- High blood pressure
- High levels of lipids and fats in the blood
- Obesity
- Heart disease

 DIAGNOSIS

WHAT THE DOCTOR LOOKS FOR

- The doctor will perform a thorough assessment of the circulatory system.
- The doctor will look for other possible causes of symptoms (e.g., arthritis or nerve disorders).
- The doctor should diagnose and treat other cardiovascular disease.

TESTS AND PROCEDURES

- Blood tests
- Noninvasive blood pressure measurements in numerous locations on the extremities
- Specialized imaging of the circulatory system (arteriography) can be done to assist in diagnosis.
- Ultrasound can be done to assess blood vessels.

 TREATMENT

GENERAL MEASURES

- Claudication is managed in the outpatient setting, except for severe cases or advanced disease.
- Conservative measures: stop smoking, initiate walking and exercise program, control of high blood fats and cholesterol
- Reduce risk factors.
- Surgical treatment may be required.

ACTIVITY

As tolerated

 MEDICATIONS

COMMONLY PRESCRIBED DRUGS

- Aspirin
- Pentoxifylline (Trental)

CONTRAINDICATIONS

Read drug product information.

PRECAUTIONS

First, try to reduce risk factors before taking medications.

SIGNIFICANT POSSIBLE INTERACTIONS

Read drug product information.

OTHER DRUGS

- Ticlopidine
- Vasodilators
- Calcium channel blockers
- Blood thinners (anticoagulants)

 FOLLOW-UP

PATIENT MONITORING

- See the doctor as often as necessary.
- Imaging of blood vessels should be repeated twice a year.

PREVENTION

- Start a walking program of 4 to 5 miles per day.
- Avoid smoking

COMPLICATIONS

A few people with claudication ultimately may require amputation of the affected leg.

WHAT TO EXPECT

The condition can gradually improve or get progressively worse.

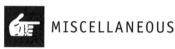 MISCELLANEOUS

GERIATRIC

Claudication is more common with advancing age.

Claudication

Doctor
Office
Phone
Pager

Special notes to patient:

Common Cold

 ## BASICS

DESCRIPTION
The common cold is an inflammation of the nasal passages caused by any number of respiratory viruses. The common cold is usually not serious; most cold sufferers treat themselves.

SIGNS AND SYMPTOMS
- Nasal stuffiness
- Sneezing
- Scratchy throat
- Cough
- Hoarseness
- Malaise
- Headache
- Fever

CAUSES
- Usually caused by 1 of 200 strains of virus
- In 40% of cases, no cause can be identified.

SCOPE
Preschool children average 6 to 10 colds annually; children in kindergarten average 12 colds annually; school children average 7 colds annually; adolescents and adults average 2 to 4 colds annually. About 31 episodes of cold occur per 100 persons annually.

MOST OFTEN AFFECTED
- Children get colds more frequently than adults. Males and females are affected in equal proportions.
- American Indians and Eskimos are at higher risk than other ethnic groups and have more frequent complications, such as ear infection.
- Certain genetic traits may make a person unusually susceptible to the common cold.

RISK FACTORS
- Exposure to infected individuals
- Touching the nose or eyes with contaminated fingers

 ## DIAGNOSIS

WHAT THE DOCTOR LOOKS FOR
The doctor will look for other conditions that can cause similar signs and symptoms (e.g., allergies or other viral infections).

TESTS AND PROCEDURES
- Blood tests
- Fluid from the nose or throat may be analyzed in the laboratory.
- In rare cases, virus can be cultured.

 ## TREATMENT

GENERAL MEASURES
- Colds are usually managed by self-care
- Rest, fluids, and relief of symptoms
- The usual course of the common cold is 6 to 10 days.
- Use a vaporizer or humidifier.
- Stop smoking and drinking alcohol.
- In infants, nasal passages may be cleared with a bulb syringe; incline mattress at 45°; use saline nasal drops.

ACTIVITY
Resume activity, as tolerated, but rest more frequently the first few days after resuming activity.

DIET
Increase fluid intake.

 ## MEDICATIONS

COMMONLY PRESCRIBED DRUGS
No cure or practical preventive measure exists for the common cold. Avoid "shotgun" medications (those that claim to treat all the symptoms of the common cold). Instead, target specific symptoms, an approach that may reduce the risk of adverse effects from medications.

- Topical sprays: oxymetazoline (for stuffy nose), ipratropium (for runny nose)
- Oral decongestants: pseudoephedrine (for stuffy nose)
- Oral antihistamines: chlorpheniramine (for sneezing, runny nose)
- Cough suppressants: codeine, dextromethorphan
- Expectorants: guaifenesin (effectiveness not yet proved)

CONTRAINDICATIONS
Oral decongestants are contraindicated in patients taking monoamine oxidase (MAO) inhibitors and selegiline.

PRECAUTIONS
- Oral decongestants
  - Can increase blood pressure, irregular heart rhythm, and may interfere with diabetes management
  - Other adverse effects include headache, nervousness, sleeplessness, and dizziness.
  - Use with caution if taking guanethidine.
- Antihistamines: can worsen nasal blockage and sinus congestion
- Cough suppressants: codeine and dextromethorphan can be abused.
- Expectorants
  - Liquid preparations may contain high concentrations of alcohol.
  - Nausea, vomiting, or abdominal pain are common adverse effects.
- Vitamin C: Use is generally safe, but can cause kidney stones and interfere with urine glucose monitoring in people with diabetes.

DRUG INTERACTIONS
Read drug product information.

OTHER DRUGS
- Many mouthwashes, gargles, and lozenges are promoted to relieve the pain of sore throat.
- Hard candy, gargling with warm saline, and products containing anesthetics (e.g., benzocaine or phenol) can all relieve pain.
- Antibacterial gargles or lozenges are of no value in treating a viral illness.
- Aromatic oils (e.g., menthol, camphor, and eucalyptus), when applied topically or taken in a lozenge, produce a sensation of increased airflow.
- Antivirals: interferon, zinc chloride

 ## FOLLOW-UP

PATIENT MONITORING
Contact the physician for fever above 102°F (38.9°C), difficulty breathing, productive cough, or shaking chills.

PREVENTION
Frequent handwashing and avoiding touching the face may help prevent colds.

Common Cold

	Doctor
	Office
	Phone
	Pager

Special notes to patient:

Common Cold

COMPLICATIONS

- Lower respiratory tract infection
- Asthma
- Severe worsening of asthma or chronic lung disease
- Ear infection (otitis media)
- Acute sinus infection
- Pneumonia

WHAT TO EXPECT

Complete recovery can be expected within 3 to 10 days.

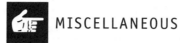 MISCELLANEOUS

PEDIATRIC

- Medications can produce toxic or adverse effects in young children.
- Do not give aspirin to children because of the risk of Reye's syndrome.
- Incidence of colds is highest among children.

GERIATRIC

Medications commonly produce adverse effects in the elderly.

PREGNANCY

- Take medications only if clearly needed.
- No clear association exists between the use of decongestants or antihistamines and birth defects.
- Indiscriminate use of codeine during pregnancy can pose a risk to the fetus.

Common Cold

Doctor
Office
Phone
Pager

Special notes to patient:

Congestive Heart Failure

BASICS

DESCRIPTION
Congestive heart failure (CHF), the principal complication of heart disease, is caused by abnormal cardiac pump function. CHF occurs at some time in all cases of severe heart disease.

SIGNS AND SYMPTOMS
- Early and mild heart failure:
  - Need to urinate during sleep hours
  - Shortness of breath on exertion
  - Diminished exercise capacity
  - Fatigue
  - Difficulty breathing
  - Weakness
  - Rapid heart rate with mild exertion
- Moderate heart failure:
  - Cough during sleep
  - Easier to breathe sitting up
  - Acute episodes of breathing difficulty during sleep
  - Wheezing, especially at night
  - Loss of appetite
  - Sensation of fullness or dull pain in abdomen
  - Rapid heart rate at rest
  - Anxiety
  - Coolness of the arms and legs
  - Swelling of the feet and ankles
- Severe heart failure:
  - Mental impairment
  - Abdominal bloating
  - A bluish discoloration around the mouth, eyes, or ears (cyanosis)
  - Low blood pressure
  - Frothy and/or pink sputum

CAUSES
- Heart attack
- Pulmonary embolism
- Metabolic disorders (hyperthyroidism, fever, stress)
- Other heart disease

SCOPE
Heart failure is the most common diagnosis in hospitalized persons above 65 years of age.

MOST OFTEN AFFECTED
Varies depending on cause. More common in men between the ages of 40 and 70; equal frequency with females 75 years of age or older.

RISK FACTORS
- Noncompliance with therapy
- Irregular heart rhythm
- Drug side effects
- Inappropriate physical, emotional, or environmental stress
- Other medical conditions

DIAGNOSIS

WHAT THE DOCTOR LOOKS FOR
- The doctor will perform a physical examination, in particular assessing heart function.
- The doctor should identify and treat correctable conditions (e.g., heart attack).

TESTS AND PROCEDURES
- A number of blood tests can be performed to assist in diagnosis.
- Urinalysis
- Chest x-ray study
- The function of the heart can be studied with echocardiograhy.
- The heart can be assessed by cardiac catheterization.

TREATMENT

GENERAL MEASURES
- Severe heart failure may require hospitalization.
- Underlying correctable conditions should be identified and treated.
- Surgery or transplantation may be required.

ACTIVITY
- During severe stage, bed rest with elevation of head of bed and antiembolism stockings to help control leg swelling
- Gradual increase in activity with walking helps increase strength.

DIET
- Sodium restriction
- Weight reduction diet, if overweight
- Low-fat diet to slow coronary artery disease

MEDICATIONS

COMMONLY PRESCRIBED DRUGS
- Digoxin
- Diuretics: furosemide (Lasix), metolazone (Zaroxolyn), Spironolactone
- Angiotensin-converting enzyme (ACE) inhibitors
- Beta-blockers: carvedilol (Coreg), bisoprolol (Zebeta)
- Vasodilators: nitroglycerin, hydralazine, prazosin, isosorbide dinitrate

CONTRAINDICATIONS
Read drug product information.

PRECAUTIONS
ACE inhibitors can cause low blood pressure (rare).

SIGNIFICANT POSSIBLE INTERACTIONS
Read drug product information.

OTHER DRUGS
Dopamine, dobutamine

FOLLOW-UP

PATIENT MONITORING
- See the doctor as often as necessary, depending on health status.
- Initially, the doctor may be seen every 2 to 3 weeks after stabilization.

PREVENTION
Treatment of underlying disorders, when possible

COMPLICATIONS
- Electrolyte disturbance
- Irregular heart rhythms
- Circulatory problems
- Digitalis toxicity

WHAT TO EXPECT
- Result of initial treatment is usually good, whatever the cause.
- The long-term outcome is variable. Death rates range from 10% with mild symptoms to 50% with advanced, progressive symptoms.

Congestive Heart Failure

Doctor
Office
Phone
Pager

Special notes to patient:

Congestive Heart Failure

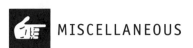 **MISCELLANEOUS**

PEDIATRIC
Heart failure in children is usually associated with congenital heart disease.

GERIATRIC
Medications may need dosage adjustment

PREGNANCY
Heart failure during pregnancy requires special care.

FURTHER INFORMATION
- American Heart Association, 7320 Greenville Avenue, Dallas, TX 75231, (214) 373-6300
- American College of Cardiology, 911 Old Georgetown Road, Bethesda, MD 20814, (301) 897-5400

Congestive Heart Failure

Doctor
Office
Phone
Pager

Special notes to patient:

Constipation

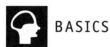 ## BASICS

DESCRIPTION

Constipation is a combination of changes in the frequency, size, consistency, and ease of stool passage, which leads to an overall decrease in the volume of bowel movements. "Normal" toilet habits vary over a wide range; occasional episodes of constipation are to be expected.

SIGNS AND SYMPTOMS

- Less frequency of defecation than usual
- Harder stool than usual
- Smaller stools than usual
- Impaction of stool
- Thickening of stool
- Lack of consistent urgency to stool
- Difficulty expelling feces
- Painful evacuation of feces
- Sensation of incomplete emptying of the bowel
- Abdominal fullness
- Painful spasm of the rectum

CAUSES

- Electrolyte disturbance
- Hormonal disturbance (hypothyroidism, diabetes)
- Congenital conditions
- Other illness, injury, or debility
- Other bowel conditions
- Inadequate fluid intake
- Side effect of drugs (e.g., anticholinergic agents, opiates)
- Chronic abuse of laxatives or cathartics
- Psychiatric, cultural, emotional, environmental factors

SCOPE

- Constipation is common, affecting most persons at some point.
- More frequent among the very young and the very old

MOST OFTEN AFFECTED

- All ages can be affected by constipation, but it is more frequent in infancy and old age.
- May affect more than one member of a family
- More frequent in females than males

RISK FACTORS

- Age (very young or very old)
- Neurosis
- Drug use
- Sedentary life style or condition

 ## DIAGNOSIS

WHAT THE DOCTOR LOOKS FOR

- The doctor will evaluate the patient and identify and treat the cause of constipation.
- The doctor should evaluate for other signs of debility or aging (e.g, arthritis).

TESTS AND PROCEDURES

- Blood tests can be done to assist in diagnosis.
- Abdominal x-ray study
- Specialized tests can be done to assess digestion (e.g., timing the passage of material through the tract).
- Digital rectal examination to rule out cancer and check for blood in the stool
- The lower intestinal tract can be visually examined by sigmoidoscopy or colonoscopy.

 ## TREATMENT

GENERAL MEASURES

- Constipation is usually managed in the outpatient setting, except when an underlying lesion or obstruction requires hospitalization.
- Attempt to eliminate medications that can cause or worsen constipation.
- Increase fluid intake.
- Modify diet.
- Use enemas if other remedies fail.
- Allow adequate time for bowel evacuation in a quiet, unhurried environment.
- Use commode with thighs drawn toward abdomen.

ACTIVITY

Exercise is encouraged.

DIET

Increase fiber (bran, fruit, green vegetables, and whole grain cereals and breads) to approximately 15 g/day. Liberal intake of fluids is encouraged.

 ## MEDICATIONS

COMMONLY PRESCRIBED DRUGS

- Bulk-forming agents: psyllium (Konsyl, Metamucil, Perdiem), methylcellulose (Citrucel), polycarbophil (Mitrolan, FiberCon)
- Laxatives: milk of magnesia, magnesium citrate, phosphate of soda, lactulose (Chronulac), sorbitol, alumina-magnesia (Maalox, Mylanta); appropriate for short-term use
- Stool softeners: docusate sodium (Colace)

CONTRAINDICATIONS

- Any obstruction or impediment to transit in the bowel; laxatives can cause distension or perforation
- Acute abdominal inflammation
- Kidney and heart failure are relative contraindications.

PRECAUTIONS

Chronic use of laxatives can cause serious problems.

DRUG INTERACTIONS

Magnesium-containing laxatives interact with tetracycline, digitalis, and phenothiazine.

OTHER DRUGS

- Lubricants (e.g., mineral oil)
- Emollient suppositories: may relieve soreness
- Cathartics (stimulants): ricinoleic acid, castor oil (Neoloid), phenolphthalein (Ex-Lax, Modane), bisacodyl (Dulcolax)
- Anthraquinone: senna (Senokot)
- Enemas: Phospho soda (Fleets); avoid soap suds (can cause colitis)
- Suppositories: sodium phosphate, glycerin, bisacodyl

 ## FOLLOW-UP

PATIENT MONITORING

See doctor if constipation persists.

PREVENTION

Some people have a tendency toward constipation. Proper diet, bowel training, and use of bulk-forming supplements are important.

Constipation

Doctor
Office
Phone
Pager

Special notes to patient:

Constipation

COMPLICATIONS

- Serious bowel disorders
- Conditions caused by repeated laxative abuse
- Fluid and electrolyte depletion

WHAT TO EXPECT

Constipation that is occasional, brief, and responsive to simple measures is harmless. Habitual constipation can be a lifelong nuisance.

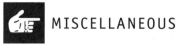 MISCELLANEOUS

GERIATRIC

- Elderly persons who have had regular bowel action throughout their lives seldom develop constipation because of age alone.
- Persons with a lifelong tendency to constipation often encounter increasing difficulty with advancing age.
- An increased risk of colorectal cancer may be associated with constipation.

PREGNANCY

Women with a tendency toward constipation may find the condition more troublesome in the third trimester and require dietary adjustment and fiber supplements.

Constipation

Doctor
Office
Phone
Pager

Special notes to patient:

Contraception

 ## BASICS

DESCRIPTION

Contraception is defined as practices designed to prevent pregnancy. Contraceptive practices either (1) prevent ovulation, (2) prevent implantation, (3) are spermicidal, or (4) prevent sperm from reaching the egg. Natural family planning aims to avoid intercourse at the time of expected ovulation. Failure rates vary among methods. The most effective form of contraception is permanent sterilization, either tubal sterilization in the female or vasectomy in the male. Neither is to be considered reversible, but can be reversed under certain circumstances. Surgical attempts at reversal are often unsuccessful.

SCOPE

About two thirds of women at risk for unwanted pregnancies use contraception.

MOST OFTEN AFFECTED

- Females: 11 to 52 years of age
- Males: any age after puberty

RISK FACTORS

- Pregnancy can occur in any woman who is ovulating and having intercourse with a fertile male.
- Young adolescents are at increased risk for unplanned pregnancy.
- Socioeconomic factors (e.g., less access to medical care, limited knowledge about reproduction) can increase the risk for unplanned pregnancy.

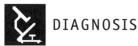 ## DIAGNOSIS

TESTS AND PROCEDURES

- Cells from the cervix can be examined by microscope (Pap smear).
- Cultures for sexually transmitted disease (gonorrhea and chlamydia)
- Blood tests
- Pregnancy test for females
- Males may have a semen analysis after vasectomy.

 ## TREATMENT

GENERAL MEASURES

- Latex condom: Use water-based lubricants; check for holes before using; leave space at tip to act as reservoir for the semen; withdraw from vagina before penis becomes flaccid; use a spermicide in addition to a condom to increase effectiveness.
- IUD: Frequently check for the presence of the string.
- Diaphragm: A diaphragm must be fitted by a physician. Before inserting, place one tablespoon of spermicidal gel or cream into the dome of diaphragm and line entire rim of the diaphragm with it; insert the diaphragm and check for proper placement; leave in for at least 8 hours after intercourse. Then remove and clean according to directions; check for holes. If another act of intercourse occurs before 8 hours, insert additional spermicidal gel or cream into vagina with an applicator device without displacing the diaphragm.
- Female condom (Reality): The female condom is available over the counter. Use new condom for each sex act; insert properly so that inner ring is well into vagina and outer ring lies against vulva; make sure that penis enters inside the sheath; remove condom after intercourse, being careful not to spill semen.
- Periodic abstinence
  - Need accurate record of menstrual cycles for at least 12 months before use
  - Problem for women with variable cycle length
  - Added effectiveness from observing cervical mucus for disappearance of abundant clear mucus and by observing basal temperature rise of about 1°F for 3 days. Both signs usually indicate ovulation.
- Permanent sterilization
  - Tubal sterilization in the female
  - Vasectomy in the male

 ## MEDICATIONS

COMMONLY PRESCRIBED DRUGS

- Oral contraceptives: Take pill daily at approximately same time; if a pill is missed, take two the following day but use an additional method of protection, such as a barrier method, until next menstrual period; if two menstrual periods are missed, seek medical care to rule out pregnancy. Do not stop pills if a period is missed.
- Spermicides: All contain nonoxynol-9. Choice depends on personal preference; foams and creams disperse well; suppositories or tablets must first dissolve.
- Implantable contraceptive: Levonorgestrel (Norplant) consists of six tubes implanted into the upper arm by a physician; effective for up to 5 years.
- Injectable contraceptive: medroxyprogesterone acetate (Depo-Provera); effective for up to 4 months

CONTRAINDICATIONS

- Implantable or injectable contraceptives
  - Active liver disease
  - Thrombophlebitis
  - Pregnancy
  - Unexplained, abnormal, uterine bleeding
  - High blood levels of fats and lipids
- Oral contraceptives
  - Same as implantable contraception plus noncompliance and estrogen-dependent cancer
  - May be inadvisable for women with high blood pressure, insulin-dependent diabetes mellitus, and migraine headaches
  - Not recommended for women 35 years of age or older who smoke, because of increased risk of heart attack.

PRECAUTIONS

Read drug product information.

DRUG INTERACTIONS

Add a barrier method if taking phenytoin (Dilantin) or antibiotics.

Contraception

Doctor
Office
Phone
Pager

Special notes to patient:

Contraception

 FOLLOW-UP

PATIENT MONITORING

- See the doctor annually for a pelvic examination and Pap smear.
- Report side effects or problems to the doctor.
- The doctor should check for presence of an IUD 1 month after insertion.

COMPLICATIONS

- Oral contraceptives
  - Clotting disorders
  - High blood pressure
  - Heart attack: main risk is in smoker, particularly after age 35
  - Nausea and vomiting: take pill on full stomach
  - Breakthrough bleeding: usually self-limiting after 3 months
  - Absence of menstrual period
  - Cyclic weight gain
  - Breast tenderness: rare with low-dose pill
  - Depression: rare with low-dose pill
  - Brown patches on skin
  - Acne or excessive hair growth
  - Jaundice
  - Weight gain throughout cycle
- Implantable contraceptive (Norplant)
  - Amenorrhea (absence of menstrual period): about 33%
  - Irregular bleeding: about 33%
  - Both are self-limited after about 1 year.
- Injectable contraceptive (Depo-Provera)
  - Irregular bleeding during first few months
  - Not readily reversible
  - Absence of menstrual periods common after 1 year of use
- IUD
  - Pelvic inflammatory disease
  - Heavy bleeding and cramps
- Pregnancy can occur with any method.

 MISCELLANEOUS

OTHERS

Healthy nonsmokers can use oral contraceptives until age 50 years.

PREGNANCY

See above

FURTHER INFORMATION

Printed materials available from American College of Obstetrics and Gynecology (800) 673-8444

Contraception

Doctor
Office
Phone
Pager

Special notes to patient:

Crohn's Disease

 ## BASICS

DESCRIPTION

Crohn's disease is a slowly progressive inflammatory disease of unknown cause that affects the small or large intestine.

SCOPE

Crohn's disease affects 20 to 100 of 100,000 persons in the United States. It is more common in whites and Jews than African-Americans or Asians.

MOST OFTEN AFFECTED

- Most initial cases of Crohn's disease occur in people 15 to 25 years of age. It is also relatively common among individuals 55 to 65 years of age. Females are affected slightly more often than males.
- About 15% of affected persons have a member of the immediate family with the disease, with a similar pattern of symptoms and age of onset.

SIGNS AND SYMPTOMS

- Diarrhea
- Weight loss
- Pain, tenderness, or feeling of fullness in the abdomen
- Lesion of the rectum, bladder, skin, or vagina
- Disease elsewhere in the body (e.g., skin disease, arthritis)
- Bleeding

CAUSES

Unknown; condition is aggravated by infection or inflammation and by smoking cessation.

RISK FACTORS

Smoking

 ## DIAGNOSIS

WHAT THE DOCTOR LOOKS FOR

- The doctor will perform a physical examination to rule out other possible conditions (e.g., ulcerative colitis, intestinal infection, or cancer).
- The doctor identifies and treats other conditions known to be associated with Crohn's disease (e.g., arthritis and skin lesions).

TESTS AND PROCEDURES

- Blood tests
- Barium x-ray study may be done to visualize the intestinal tract.
- The intestinal tract can be visually examined by colonoscopy.
- A sample of tissue can be obtained by biopsy for analysis.
- Plain x-ray film or computed tomography (CT) scan of the abdomen

 ## TREATMENT

GENERAL MEASURES

- Crohn's disease is customarily treated in an outpatient setting.
- Hospitalization may be required for complications or special treatments.
- The disease is progressive and often requires surgery.
- Attention to maintaining weight and nutrition is important.
- Use a sitz bath at the direction of the doctor.
- Clean anal area with soap and water after bowel movements.

ACTIVITY

Full activity as tolerated

DIET

- Usually no restrictions
- If fat malabsorption is a problem, reduce dietary fat.
- Avoid highly fibrous substances if scarring or recurring obstructions develop.
- Increase dietary fiber if diarrhea is prominent; reducing dietary fat sometimes is also recommended.

 ## MEDICATIONS

COMMONLY PRESCRIBED DRUGS

- Mesalamine (5-aminosalicylic acid), methotrexate, azathioprine (Imuran), prednisone, sulfasalazine
- Prednisone, hydrocortisone (Cortenema), or mesalamine enemas
- Metronidazole (Flagyl), olsalazine (Dipentum)

CONTRAINDICATIONS

Drug allergy

PRECAUTIONS

- Sulfasalazine may not be tolerated because it frequently causes nausea, vomiting, and other gastrointestinal distress.
- Drug allergies are common.
- Male sterility is a problem with chronic use.

SIGNIFICANT POSSIBLE INTERACTIONS

- Folic acid supplements are needed with mesalamine use.
- Read drug product information.

OTHER DRUGS

- Antibiotics
- Mercaptopurine (6-mercaptopurine)

 ## FOLLOW-UP

PATIENT MONITORING

- See the doctor every 3 to 6 months if symptoms are stable or as often as necessary based on health status.
- Contact the doctor about changes in condition.
- The digestive tract may be periodically examined by endoscopy.

PREVENTION

An individual with Crohn's disease should receive good medical care, including ongoing care with a regular physician and consults with a specialist when necessary.

COMPLICATIONS

- Progression of Crohn's disease is nearly certain, even after surgery.
- About 15% of patients develop an ulcer or lesion.
- About 10% of patients have disease elsewhere in the body (e.g., skin disease or arthritis).
- Extensive colon disease is associated with an increased risk of cancer.
- Colon can become severely diseased or perforated, which can lead to massive bleeding.

WHAT TO EXPECT

- The average patient has surgery every 7 years.
- Short-bowel syndrome may develop after four surgeries.
- Expect the disease to recur.
- Most people have a normal life with work, children, and full activities, but overall lifespan is shortened.

Crohn's Disease

Doctor
Office
Phone
Pager

Special notes to patient:

Crohn's Disease

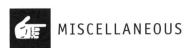 **MISCELLANEOUS**

PEDIATRIC
Crohn's disease is rare in children.

OTHERS
Occurs at any age

PREGNANCY
- Long-time use of sulfasalazine can cause sterility in males that resolves when the person stops taking medication.
- Crohn's disease is not a contraindication to pregnancy.

FURTHER INFORMATION
Crohn's and Colitis Foundation of America Inc., 11th floor, Park Ave South, NY 10016, Phone (800) 343-3637

Crohn's Disease

Doctor
Office
Phone
Pager

Special notes to patient:

Croup

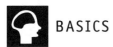 BASICS

DESCRIPTION
Croup, a viral illness characterized by barking cough, high-pitched breathing, and fever, often causes upper airway obstruction in children.

SIGNS AND SYMPTOMS
- Barking, spasmodic cough
- Noisy, high-pitched breathing
- Low-grade to moderate fever
- Bluish discoloration around eyes, mouth, and nail beds (cyanosis)
- Fatigue

CAUSES
Viral infection

SCOPE
About 15,000 to 40,000 cases of croup occur per 100,000 persons in the United States.

MOST OFTEN AFFECTED
Children; males and females in equal proportion

RISK FACTORS
- History of croup
- Recurring upper respiratory infections

 DIAGNOSIS

WHAT THE DOCTOR LOOKS FOR
- The doctor will perform a physical examination to assess for the presence of croup.
- Conditions that can cause similar signs and symptoms include epiglottitis, foreign body aspiration, and other types of infection.

TESTS AND PROCEDURES
- Blood tests
- Fluid from the throat can be sent for laboratory analysis.
- X-ray study of the neck
- The airway can be examined by laryngoscopy or bronchoscopy.

 TREATMENT

GENERAL MEASURES
- Mild cases of croup can be managed in the outpatient setting.
- Severe cases may require intensive care.
- Humidification ("croup tent")
- Intravenous (IV) fluids
- Intubation may be required.
- Tracheotomy (rarely)

ACTIVITY
Must keep patient quiet; crying can worsen symptoms.

DIET
- Nothing by mouth for severe cases
- Frequent small feedings with increased fluids for mild cases

 MEDICATIONS

COMMONLY PRESCRIBED DRUGS
- Dexamethasone
- Racemic epinephrine (Vaponefrin)
- Antibiotics
- Oxygen as needed

PRECAUTIONS
Read drug product information.

CONTRAINDICATIONS
Read drug product information.

DRUG INTERACTIONS
Read drug product information.

OTHER DRUGS
- Budesonide
- Ribavirin
- Amantadine

FOLLOW-UP

PATIENT MONITORING
- Patients in the hospital will be seen often by the doctor and other healthcare professionals.
- See the doctor as often as necessary.
- Contact doctor immediately for any severe worsening of condition, or call 911.

COMPLICATIONS
- Bacterial infection
- Cardiopulmonary arrest
- Pneumonia

WHAT TO EXPECT
- If required, intubation is maintained for 3 to 5 days.
- If required, tracheotomy is maintained for 3 to 7 days.
- Recovery is usually complete, without lasting effects.

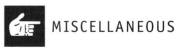 MISCELLANEOUS

PEDIATRIC
Croup is common in children under 3 years of age.

Croup

Doctor
Office
Phone
Pager

Special notes to patient:

Cutaneous (Skin) Drug Reactions

 ## BASICS

DESCRIPTION

Cutaneous (skin) rashes or eruptions are the most common adverse reactions to drug therapy. Most reactions develop within 1 week of initiation of drug therapy but can occur up to 4 weeks later.

SCOPE

- About 144 cases of drug reaction occur among 100,000 hospitalized persons.
- Overall prevalence is unknown among the 125 million nonhospitalized Americans who regularly use prescription drugs as outpatients.

MOST OFTEN AFFECTED

All ages affected; females more often than males

SIGNS AND SYMPTOMS

- Eruptions of skin: most frequent skin reaction; reddened pimples or bumps that often itch; onset is typically 7 to 10 days after initiation of drug; can last 1 to 2 weeks
- Rash: itchy red spots; may fade within 24 hours, but new rash may develop
- Acne-like eruptions
- Eczema-like reactions: itchy, scaling skin on inner surfaces of arms or legs
- Patches of dry skin or hair loss
- Sensitivity to light

CAUSES

Exposure to medication

RISK FACTORS

Drug therapy, especially with antibiotics

 ## DIAGNOSIS

WHAT THE DOCTOR LOOKS FOR

- The doctor performs an examination and looks for other diseases that cause similar signs.
- The doctor will look for other conditions known to be associated with drug reactions (e.g., severe allergies, swelling, or bone marrow disorders).

TESTS AND PROCEDURES

- Routine blood tests are usually not helpful.
- A sample of tissue can be obtained by biopsy for laboratory analysis.
- Skin testing for allergies may be performed.

 ## TREATMENT

GENERAL MEASURES

- The doctor should evaluate a person with rash or swelling as soon as possible.
- Hospitalization may be required for severe allergies or other acute reactions.
- Stop taking the drug that causes reactions.
- Avoid further use of the drug that caused the reaction.

ACTIVITY

- No specific restrictions in general
- For acute dry scaly skin or rash, bathe with tepid water and avoid activities that cause sweating.

DIET

No dietary restrictions

 ## MEDICATIONS

COMMONLY PRESCRIBED DRUGS

- Most cases require no specific therapy.
- Antihistamines may relieve symptoms of rash, swelling, and inflammation.
- Skin creams or lotions can be used for dry skin.
- Topical corticosteroids

CONTRAINDICATIONS

Read drug product information.

PRECAUTIONS

Read drug product information.

DRUG INTERACTIONS

Read drug product information.

 ## FOLLOW-UP

PATIENT MONITORING

- See the doctor often to ensure that the reaction is not progressing.
- Patients with severe reactions may require hospitalization.

PREVENTION

Avoid drugs that cause reaction.

WHAT TO EXPECT

- Eruptions generally fade within days after stopping drug therapy.
- Rash, swelling, and other severe reactions are potentially more serious and can even be life-threatening.

 ## MISCELLANEOUS

GERIATRIC

- Reactions are more likely to occur among elderly who take a greater number of medications.
- Severe reactions are less tolerated in the elderly.

FURTHER INFORMATION

American Academy of Dermatology, 930 N. Meacham Rd., P.O. Box 4014, Schaumberg, IL 60168-4014; (708) 330-0230

Cutaneous (Skin) Drug Reactions

Doctor
Office
Phone
Pager

Special notes to patient:

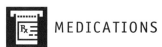

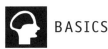 BASICS

DESCRIPTION

Cystic fibrosis (CF) is a generalized disorder of infants, children, and young adults. Characteristics include chronic pulmonary disease, pancreatic disease, and abnormally high levels of salts in the sweat.

SIGNS AND SYMPTOMS

- Sweat glands
  - Increased concentrations of salt
  - Dehydration with heat and infections
- Respiratory system:
  - Wheezing
  - Chronic cough
  - Difficulty breathing
  - Rapid breathing
  - Barrel chest
  - Repeated bouts of bronchitis or pneumonia
- Gastrointestinal system:
  - Failure to thrive
  - Chronic, recurrent abdominal pain
  - Gastroesophageal reflux
  - Voracious appetite before treatment
  - A sensation of fullness in the abdomen
  - Frequent, bulky, foul-smelling, pale stool
- Others:
  - Delayed weight gain during growth and development
  - Retarded bone growth
  - Delayed sexual development
  - Infertility in males
  - Decrease in female fertility

CAUSES

Genetic defect

SCOPE

CF is the most common lethal genetic disease. It affects about 1 of 2,500 white. It is less common in African-Americans, Native Americans, and Asians.

MOST OFTEN AFFECTED

Infants, children, and young adults are most often affected, as the average age of survival is 29 years. Males and females are affected equally. CF tends to run in families.

RISK FACTORS

Family history of CF

DIAGNOSIS

WHAT THE DOCTOR LOOKS FOR

- The doctor will perform a thorough physical examination to look for specific signs and symptoms of CF.
- Other possible causes of signs and symptoms will be investigated (e.g., immune system disorders, recurring pneumonia, or asthma).
- The doctor will look for known complications of CF (e.g., collapsed lung, heart failure, or other serious conditions).

TESTS AND PROCEDURES

Blood tests
Sweat tests
Genetic screening
Stool studies
Fluid from airway can be cultured for laboratory analysis.
Pulmonary function tests
Exercise testing may be performed.
The structures and function of the heart can be evaluated by ultrasound.
Chest x-ray study

TREATMENT

GENERAL MEASURES

- CF is usually managed in the outpatient setting.
- Infections or other crisis may require hospitalization.
- Intravenous (IV) antibiotics to prevent infection may be provided at home.
- Care by experienced physician and team (respiratory therapist, nurse, nutritionist, physical therapist, counselor, social worker) is crucial.
- Goals are to prevent and treat respiratory failure and pulmonary complications.
- Respiratory therapy
- Regular exercises for fitness
- Emphasis on good nutrition; supplements may be needed
- Medication for treatment of symptoms
- Insulin, if diabetes develops
- Surgery may be needed for some complications
- Organ transplants possible for lung, liver, and endocrine pancreas

ACTIVITY

Physical conditioning to the extent possible for cardiorespiratory fitness

DIET

- Allow liberal salting of foods, if desired
- High dietary protein, calories, fat
- Vitamin supplements (double the recommended daily allowance)

MEDICATIONS

COMMONLY PRESCRIBED DRUGS

- Antibiotics: may be oral, IV, or aerosolized
- Other therapies: pancreatic enzyme replacement, bronchodilators, dornase alfa (DNase), ibuprofen, oxygen therapy, annual flu vaccine

CONTRAINDICATIONS

Read drug product information.

PRECAUTIONS

Read drug product information.

SIGNIFICANT POSSIBLE INTERACTIONS

Read drug product information.

OTHER DRUGS

Other antibiotics

FOLLOW-UP

PATIENT MONITORING

See the doctor at least three times a year; management at a cystic fibrosis center is recommended.

PREVENTION

- Genetic counseling
- Prenatal diagnosis for future pregnancies
- For respiratory infections: vaccines, avoidance of general anesthesia, management by a good medical team

COMPLICATIONS

- Collapsed lung
- Heart failure
- Pulmonary hypertension
- Emphysema
- Other circulatory and respiratory problems
- Diabetes
- Metabolic disorders
- Bleeding esophageal varices
- Liver and intestinal disorders
- Sterility in females
- Numerous psychosocial aspects
- Malnutrition
- Retarded growth

Cystic Fibrosis

Doctor
Office
Phone
Pager

Special notes to patient:

Cystic Fibrosis

WHAT TO EXPECT

- The outcome largely depends on the involvement of the lungs.
- The prognosis is improving because of early detection and aggressive treatment.
- Average survival is to 29 years of age.

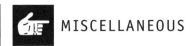 MISCELLANEOUS

PEDIATRIC

Diagnosis is usually confirmed in infancy or early childhood but some cases go undetected until adolescence.

PREGNANCY

If physical condition is good at the start of pregnancy, the mother usually returns to that level following birth. If health is poor before pregnancy, health status may worsen following birth.

PATIENT EDUCATION

Cystic Fibrosis Foundation, 6931 Arlington Road, Ste. 2000, Bethesda, MD 20814, (800) 3444823.

Cystic Fibrosis

	Doctor
	Office
	Phone
	Pager

Special notes to patient:

Dehydration

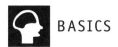 ## BASICS

DESCRIPTION
Dehydration is a depletion of body fluids that occurs when fluids are lost from the gastrointestinal tract, urinary tract, and skin.

SIGNS AND SYMPTOMS
- Skin that "tents" when pinched
- Dry, shrunken tongue
- Dizziness when standing
- Rapid heart rate
- Disorientation
- Shock

CAUSES
Excessive fluid loss from the gastrointestinal tract, urinary tract, and skin. Can result from vomiting, diarrhea, excessive sweating, dialysis, chronic kidney disease, diuretic ("water pill") therapy, diabetes mellitus, and other disorders.

 ## TREATMENT

GENERAL MEASURES
- Replacement of fluids and salts
- Discontinue diuretics
- Dehydration and ongoing fluid losses from infections gastroenteritis can be treated with oral feeding of special solutions. These solutions are balanced for maximum fluid absorption. Example fluids include:
  - WHO-ORS
  - Rehydralyte
  - Pedialyte
  - Kaolectro
  - Beech Nut Pedi. Electrolyte
- The World Health Organization distributes a solution (WHO-ORS) whose recipe is similar to the following:
  - 1 liter (quart) of clean water
  - 1/2 tsp table salt
  - 1/2 tsp baking soda
  - 1/4 tsp salt substitute (potassium chloride)
  - 2 Tbsp table sugar

This solution should only be used for rehydration. Its high salt content makes it unsuitable as a sole source of fluid.

Dehydration

Doctor
Office
Phone
Pager

Special notes to patient:

Dementia

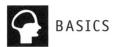 ## BASICS

DESCRIPTION

- Dementia, also called "senility," is the persistent impairment of intellectual functioning.
- Alzheimer's disease, the most common form of dementia, is characterized by a relentless deterioration of higher brain functioning. The rate of deterioration varies.
- Multiinfarct dementia (MID) results from strokes or "mini-strokes."
- Some forms of dementia can be reversed.

SIGNS AND SYMPTOMS

- Impaired memory, abstract thinking, and judgment
- Difficulty with language or speaking
- Personality change, emotional outbursts, wandering, restlessness, hyperactivity
- Sleep disturbances
- Mood disturbances
- Urinary incontinence
- Fecal incontinence (late)
- Tremor
- Hallucinations, delusions
- Paranoia
- Weight loss
- Seizures

CAUSES

- Alzheimer's disease
- Stroke or "mini-strokes" caused by atherosclerosis (hardening) of brain arteries
- Other brain disorders

SCOPE

- About 1.2 million people in the United States have severe dementia, and another 2.5 million have moderate illness.
- Of all persons above 65 years of age, 10% have clinically important dementia.
- At least 15% of those with Alzheimer's disease have a family history of the disease.

MOST OFTEN AFFECTED

The incidence of dementia increases with age. Males and females are affected in equal proportion. Some forms can occur in younger persons.

RISK FACTORS

- Increasing age
- Atherosclerotic disease
- Trisomy 21 (Down syndrome)
- History of head trauma
- History of central nervous system infection

 ## DIAGNOSIS

WHAT THE DOCTOR LOOKS FOR

- The doctor will perform a physical examination to identify any medical problems.
- Psychologic functioning will be evaluated.
- Possible causes of dementia will be identified and treated.

TESTS AND PROCEDURES

- Blood tests
- Syphilis test
- Mental status testing
- Electroencephalogram (EEG) can be performed to assist in diagnosis.
- Computed tomography (CT) scan, magnetic resonance imaging (MRI), or positron emission tomography (PET) can be done to evaluate brain structures and function.

 ## TREATMENT

GENERAL MEASURES

- Dementia is managed in the outpatient setting, except when complications require hospitalization.
- Nursing home care or adult daycare may be necessary.
- Daily schedules and written directions can be helpful.
- Emphasis is on nutrition, personal hygiene, personal safety (accident-proofing the home), and supervision
- Provide sensory stimulation (prominent displays of clocks and calendars).

ACTIVITY

Fully active with direction and supervision

DIET

No special diet

 ## MEDICATIONS

COMMONLY PRESCRIBED DRUGS

- Antipsychotics: haloperidol (Haldol), thioridazine (Mellaril)
- Depression: nortriptyline (Pamelor), desipramine (Norpramin), sertraline (Zoloft), fluoxetine (Prozac), paroxetine (Paxil), fluvoxamine (Luvox)
- Sleep disturbance: temazepam (Restoril), zolpidem (Ambien), trazodone (Desyrel), chloral hydrate
- Tacrine (Cognex)
- Donepezil (Aricept)

CONTRAINDICATIONS

- Antipsychotics (haloperidol, thioridazine): severe depression, Parkinson's disease, hypo- or hypertension
- Tricyclic antidepressants (nortriptyline, desipramine): heart attack, acute narrow-angle glaucoma
- Acute active liver disease; active, untreated peptic ulcers

PRECAUTIONS

Drugs have numerous precautions; read drug product information.

DRUG INTERACTIONS

Drugs have numerous interactions; read drug product information.

OTHER DRUGS

- Lithium carbonate
- Carbamazepine (Tegretol)

 ## FOLLOW-UP

PATIENT MONITORING

The patient should see the doctor as often as needed for evaluation of health and mental function and monitoring of drug therapy.

COMPLICATIONS

- Drug side effects
- Falls
- Pressure sores
- Malnutrition
- Constipation
- Infections

WHAT TO EXPECT

- Alzheimer's disease: the progression of this disease varies, but it inevitably leads to profound impairment.
- Some forms of dementia can be treated, but the course of most dementia varies.

 ## MISCELLANEOUS

FURTHER INFORMATION

Alzheimer's Association, (800) 621-0379

Dementia

Doctor
Office
Phone
Pager

Special notes to patient:

Depression

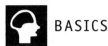 BASICS

DESCRIPTION

Depression results when a person experiences more frustration and anger than can be personally handled. Each person is capable of handling a different amount of frustration or anger.

SIGNS AND SYMPTOMS

- Depressed mood
- Poor appetite: either weight gain or loss (may eat or drink out of boredom or reasons other than appetite)
- Sleep disorder: either insomnia or excessive sleepiness
- Fatigue: tiredness out of proportion to the amount of energy expended
- Agitation, restlessness, irritability, or withdrawal
- Lack of interest in pleasure, decreased sexual appetite, lack of pleasure in activities or things the person used to enjoy
- Poor self-image: self-reproach, excessive guilt
- Difficulty concentrating, poor memory, inability to make decisions
- Suicidal thoughts

CAUSES

- Neurotransmitter imbalance
- Many life stressor and losses

SCOPE

Estimates indicate that 5% to 20% of the population will experience a significant depression at some time.

MOST OFTEN AFFECTED

Average age is 30 to 40 years; women more often than men. A tendency to depression may be inheritable.

RISK FACTORS

- Female gender
- Family history (depression, suicide, alcoholism, other substance abuse)
- Chronic disease, especially multiple diseases
- Migraine headaches
- Chronic pain
- Recent heart attack
- Peptic ulcer disease
- Menopause
- Losses
- Substance abuse
- Insomnia
- Stressful situations
- Adolescence
- Advancing age
- Retirement
- Children with behavioral disorders, especially hyperactivity

 DIAGNOSIS

WHAT THE DOCTOR LOOKS FOR

The doctor will evaluate the patient to identify causes of depression (e.g., brain disease, hormone disorders, or other conditions).

TESTS AND PROCEDURES

- Blood tests
- Urinalysis
- Electrocardiogram (ECG)
- Measurement of brain activity may be performed, called electroencephalography (EEG).
- Computed tomography (CT) scan or magnetic resonance imaging (MRI) may be performed to assist in diagnosis.
- Psychologic testing may be given.

 TREATMENT

GENERAL MEASURES

- Depression is normally managed in the outpatient setting. Inpatient care is indicated for seriously depressed or suicidal patients.
- Psychotherapy is helpful in solving the problems caused by depression.
- Consider support groups.

ACTIVITY

No restrictions

DIET

No special diet

 MEDICATIONS

COMMONLY PRESCRIBED DRUGS

- Anxiety, restlessness, irritability or sleeplessness: amitriptyline (Elavil, Endep), nortriptyline (Pamelor, Aventyl), doxepin (Adapin, Sinequan), trazodone (Desyrel), trimipramine (Surmontil)
- Fatigue, excessive sleepiness, indecisiveness, or difficulty in concentration: imipramine (Tofranil), desipramine (Norpramin, Pertofrane), fluoxetine (Prozac), sertraline (Zoloft), paroxetine (Paxil), protriptyline (Vivactil), bupropion (Wellbutrin)
- Venlafaxine (Effexor)

CONTRAINDICATIONS

Read drug product information.

PRECAUTIONS

- Medications have sedating side effects.
- Most common side effects are dry mouth, constipation, profuse sweating, and sleepiness. Most side effects decrease or disappear in 2 to 3 weeks.

DRUG INTERACTIONS

- Read drug product information.
- Avoid nonprescription drugs containing pseudoephedrine, phenylephrine, or phenylpropanolamine (cold medicines).

OTHER DRUGS

- Clomipramine (Anafranil)
- MAO inhibitors
- St. John's wort
- Fluvoxamine (Luvox)

 FOLLOW-UP

PATIENT MONITORING

- See the doctor within 2 weeks after starting medication. Do not expect to feel greatly improved at this visit.
- Office visits about every 2 weeks until improvement begins
- If treatment is adequate, depression should improve within 4 weeks.

Depression

	Doctor
	Office
	Phone
	Pager

Special notes to patient:

Depression

- The doctor should be seen 3 months thereafter.
- Treatment must continue even after improvement.

PREVENTION

See *Causes* and *Risk Factors*

COMPLICATIONS

- Suicide
- Failure to improve

WHAT TO EXPECT

Properly treated, depression almost always improves.

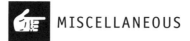 MISCELLANEOUS

PEDIATRIC

Depression occurs in children.

GERIATRIC

Depression is more common among the elderly.

PREGNANCY

Medications should be used with caution during pregnancy. Rely on psychotherapy and support groups until pregnancy is completed.

FURTHER INFORMATION

National Depression Manic Depression Association (DMDA), (800) 82-MDMDA

Depression

Doctor
Office
Phone
Pager

Special notes to patient:

Dermatitis, Contact

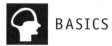 ## BASICS

DESCRIPTION

Contact dermatitis is an inflammatory reaction of the skin to an external substance. Primary dermatitis is caused by skin injury by specific irritants, generally producing discomfort immediately after exposure. Allergic contact dermatitis affects individuals previously sensitized to the substance. It is a delayed reaction, developing over several hours.

SIGNS AND SYMPTOMS

- Bumps, blisters, or rash surrounded by reddened skin
- Crusting or oozing
- Itching
- Thickening of skin
- Flaking, scaling
- Fissuring
- Can occur in areas where skin is thinner (eyelids, genitalia)
- Usually occurs in areas that have been in contact with the offending agent (e.g., nails and nail polish)
- Linear lesions or welts
- Lesions with sharp borders and sharp angles

CAUSES

- Plants (poison ivy, oak, sumac)
- Chemicals (hair dyes, industrial chemicals, detergents, waxes)
- Nickel (jewelry, zippers)
- Topical medicines (antibiotics, benzocaine)

MOST OFTEN AFFECTED

Contact dermatitis occurs in people of all ages, males and females in equal proportion. Allergic dermatitis is more common in families with a history of allergies.

RISK FACTORS

- Occupation
- Hobbies
- Travel
- Cosmetics
- Jewelry

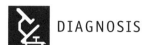 ## DIAGNOSIS

WHAT THE DOCTOR LOOKS FOR

The doctor will look for signs and symptoms of contact dermatitis.

TESTS AND PROCEDURES

Patch tests for allergies

GENERAL MEASURES

- Contact dermatitis is managed in the outpatient setting.
- Remove the offending agent.
- Avoid irritating substances.
- Topical soaks
- Lukewarm water baths for itching
- Aveeno (oatmeal) baths
- Emollients (white petrolatum, Eucerin)

ACTIVITY

Stay active, but avoid overheating.

DIET

No special diet

 ## MEDICATIONS

COMMONLY PRESCRIBED DRUGS

- Topical
  - Lotion of zinc oxide, talc, menthol (0.25%), phenol (0.5%)
  - Corticosteroids: fluocinonide (Lidex)
  - Calamine lotion
  - Topical antibiotics for secondary infection: bacitracin, gentamicin, erythromycin
- Systemic
  - Antihistamine: hydroxyzine, diphenhydramine
  - Corticosteroids: prednisone
  - Antibiotics: erythromycin

PRECAUTIONS

- Drowsiness from antihistamines
- Local skin effects from prolonged use of potent topical steroids

OTHER DRUGS

Other topical antibiotics

 ## FOLLOW-UP

PATIENT MONITORING

See the doctor as often as necessary.

PREVENTION

Avoid causative agents. Use of protective gloves (with cotton lining) when handling agents may be helpful.

COMPLICATIONS

- Severe eruption
- Secondary bacterial infection

WHAT TO EXPECT

Contact dermatitis is harmless and usually goes away by itself.

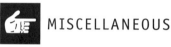 ## MISCELLANEOUS

GERIATRIC

The elderly have an increased incidence of dermatitis because of dry skin.

PREGNANCY

Usual cautions with medications.

Dermatitis, Contact

Doctor
Office
Phone
Pager

Special notes to patient:

Diabetes Mellitus, Insulin-Dependent (IDDM or Type I)

 ## BASICS

DESCRIPTION

Insulin-dependent diabetes mellitus (IDDM) is a chronic disease caused by the insufficient production of insulin. It requires the regular administration of insulin. Individuals with poorly controlled IDDM are at risk for several complications, including eye, nerve, kidney, and cardiovascular problems.

SIGNS AND SYMPTOMS

- Frequent urination
- Severe thirst, frequent drinking
- Excessive eating
- Loss of appetite
- Weight loss
- Fatigue, lethargy
- Muscle cramps
- Irritability and mood swings
- Vision changes, such as blurriness
- Altered school or work performance
- Headaches
- Anxiety attacks
- Chest pain and occasional difficult breathing
- Abdominal discomfort and pain
- Nausea
- Diarrhea or constipation

CAUSES

- Inherited genetic defect
- Environmental factors (e.g., viruses, diet, toxins, and stress) can be involved.

SCOPE

Insulin-dependent diabetes mellitus affects 15 of 100,000 persons annually.

MOST OFTEN AFFECTED

The average age of onset is 8 to 12 years. Males and females are affected in equal numbers. IDDM is more common in whites, less common in African-Americans. It may be inherited.

RISK FACTORS

Genetic factors

 ## DIAGNOSIS

WHAT THE DOCTOR LOOKS FOR

- The doctor will obtain a history and perform a physical examination to identify the signs and symptoms of diabetes.
- A cause of diabetes will be identified, if possible.

TESTS AND PROCEDURES

- A number of blood tests can be performed to assist in diagnosis.
- Electrolytes
- Urinalysis
- A procedure called an oral glucose tolerance test can be done to assess how the body metabolizes sugar.

 ## TREATMENT

GENERAL MEASURES

- Initial care may require hospitalization.
- Diabetes is usually managed on an outpatient basis, preferably in a diabetes clinic where a team approach is used.
- Routine care is provided by the family at home. The child is encouraged to do as much self-care as possible.
- For the very young child, treatment is aimed at maintaining blood sugar levels within a normal range. "Tight control" of blood glucose levels, in which the individual strives to maintain normal blood glucose levels at all times, may be dangerous for the very young child. For adults, tight control may prevent or reduce the severity of diabetes complications. However, it can increase the frequency of hypoglycemia (low blood sugar levels).
- Prevention of complications is a goal of treatment.

ACTIVITY

- All normal activities, including full participation in sports activities
- Regular, rather than periodic, aerobic exercise is preferable.

DIET

A well-balanced diet is important in the management of diabetes. Meals and snacks must be coordinated with insulin injections. The advice of a nutritionist is helpful in the management of IDDM.

 ## MEDICATIONS

COMMONLY PRESCRIBED DRUGS

Insulin

CONTRAINDICATIONS

None

PRECAUTIONS

Patients will receive extensive education about how to avoid hypoglycemia and rebound hyperglycemia (high blood sugar levels).

OTHER DRUGS

- Immunosuppressants: cyclosporine
- Other experimental drugs: azathioprine, steroids, nicotinamide

 ## FOLLOW-UP

PATIENT MONITORING

- Initially, the doctor should be seen frequently until stable; then every 2 to 3 months thereafter.
- Daily home blood glucose monitoring with home blood glucose meter (e.g., One-Touch, Accuchek, Glucometer, Exactech, Answer) three to four times daily, with adjustment or supplementation of insulin dose based on blood glucose levels
- Periodic (about every 3 months) blood tests to assess overall glycemic control
- Dietary management should be regularly reviewed and updated.

PREVENTION

None known

Diabetes Mellitus, Insulin-Dependent (IDDM or Type I)

Doctor
Office
Phone
Pager

Special notes to patient:

Diabetes Mellitus, Insulin-Dependent (IDDM or Type I)

COMPLICATIONS

- Vascular disease
- High levels of fats in the bloodstream
- Foot problems
- Low blood sugar
- Diabetic ketoacidosis
- Excessive weight gain
- Psychologic problems related to chronic disease

WHAT TO EXPECT

- Initial remission or "honeymoon" phase with decreased insulin needs and easier overall control; usually lasts 3 to 6 months and rarely beyond a year
- Progression to "total diabetes" is usually gradual, but a major stress or illness may bring it on more acutely.
- Longevity and quality of life are increasing with careful blood glucose monitoring and improvements in insulin delivery
- Currently, people with IDDM probably have a reduced life expectancy, but it has improved dramatically over the past 20 years.
- Advances in understanding diabetes may prevent or minimize complications.

 MISCELLANEOUS

PEDIATRIC

IDDM is more prevalent among children. For this reason, it is sometimes called "juvenile onset diabetes."

PREGNANCY

- Planning the pregnancy and tightly controlling blood sugar levels before conception is important.
- It is now possible to have a safe pregnancy, with vaginal delivery of a term baby (with care by a physician skilled in managing pregnant diabetic patients).

FURTHER INFORMATION

American Academy of Family Physicians Foundation, P.O. Box 8418, Kansas City, MO 64114, (800) 274-2237, ext. 4400

Diabetes Mellitus, Insulin-Dependent (IDDM or Type I)

Doctor
Office
Phone
Pager

Special notes to patient:

Diabetes Mellitus, Non–Insulin-Dependent (NIDDM)

 ## BASICS

DESCRIPTION

Non–insulin-dependent diabetes mellitus (NIDDM) is a defect of insulin secretion and action, accounting for 80% of diabetic cases. People with poorly controlled NIDDM are at risk for a variety of complications, including eye, nerve, kidney, and cardiovascular problems. Despite its name, NIDDM is sometimes managed with insulin. However, many people with NIDDM manage their disease with oral medications, diet, and exercise.

SIGNS AND SYMPTOMS

- Kidney, nerve, and retinal diseases
- Frequent urination
- Excessive thirst, frequent drinking
- Excessive eating
- Weight loss
- Weakness
- Fatigue
- Frequent infections

CAUSES

Genetic factors and obesity are important.

SCOPE

NIDDM affects about 5,000 of 100,000 persons in the United States.

MOST OFTEN AFFECTED

Typically occurs after age 40. Females are affected more frequently than males in white populations. May be inherited.

RISK FACTORS

- Family history
- Gestational diabetes
- Obesity

 ## DIAGNOSIS

WHAT THE DOCTOR LOOKS FOR

The doctor will perform a physical examination to identify the signs and symptoms of NIDDM.

TESTS AND PROCEDURES

Blood tests, including several measurements of blood sugar levels

 ## TREATMENT

GENERAL MEASURES

- NIDDM is managed in the outpatient setting, except for complicating emergencies requiring hospitalization.
- Home monitoring of blood or urine glucose
- Regular examination for complications

ACTIVITY

Regular aerobic exercise can improve glucose tolerance and decrease medication requirements.

DIET

- American Diabetes Association (ADA) provides dietary recommendations for NIDDM. The most important part of this diet is weight loss in obese patients. The diet is similar to that recommended by the American Heart Association and includes increased complex carbohydrate, decreased fat, and moderation in salt and alcohol.
- Dietary treatment alone can often result in adequate metabolic control in NIDDM.

 ## MEDICATIONS

COMMONLY PRESCRIBED DRUGS

- Oral medications to lower blood sugar levels (hypoglycemic drugs): tolbutamide, tolazamide, chlorpropamide, glyburide (Diabeta, Micronase), glipizide (Glucotrol), pioglitazone (Actos), rosiglitazone (Avandia)
- Insulin

CONTRAINDICATIONS

Oral medications: IDDM, pregnancy, history of allergy; use caution in liver or renal disease and acute infection or stress.

PRECAUTIONS

Home glucose monitoring (one to four times per day) is recommended for most patients taking insulin.

DRUG INTERACTIONS

- Drugs that enhance the effect of oral hypoglycemic drugs: salicylates, clofibrate, warfarin (Coumadin), chloramphenicol, ethanol
- Beta-blockers can mask symptoms of hypoglycemia and delay return to normal blood sugar levels.

OTHER DRUGS

- Metformin
- Phenformin
- Acarbose

Diabetes Mellitus, Non–Insulin-Dependent (NIDDM)

Doctor
Office
Phone
Pager

Special notes to patient:

Diabetes Mellitus, Non–Insulin-Dependent (NIDDM)

 FOLLOW-UP

PATIENT MONITORING

- See the doctor as often as necessary for control of blood sugar levels. Visits every 2 to 4 months are typical.
- Annual physical examination

PREVENTION

Avoid weight gain and obesity. Maintenance of regular physical activity may prevent or delay NIDDM.

COMPLICATIONS

- Nerve disease
- Eye disease
- Kidney disease
- Cardiovascular disease
- Coma
- Gangrene of extremities
- Blindness
- Skin ulcers

WHAT TO EXPECT

- Maintenance of normal blood sugar levels may delay or prevent complications of diabetes.
- In susceptible individuals, complications begin to appear 10 to 15 years after onset, but they can also be present at time of diagnosis.

 MISCELLANEOUS

PEDIATRIC

Occasional cases of NIDDM have been seen in children.

GERIATRIC

NIDDM, which is common in the elderly, is a significant contributing factor to blindness, renal failure, and lower limb amputations.

OTHERS

NIDDM is generally a disease of adults, appearing after 40 years of age.

PREGNANCY

Diabetes can cause significant maternal complications and fetal wasting. Intensive management by those skilled in this area has improved the outcome dramatically.

FURTHER INFORMATION

American Diabetes Association, 430 North Michigan Ave., Chicago, IL 60611

Diabetes Mellitus, Non–Insulin-Dependent (NIDDM)

Doctor
Office
Phone
Pager

Special notes to patient:

Diaper Rash

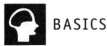 ## BASICS

DESCRIPTION

Diaper rash, also called "diaper dermatitis," is a rash occurring under the covered area of a diaper.

SIGNS AND SYMPTOMS

- Prominent rash on buttocks and pubic skin
- Folds of skin may or may not be affected.
- Genitalia may or may not be affected.
- Child scratches vigorously at night.
- Skin seems chapped.
- Weeping or crusting
- Swelling

CAUSES

Irritation to skin from prolonged contact with urine or feces

SCOPE

Diaper rash is common.

MOST OFTEN AFFECTED

Infants; males and females in equal proportion

RISK FACTORS

- Infrequent diaper changes
- Waterproof diapers
- Improper laundering
- Family history of dermatitis
- Hot, humid weather
- Recent treatment with oral antibiotics
- Diarrhea

 ## DIAGNOSIS

WHAT THE DOCTOR LOOKS FOR

- The doctor will perform a physical examination to look for signs of diaper rash.
- Other causes of rash should be identified and treated (e.g., contact dermatitis or infection).

TEST AND PROCEDURES

Rash can be cultured for laboratory analysis.

 ## TREATMENT

GENERAL MEASURES

- Diaper rash is managed in the outpatient setting.
- Expose the buttocks to air as much as possible:
- Do not use waterproof pants during treatment day or night. They keep skin wet, making it susceptible to rash or infection.
- Change diapers frequently, even at night if the rash is extensive.
- Super absorbable diapers are beneficial.
- Discontinue use of baby lotion, powder, ointment, or baby oil (except zinc oxide).
- Apply zinc oxide ointment to the rash at the earliest sign of diaper rash, and two or three times a day thereafter (apply to clean, thoroughly dry skin).
- Use mild soap and pat dry.

ACTIVITY

Protect from overheating

DIET

No special diet

 ## MEDICATIONS

COMMONLY PRESCRIBED DRUGS

- Antifungal medications: miconazole nitrate (2%) cream, miconazole powder, econazole (Spectazole), clotrimazole (Lotrimin), ketoconazole (Nizoral)
- Steroid creams: hydrocortisone (0.5% to 1%), clioquinol-hydrocortisone (Vioform-Hydrocortisone)
- Antibiotics

 ## FOLLOW-UP

PATIENT MONITORING

The doctor should be seen weekly until diaper rash is cleared, then at times of recurrence.

PREVENTION

See *General Measures*

COMPLICATIONS

Infection

WHAT TO EXPECT

Quick, complete recovery with appropriate treatment

 ## MISCELLANEOUS

PEDIATRIC

Diaper rash is most common among children.

GERIATRIC

Diaper rash can affect incontinent elderly persons.

Diaper Rash

Doctor
Office
Phone
Pager

Special notes to patient:

Diarrhea, Acute

 ## BASICS

DESCRIPTION

Acute (of short duration) diarrhea of abrupt onset in a healthy individual is most often caused by an infectious process. A variety of symptoms are often observed, including frequent passage of loose or watery stools, fever, chills, anorexia, vomiting, and malaise.

- Acute viral diarrhea: most common form, usually occurs for 1 to 3 days, is self-limited
- Bacterial diarrhea: develops within 12 hours of eating bacteria-contaminated food
- Protozoal infections: prolonged, watery diarrhea that often afflicts travelers returning from areas where the water supply has been contaminated
- Traveler's diarrhea: typically begins 3 to 7 days after arrival in a foreign location and is generally acute

SIGNS AND SYMPTOMS

- Loose, liquid stools
- Blood or mucus
- Fever
- Abdominal pain and distension
- Headache
- Loss of appetite
- Malaise, fatigue
- Vomiting
- Muscle ache
- Cramping, pale-greasy stools, fatigue, weight loss

CAUSES

Infection with bacteria, virus, or parasite

MOST OFTEN AFFECTED

All ages

RISK FACTORS

- Visiting a developing country
- Immune system disorders

 ## DIAGNOSIS

WHAT THE DOCTOR LOOKS FOR

- The doctor will perform a thorough physical examination.
- Causes of diarrhea should be identified and treated (e.g., ulcerative colitis).

TESTS AND PROCEDURES

- Blood tests
- A sample of stool may be obtained for culture and laboratory analysis.
- Abdominal x-ray study
- The intestinal tract may be visually examined by sigmoidoscopy.

 ## TREATMENT

GENERAL MEASURES

- Diarrhea is managed in the outpatient setting, except for dehydration or other complicating emergencies requiring hospitalization.
- Replacement of lost fluid and salts
- Clear liquids such as tea, broth, carbonated beverages (without caffeine), and rehydration fluids (e.g., Gatorade) to replace lost fluid

ACTIVITY

Bed rest

DIET

- During periods of active diarrhea, avoid coffee, alcohol, dairy products, most fruits, vegetables, red meats, and heavily seasoned foods.
- After 12 hours with no diarrhea, begin eating clear soup, salted crackers, dry toast or bread, and sherbet.
- As stooling rate decreases, slowly add rice, baked potato, and chicken soup with rice or noodles to diet.
- As stool begins to retain shape, add baked fish, poultry, applesauce, and bananas to diet.

 ## MEDICATIONS

COMMONLY PRESCRIBED DRUGS

- Loperamide, bismuth subsalicylate
- Antibiotics: metronidazole, trimethoprim-sulfamethoxazole, ciprofloxacin (Cipro)

CONTRAINDICATIONS

Avoid alcoholic beverages when taking metronidazole.

PRECAUTIONS

- Antidiarrhea medications should be used with caution in cases of infectious diarrhea or antibiotic-associated colitis.
- Doxycycline, sulfamethoxazole-trimethoprim, and ciprofloxacin can cause photosensitivity. Use sunscreen.

DRUG INTERACTIONS

- Bismuth subsalicylate can cause toxicity in patients taking aspirin and may alter anticoagulation control in patients taking coumadin.
- Ciprofloxacin and erythromycin increase theophylline levels.

OTHER DRUGS

- Doxycycline
- Diphenoxylate-atropine
- Tinidazole, secnidazole
- Vancomycin

 ## FOLLOW-UP

PATIENT MONITORING

Contact the doctor if the diarrhea continues for 3 to 5 days with or without blood or mucus.

PREVENTION

- Avoid brushing teeth with contaminated water, ingesting ice cubes, or eating cold salads or meats when traveling.
- Avoid uncooked or undercooked seafood or meat, buffet meals left out for several hours, or food served by street vendors.

COMPLICATIONS

- Dehydration
- Sepsis
- Shock
- Anemia

WHAT TO EXPECT

Diarrhea is a common problem that is rarely life-threatening if attention is given to maintaining adequate hydration.

 ## MISCELLANEOUS

PEDIATRIC

May be caused by overfeeding, medications, cystic fibrosis, and malabsorption disorders

GERIATRIC

Watery diarrhea in elderly patient with chronic constipation can result from fecal impaction or cancer.

PREGNANCY

Dehydration can lead to premature labor.

Diarrhea, Acute

Doctor
Office
Phone
Pager

Special notes to patient:

Dissociative Disorders

 ## BASICS

DESCRIPTION

Dissociative disorders are characterized by a sudden change in state of consciousness, identity, behavior, thoughts, feelings, and perception of external reality. These disorders include amnesia, identity disorder, fugue states, sleep-walking, conversion reactions, and others.

SIGNS AND SYMPTOMS

- Symptoms cause significant distress or impairment in social, occupational, or other important areas of functioning.
- Dissociative amnesia:
  - Episodes of inability to recall important personal information that is too extensive to be explained by ordinary forgetfulness
  - Not caused by other illness or substance abuse
- Dissociative fugue:
  - Sudden unexpected travel away from home or one's customary place of work with an inability to recall one's past
  - Confusion about personal identity or assumption of a new identity (partial or complete)
- Dissociative identity disorder:
  - The presence of two or more distinct personality states
  - Inability to recall important personal information
  - Reports of time distortion
  - Hearing voices
  - Chronic headaches
  - History of severe emotional or physical abuse as a child
  - Referring to self as "he or she," "we," "us"
  - Eating disorders
  - Flashbacks
  - Unreal feelings
  - Amnesia about important childhood events
  - Personal objects and belongings that cannot be accounted for
  - Denying behavior not remembered
  - Different handwriting styles
  - Sudden mood changes
  - Sudden behavioral changes (e.g., from adult to young child)
  - Feeling controlled by "another person" from within
  - Self-inflicted violence such as wrist cutting
- Depersonalization disorder: Persistent or recurrent experiences of feeling detached from one's mental processes or body (e.g., feeling like one is in a dream).

CAUSES

- Physical, emotional, verbal, or sexual abuse in childhood
- Sudden and severe trauma or threat to one's psychological or physical integrity
- Witnessing a traumatic event (e.g., an industrial or car accident)
- Other psychological factors

SCOPE

Dissociative disorder affects 8% to 10% of the general psychiatric population. As many as 70% of young adults report short periods of dissociative experiences that are self-limiting and resolve spontaneously.

MOST OFTEN AFFECTED

Adolescents and young to middle-aged adults. Rare as a new illness in the elderly. If untreated, may linger from childhood into adult and old age: Females affected twice as frequently as males.

RISK FACTORS

- Exposure to neglect, abuse, and trauma in one's childhood
- Tendency to cope with life stresses by excessively using an escape mechanism of day dreaming or dissociation

 ## DIAGNOSIS

WHAT THE DOCTOR LOOKS FOR

- The doctor will obtain a history and perform a thorough physical examination.
- Other mental, nervous system, or medical disorders should be identified and treated.

TESTS AND PROCEDURES

- Toxicology screening
- An electroencephalogram (EEG) can be done to rule out epilepsy and sleep disorders.
- Sleep study, called polysomnogram, can be done to rule out sleep apnea.
- Computed tomography (CT) scan and magnetic resonance imaging (MRI) can be performed to assist in diagnosis.
- Psychologic testing can be done.

 ## TREATMENT

GENERAL MEASURES

- Dissociative disorders are usually managed in an outpatient setting.
- Hospitalization may be required during a crisis.
- Individual psychotherapy plus behavior modification and other therapy
- Support groups, group therapy, expressive art therapy, occupational and recreational therapy, reading therapy, and writing therapy
- Self-hypnosis, relaxation exercises, and guided imagery

ACTIVITY

Based on patient's condition

 ## MEDICATIONS

COMMONLY PRESCRIBED DRUGS

- No specific cures
- Antidepressants
- Benzodiazepines
- Propranolol
- Neuroleptics: thioridazine, haloperidol, chlorprothixene, perphenazine, risperidone
- Droperidol

CONTRAINDICATIONS

Read drug product information.

Dissociative Disorders

Doctor
Office
Phone
Pager

Special notes to patient:

Dissociative Disorders

PRECAUTIONS
Read drug product information.

DRUG INTERACTIONS
Read drug product information.

OTHER DRUGS
- Buspirone
- Clomipramine, fluvoxamine
- Risperidone (Risperdal)
- Olanzapine (Zyprexa)
- Quetiapine (Seroquel)

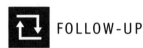 FOLLOW-UP

PATIENT MONITORING
- See the doctor for at least an hour of psychotherapy up to three to four sessions per week to avoid hospitalizations.
- Hospitalized patients require more intensive treatment.

PREVENTION
- Child abuse prevention
- Crisis intervention following individual trauma and natural or man-made disasters is crucial to prevent chronic illness or disability.

COMPLICATIONS
Self-inflicted violence; suicide attempts; substance abuse and chemical dependency

WHAT TO EXPECT
- Without treatment, the outcome ranges from spontaneous improvement or recovery to acute and chronic disease.
- Effective treatment produces partial or full recovery for many patients.

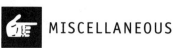 MISCELLANEOUS

PEDIATRIC
Suspect abuse or neglect.

GERIATRIC
Dissociative disorders are less common among the elderly; drug side effects are a more likely cause of symptoms.

Dissociative Disorders

Doctor
Office
Phone
Pager

Special notes to patient:

Diverticular Disease

 ## BASICS

DESCRIPTION
Diverticular disease is caused by an abscess in (or inflammation of) abnormal outpouchings of the intestine.

SIGNS AND SYMPTOMS
- Symptoms may be mild or absent
- Pain
- Diarrhea or constipation
- Bloated abdomen
- Dark, tarry stool
- Fever with chills as severity increases
- Loss of appetite, nausea, vomiting
- Difficult urination

SCOPE
Diverticular disease affects up to 20% of the general population. However, the incidence increases to 40% to 50% among individuals 50 to 70 years of age.

MOST OFTEN AFFECTED
Diverticular disease is rare in people younger than 40 years of age; it is most common in those 50 to 70 years of age. Males and females are equally affected.

CAUSES
- Causes are not clearly proved
- Low-fiber diet

RISK FACTORS
- Age above 40 years
- Low-fiber diet
- Previous diverticular disease

 ## DIAGNOSIS

WHAT THE DOCTOR LOOKS FOR
The doctor will perform a physical examination to identify causes of similar symptoms (e.g., irritable bowel syndrome, lactose intolerance, or cancer).

TESTS AND PROCEDURES
- Blood tests
- Urinalysis and culture
- Abdominal x-ray study, barium enema
- Computed tomography (CT) scan can be done to assist in diagnosis.
- Blood vessels can be assessed by a radiologic procedure called "angiography".
- Other special imaging procedures may be done.
- The digestive tract or urinary system can be examined by endoscopy.

 ## TREATMENT

GENERAL MEASURES
- Diverticular disease is usually managed in the outpatient setting.
- A few people with diverticular disease require hospitalization.
- Surgery may be necessary.

ACTIVITY
Depends on condition; activity may be restricted

DIET
- Nothing by mouth during acute episode, progress to fluids, then to high-fiber diet as normal bowel function returns.
- Increase dietary fiber with high-fiber foods or fiber supplement, if appropriate.

 ## MEDICATIONS

COMMONLY PRESCRIBED DRUGS
- Antispasmodics: hyoscyamine (Levsin), buspirone (BuSpar), meperidine (Demerol), high-fiber diet
- Antibiotics: metronidazole (Flagyl), amoxicillin, ciprofloxacin, gentamicin, clindamycin
- Pain reliever
- Bleeding: vasopressin

CONTRAINDICATIONS
Allergic reaction

PRECAUTIONS
Morphine and other opiates should be avoided.

DRUG INTERACTIONS
Read drug product information.

OTHER DRUGS
Tobramycin, metronidazole, cephalosporins

 ## FOLLOW-UP

PATIENT MONITORING
See the doctor as often as necessary, based on symptoms and health status.

PREVENTION
High-fiber diet and use of soluble fiber supplements (e.g., psyllium, agar, and methylcellulose)

COMPLICATIONS
- Bleeding
- Perforation
- Inflammation of the abdominal lining
- Bowel obstruction
- Abscess
- Fistula

WHAT TO EXPECT
- Outcome is good with early detection and treatment of complications.
- After successful treatment of initial episode, up to 67% of patients have no repeat attacks that require hospitalization.
- Of those with bleeding, up to 20% will rebleed in a period of months to years.

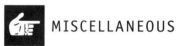 ## MISCELLANEOUS

PEDIATRIC
Very rare among children

GERIATRIC
More common among the elderly

PREGNANCY
Could be confused with ectopic pregnancy

FURTHER INFORMATION
National Digestive Diseases Information Clearinghouse, Box NDDIC, Bethesda, MD 20892, (301) 468-6344

Diverticular Disease

Doctor

Office

Phone

Pager

Special notes to patient:

Dysfunctional Uterine Bleeding

 ## BASICS

DESCRIPTION
Dysfunctional uterine bleeding is abnormal uterine bleeding in the absence of a detected disease. It is also called "breakthrough bleeding" or "estrogen withdrawal bleeding."

SIGNS AND SYMPTOMS
- Uterine bleeding:
  - Unrelated to menstrual cycle
  - Heavier than normal menstrual flow
  - Occurs in an irregular pattern
  - Rarely painful
- Absence of other systemic symptoms or bleeding elsewhere

CAUSES
- Hormonal disturbance
- Other: uterine lesions, cancer, vaginal infection, foreign body, ectopic pregnancy, other medical conditions
- Tends to run in families

SCOPE
Widespread, but exact prevalence is unknown

MOST OFTEN AFFECTED
Females 12 to 45 years of age

RISK FACTORS
See Causes

 ## DIAGNOSIS

WHAT THE DOCTOR LOOKS FOR
The doctor will perform a physical examination to identify and treat causes of uterine bleeding.

TESTS AND PROCEDURES
- Blood tests
- Pregnancy test
- Basal body temperature may be charted.
- Ultrasound may be done to assist with diagnosis.
- Pap smear
- Cells from the uterus can be obtained by biopsy for laboratory analysis.

 ## TREATMENT

GENERAL MEASURES
- Dysfunctional uterine bleeding is almost always managed as an outpatient.
- Hospitalization may be required.
- Surgery (e.g., hysterectomy, dilatation and curettage) may be required.

ACTIVITY
As tolerated

DIET
Normal; include adequate iron

 ## MEDICATIONS

COMMONLY PRESCRIBED DRUGS
- Conjugated estrogens
- Medroxyprogesterone, ethinyl estradiol
- Supplemental iron therapy
- Naproxen sodium, mefenamic acid
- Leuprolide acetate, nafarelin, goserelin

PRECAUTIONS
Read drug product information.

DRUG INTERACTIONS
Read drug product information.

OTHER DRUGS
- Progesterone
- Danazol

FOLLOW-UP

PATIENT MONITORING
- See the doctor as often as necessary.
- Maintain a menstrual calendar to document the pattern of bleeding and its relation to therapy.

PREVENTION
Avoid prolonged stress or emotional turmoil.

COMPLICATIONS
- Anemia
- Cancer
- Drug side effects

WHAT TO EXPECT
- The outcome varies.
- In young women, most cases can be treated successfully without surgery.

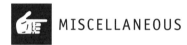 MISCELLANEOUS

GERIATRIC
Cancer should be ruled out.

OTHERS
Young women and those in their later reproductive years are most often affected.

FURTHER INFORMATION
American College of Obstetricians & Gynecologists (ACOG), 409 12th St., SW, Washington, DC 20024-2188, (800) 762-ACOG

Dysfunctional Uterine Bleeding

Doctor
Office
Phone
Pager

Special notes to patient:

Dysmenorrhea

 ## BASICS

DESCRIPTION
Dysmenorrhea is pelvic pain that occurs around the time of menstruation. It is a leading cause of absenteeism for women under 30 years of age.

SIGNS AND SYMPTOMS
- Mild: pelvic discomfort, cramping, or feeling of heaviness on first day of menstrual bleeding with no associated symptoms
- Moderate: discomfort occurring on first 2 to 3 days of menses and accompanied by mild malaise, diarrhea, and headache
- Severe: intense, cramp-like pain lasting 2 to 7 days and often with gastrointestinal upset, back pain, thigh pain, and headache

CAUSES
- Hormone disturbance
- Anatomic abnormalities
- Other physical conditions

SCOPE
About 40% of adult women have menstrual pain; 10% are incapacitated for 1 to 3 days each month.

MOST OFTEN AFFECTED
Women 20 to 30 years of age

RISK FACTORS
- Never given birth
- Positive family history
- Pelvic infection
- Sexually transmitted diseases
- Endometriosis
- Cigarette smoking
- Obesity

 ## DIAGNOSIS

WHAT THE DOCTOR LOOKS FOR
- The doctor will obtain a history and perform a physical examination.
- Causes of dysmenorrhea (e.g., infection, complications of pregnancy, endometriosis) should be identified and treated.

TESTS AND PROCEDURES
- Ultrasound can be done to assist in diagnosis.
- The reproductive system can be examined by laparoscopy.

 ## TREATMENT

GENERAL MEASURES
- Dysmenorrhea is usually managed in the outpatient setting.
- Treatment is directed at general physical conditioning.
- Infections must be treated if present.
- Transcutaneous electrical nerve stimulator (TENS) may relieve symptoms.
- Surgery may be required.

ACTIVITY
Normal

DIET
- Normal. Supplementing with vitamin B_1 has been effective when used for 90 days.
- Supplementing with a fish oil capsule has been found effective when used for 2 months

 ## MEDICATIONS

COMMONLY PRESCRIBED DRUGS
- Nonsteroidal antiinflammatory drugs (NSAIDs): ibuprofen (Motrin, Advil, Nuprin), naproxen sodium (Anaprox, Aleve), aspirin
- Other nonsteroidal antiinflammatory drugs
- Oral contraceptives

CONTRAINDICATIONS
- Platelet disorders
- Gastric ulcers or gastritis
- Blood clotting disorders
- Vascular disease
- Contraindications to oral contraceptives

PRECAUTIONS
- Can irritate gastrointestinal tract
- Can cause blood clotting disorders
- Can impair kidney function
- Can contribute to heart failure
- Can lead to liver disorder

DRUG INTERACTIONS
- Blood thinners (anticoagulants)
- Aspirin with other NSAIDs
- Methotrexate
- Furosemide
- Lithium

OTHER DRUGS
- Nafarelin acetate
- Calcium channel blockers (e.g., nifedipine)
- Hydrocodone or tramadol (Ultram)
- Other NSAIDs

 ## FOLLOW-UP

PREVENTION
- None known
- Reduce risk of sexually transmitted diseases

COMPLICATIONS
- Anxiety, depression, or both
- Infertility from underlying pathology

WHAT TO EXPECT
Dysmenorrhea often improves with age and childbirth. Some forms require therapy based on underlying cause.

Dysmenorrhea

Doctor
Office
Phone
Pager

Special notes to patient:

Eclampsia

BASICS

DESCRIPTION

Eclampsia, or toxemia of pregnancy, is the presence of seizures in a pregnant female without underlying neurologic disease who also has preeclampsia. Preeclampsia is hypertension (high blood pressure), swelling, and protein in the urine, during pregnancy. Eclampsia can also occur after birth, almost always within 24 hours.

SIGNS AND SYMPTOMS

- Seizures
- Headache, visual disturbances, and stomach pain often precede seizure.
- Seizures can occur once or repeatedly.
- After-seizure coma and bluish discoloration around mouth, eyes, and nail beds (cyanosis)
- Swelling, fluid in lungs

CAUSES

Exact cause of seizures remains unclear.

SCOPE

- Preeclampsia affects 5% of all pregnancies; incidence of eclampsia is unclear.
- Up to 2% of women with preeclampsia progress to eclampsia, a number that is decreasing with improved monitoring and care.

MOST OFTEN AFFECTED

Preeclampsia and eclampsia are more common in younger women, but the incidence of seizures is much greater among older women. Predisposition may be genetic.

RISK FACTORS

- First pregnancy
- Obstetric conditions (e.g., multiple fetuses)
- Preexisting high blood pressure or kidney disease
- Strong family history of preeclampsia or eclampsia
- Poor prenatal care
- Pregnancy weight gain over 30 pounds

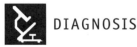 DIAGNOSIS

WHAT THE DOCTOR LOOKS FOR

- The doctor will perform a physical examination to identify the signs and symptoms of eclampsia.
- Other possible causes of seizures will be considered (e.g., epilepsy).
- Until other causes are proven, all pregnant women with seizures should be considered to have eclampsia.

TESTS AND PROCEDURES

- A variety of blood tests can be ordered to assist in diagnosis.
- Urinalysis, 24-hour urine collection

TREATMENT

GENERAL MEASURES

- The management of eclampsia requires hospitalization. Intravenous (IV) medications are given, and the patient is monitored, if necessary.
- Needs of the newborn should be considered; transfer to a specialized neonatal care facility may be required.
- Treatment consists of controlling seizures, giving oxygen, lowering blood pressure, and delivering the newborn as soon as possible.

ACTIVITY

Bed rest

DIET

Nothing by mouth until stable, then usual seizure precautions; low-salt diet is commonly recommended.

MEDICATIONS

COMMONLY PRESCRIBED DRUGS

- Magnesium sulfate
- IV fluids

CONTRAINDICATIONS

Drug allergies

OTHER DRUGS

Diazepam, lorazepam, phenytoin, phenobarbital, nifedipine

FOLLOW-UP

PATIENT MONITORING

See the doctor often to monitor the health status of mother and baby.

PREVENTION

- Adequate prenatal care
- Good control of preexisting hypertension
- Recognition and treatment of preeclampsia

COMPLICATIONS

- Temporary deficits (e.g., blindness) affect 56% of women with eclampsia.
- Most women do not suffer long-term effects.
- Death from toxemia or its complications
- Death of fetus

WHAT TO EXPECT

- One fourth of women with eclampsia have hypertension in subsequent pregnancies, but only 5% of these will have severe hypertension, and only 2% will be eclamptic again.
- Women who have been eclamptic and have many children can be at higher risk for essential hypertension later in life.
- Women who have been eclamptic and have many children are at greater risk of death in subsequent pregnancies than women who are pregnant for the first time.

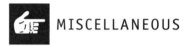 MISCELLANEOUS

PEDIATRIC

Adequate neonatal care and facilities are essential.

PREGNANCY

Eclampsia is a complication of pregnancy.

FURTHER INFORMATION

Additional materials from: American College of Obstetricians & Gynecologists, 409 12th St., SW, Washington, DC 20024-2188, (800) 762-ACOG

Eclampsia

Doctor
Office
Phone
Pager

Special notes to patient:

Endometriosis

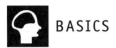 ## BASICS

DESCRIPTION
Endometriosis is a disorder of the uterus that leads to painful menstruation, infertility, and other conditions. It is caused by the misplacement of uterine lining tissue outside the uterus (e.g., on the ovaries or in the fallopian tubes). Endometriosis can also affect distant sites throughout the abdomen and chest.

SIGNS AND SYMPTOMS
- Infertility
- Painful intercourse
- Menstrual cramps
- Difficulty with defecation
- Chronic pelvic pain
- Premenstrual spotting
- Miscarriage

CAUSES
Unknown

SCOPE
Endometriosis affects 8% to 30% of women of childbearing age.

MOST OFTEN AFFECTED
Women of reproductive age

RISK FACTORS
- Hereditary or genetic predisposition
- Personality traits (achieving, egocentric, overanxious, perfectionist, intelligent, underweight; however, the validity of these observations is lacking)
- Delayed childbearing
- Hormonal disturbance (luteinized unruptured follicle syndrome)

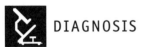 ## DIAGNOSIS

WHAT THE DOCTOR LOOKS FOR
- The doctor will perform a thorough physical examination to identify and rule out other potential causes of pelvic pain, including complications of pregnancy, urinary tract infection, irritable bowel syndrome, ulcerative colitis, Crohn's disease, ruptured ovarian cyst, and other conditions.
- The doctor will look for other conditions known to be associated with endometriosis.

TESTS AND PROCEDURES
- Blood tests, urinalysis
- Ultrasound or magnetic resonance imaging (MRI) can be done to assess the pelvic structures.
- The reproductive tract can be visually examined by laparoscopy.
- A sample of uterine tissue can be obtained by biopsy for laboratory analysis.

 ## TREATMENT

GENERAL MEASURES
- Endometriosis should be diagnosed and treated early to prevent infertility and pelvic pain.
- Prevention of disease is difficult; however, disease can be managed with oral contraceptive agents.
- Treatment of endometriosis can require hospitalization.
- Surgery may be required.

ACTIVITY
Activity may be limited, depending on severity of pelvic pain.

DIET
No special diet

 ## MEDICATIONS

COMMONLY PRESCRIBED DRUGS
- Nafarelin (Synarel), leuprolide acetate (Lupron, Depo-Lupron), goserelin (Zoladex)
- Maintenance: oral contraceptives, calcium supplements

CONTRAINDICATIONS
Any contraindication to the drug itself or low estrogen levels

PRECAUTIONS
Drugs can cause calcium loss, hot flashes, tingling sensation of face and arms. Contraception should be used by sexually active women.

SIGNIFICANT POSSIBLE INTERACTIONS
Refer to manufacturer's literature.

OTHER DRUGS
- Danazol (Danocrine)
- Medroxyprogesterone (Provera)
- Megestrol (Megace)
- "Continuous" oral contraceptives (e.g., norgestrel-ethinyl estradiol [Lo/Ovral, Ovral]) until childbearing is desired

 ## FOLLOW-UP

PATIENT MONITORING
- See the doctor every 8 to 12 weeks.
- Ultrasound should be done every 8 to 12 weeks.
- Additional surgery may be needed.

PREVENTION
- Pregnancy seems to temporarily improve the disease.
- Endometriosis is generally a recurring disorder that can persist even into early menopause.

COMPLICATIONS
- Fertility problems
- Chronic pelvic pain
- Hysterectomy

WHAT TO EXPECT
- Pregnancy can occur, but depends on the severity of the disease.
- Disease gradually improves with the onset of menopause, but can usually be controlled during the reproductive years.

 ## MISCELLANEOUS

GERIATRIC
Endometriosis can persist during early menopause and can be worsened with estrogen replacement therapy (ERT).

PREGNANCY
See a Board-certified reproductive endocrinologist or gynecologist with expertise in infertility.

FURTHER INFORMATION
The American Fertility Society, 2140 11th Ave South, Suite 200, Birmingham, AL 35205-2800, (205) 933-8494

Endometriosis

Doctor
Office
Phone
Pager

Special notes to patient:

Epididymitis

 ## BASICS

DESCRIPTION
Epididymitis is an inflammation of the epididymis, an elongated structure attached to the testicle. This condition causes pain of the scrotum, swelling and hardening of the epididymis, and eventually the formation of a fluid-filled cavity.

SIGNS AND SYMPTOMS
- Scrotal pain, sometimes extending to the groin region
- Urethral discharge
- Symptoms of urinary tract infection: frequent urination, painful urination, cloudy urine, or blood in the urine
- A swollen, firm mass within the scrotum
- Swelling of the scrotum
- Fever and chills occur with severe infection and abscess formation.

CAUSES
- Infection (e.g., chlamydia, gonorrhea, other bacteria)
- Urinary tract obstruction
- Inflammation
- Birth defect

SCOPE
Epididymitis is common in the United States.

MOST OFTEN AFFECTED
Epididymitis primarily affects younger, sexually active men or older men with urinary infection, but it can also occur in prepubertal boys (rarely).

RISK FACTORS
- Urinary tract infection
- Use of urinary catheter
- Urethral instrumentation or surgery
- Urethral scarring

 ## DIAGNOSIS

WHAT THE DOCTOR LOOKS FOR
The doctor will perform a physical examination to identify causes of scrotal pain (e.g., testicular torsion, mumps, or trauma).

TESTS AND PROCEDURES
- Urinalysis and culture
- Ultrasound can be used to evaluate the scrotum.

 ## TREATMENT

GENERAL MEASURES
- Epididymitis is usually managed on an outpatient basis.
- Hospitalization may be required for severe infection or surgery.
- Elevate the scrotum.
- Apply a cold pack to the affected area.
- Local anesthetic can be used in severe cases.
- Surgery may be required.

ACTIVITY
Bed rest for minimum of 1 to 2 days

DIET
No restrictions, but drink large amounts of fluids.

MEDICATIONS

COMMONLY PRESCRIBED DRUGS
- Antibiotics: doxycycline, tetracycline, trimethoprim-sulfamethoxazole (Bactrim, Septra), ciprofloxacin (Cipro), ofloxacin (Floxin), norfloxacin (Noroxin), ceftriaxone, gentamicin
- Pain relievers: nonsteroidal anti-inflammatory drugs (e.g., naproxen or ibuprofen), acetaminophen-codeine, oxycodone-acetaminophen

CONTRAINDICATIONS
None

PRECAUTIONS
Read drug product information.

DRUG INTERACTIONS
Read drug product information.

 ## FOLLOW-UP

PATIENT MONITORING
See the doctor often until all signs of infection have cleared.

PREVENTION
- Vasectomy
- Antibiotics
- Early treatment
- Avoid vigorous rectal examination

COMPLICATIONS
- Recurrent epididymitis
- Infertility
- Gangrene

WHAT TO EXPECT
- Pain improves within 1 to 3 days, but it can take several weeks or months to completely resolve.
- Sterility may result.

 ## MISCELLANEOUS

GERIATRIC
Diabetic patients with nerve disease may have little pain despite severe infection.

Epididymitis

Doctor
Office
Phone
Pager

Special notes to patient:

Epiglottitis

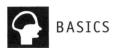 ## BASICS

DESCRIPTION
Epiglottitis is an acute inflammation of the epiglottis, a flap of tissue above the larynx, and related structures. It can cause severe airway obstruction. Epiglottitis is a medical emergency that requires prompt emergency care.

SIGNS AND SYMPTOMS
- Develops rapidly
- Fever
- Difficulty swallowing, drooling
- Sore throat
- Swollen glands in neck
- Difficulty breathing
- Muffled voice or cry
- Minimal cough
- Shock

CAUSES
Infection with *Hemophilus influenzae* (in children and adults) or group A Streptococcus in adults.

SCOPE
The incidence of epiglottitis has dropped dramatically since the introduction of the *H. influenzae* b vaccine.

MOST OFTEN AFFECTED
- Epiglottitis most commonly affects children 3 to 7 years of age, although any age can be affected.
- Infrequent in adults
- Occurs with equal frequency in males and females

 ## DIAGNOSIS

WHAT THE DOCTOR LOOKS FOR
- The doctor will perform a complete physical examination to assess the degree of symptoms.
- Other airway conditions will be identified (e.g., croup, infection, or foreign body).

TESTS AND PROCEDURES
- Blood tests
- A sample of blood can be cultured for laboratory analysis.
- Fluid from the throat may be cultured.
- X-ray study of the neck and chest can be done to assist in diagnosis.
- The airway can be visually examined by intubation.
- A sample of spinal fluid can be obtained for laboratory analysis.

 ## TREATMENT

GENERAL MEASURES
- Acute epiglottitis requires emergency care and hospitalization.
- Mechanical breathing may be required.
- A surgical opening may be made in the neck.
- Other surgery may be required.

 ## MEDICATIONS

COMMONLY PRESCRIBED DRUGS
Antibiotics: cefotaxime, ceftriaxone

CONTRAINDICATIONS
Read drug product information.

PRECAUTIONS
Read drug product information.

DRUG INTERACTIONS
Read drug product information.

OTHER DRUGS
- Ampicillin, chloramphenicol
- Antifever medication

 ## FOLLOW-UP

PATIENT MONITORING
See the doctor often during hospitalization.

PREVENTION
H. influenzae vaccine (not 100% protective) Prevention with rifampin

COMPLICATIONS
- Pneumonia, meningitis, other inflammatory conditions
- Septic shock
- Air in the chest cavity
- Death from asphyxia

WHAT TO EXPECT
The risk of death or serious illness is low with appropriate intervention.

Epiglottitis

Doctor
Office
Phone
Pager

Special notes to patient:

Fatigue

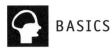 ## BASICS

DESCRIPTION
Fatigue is a state of discomfort and decreased level of energy resulting from prolonged or excessive exertion or loss of ability to respond appropriately to stimulation. Fatigue is also called lassitude, tiredness, lethargy, malaise, and ennui.

CAUSES
Drug or alcohol use, overexertion, anemia, chronic fatigue syndrome, diabetes mellitus or other medical conditions, emotional problems (e.g., depression), inadequate nutrition, inadequate rest, obesity, poor physical conditioning, and others.

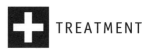 ## TREATMENT

GENERAL MEASURES
Treatment is directed at the underlying cause of fatigue.

Fatigue

Doctor
Office
Phone
Pager

Special notes to patient:

Fecal Incontinence

 ## BASICS

DESCRIPTION
Fecal incontinence (encopresis) is the regular passage of feces into clothes or other inappropriate places by a child older than 4 years of age.

SIGNS AND SYMPTOMS
- Constipation, usually
- Pasty stool found on underclothes
- Fecal or foul odor surrounds the child
- Pain around the navel
- Occasional passage of a large volume of stool
- History of painful bowel movements
- Shyness and withdrawal, acting out, or aggressive behavior
- Some have had psychotherapy.
- Some have had recurrent urinary tract infections.

CAUSES
- Psychologic (toilet training issues)
- Rectal disorders (e.g., painful defecation, poor muscle tone)
- Dietary or metabolic (lack of fiber, excessive protein or milk intake, inadequate water intake, hypothyroidism)

SCOPE
Encopresis affects 1.3% of all children above 4 years of age.

MOST OFTEN AFFECTED
Onset occurs in 70% before 5 years of age; males are affected more frequently than females.

RISK FACTORS
- Boys are more often affected.
- Difficulty with bowel training
- Unresolved defecation problems

 ## DIAGNOSIS

WHAT THE DOCTOR LOOKS FOR
- Fecal incontinence is often noticed by the doctor during the physical examination; many parents and children do not mention the problem to their doctors.
- Underlying causes of constipation should be identified and treated.

TESTS AND PROCEDURES
- Urinalysis and urine culture
- Blood tests
- X-ray study of the abdomen
- A barium enema can be done to assess the digestive tract.
- A sample of colon tissue can be obtained by biopsy for laboratory analysis.

 ## TREATMENT

GENERAL MEASURES
- Hospital admission may be necessary.
- If impaction is present, it must be treated.
- Avoid development of impaction.
- Avoid frequent and repeated digital examinations, enemas, and suppositories.
- Biofeedback training can be used as alternative therapy or when conventional therapy has been unsuccessful.
- Child should sit on the toilet twice a day at the same times each day for 10 to 15 minutes and 10 to 15 minutes after a meal.

ACTIVITY
Unrestricted

DIET
- Avoid excessive milk, bananas, apples, gelatin.
- Increase fiber.

 ## MEDICATIONS

COMMONLY PRESCRIBED DRUGS
- Stool impaction: mineral oil, enemas, polyethylene glycol (Colyte, NULYTELY)
- Maintenance: mineral oil, lactulose, methylcellulose (Citrucel), psyllium (Metamucil, Perdiem), polycarbophil (Mitrolan), malt soup extract (Maltsupex), fiber wafers, multivitamins

CONTRAINDICATIONS
Read drug product information.

PRECAUTIONS
Avoid mineral oil at bedtime. Read drug product information.

DRUG INTERACTIONS
Read drug product information.

FOLLOW-UP

PATIENT MONITORING
- Maintenance treatment program should be followed for at least 6 months and maybe for as long as 1 to 2 years.
- See the doctor every 4 to 10 weeks.
- Contact doctor as needed by telephone.

PREVENTION
- Improve feeding practices.
- Bowel training
- Early detection
- Use dark Karo syrup and fiber for hard stools.
- Prompt treatment of skin problems to avoid painful defecation.
- Look for signs of relapse, which include large caliber stools, decrease in frequency of defecation, soiling.

COMPLICATIONS
- Excessive enemas or suppositories can cause colitis.
- Dermatitis around the anal area
- Anal fissure

WHAT TO EXPECT
- The outcome is usually good, although relapses can occur.
- Children with psychosocial or emotional problems preceding the fecal incontinence are more resistant to treatment.

Fecal Incontinence

Doctor
Office
Phone
Pager

Special notes to patient:

Fertility Problems

 ## BASICS

DESCRIPTION

Fertility problems are usually suspected if a couple fails to conceive after 1 year of unprotected intercourse.

SIGNS AND SYMPTOMS

- Hormone disorder (e.g., hypothyroidism, abnormal puberty)
- Sexual dysfunction (e.g., premature ejaculation)
- Irregular ovulation
- Excessive body hair (hirsutism)
- Endometriosis
- Obesity
- Acne

CAUSES

- Most couples have more than one factor.
- Male factors are responsible for 30% to 40% of fertility problems.
- Ovulation factors are responsible for 15% of fertility problems.
- Cervical and uterine factors are responsible for 10% of fertility problems; fallopian tube and other anatomic problems are responsible for 25% to 30%.
- Immune factors are responsible for 5% of fertility problems.
- Psychological, nutritional, or metabolic factors are responsible for 5% of fertility problems.

SCOPE

Fertility problems affect 10% to 15% of all couples.

MOST OFTEN AFFECTED

Fertility problems increase with age. They affect 14% of individuals 30 to 34 years of age, 20% of those aged 35 to 39, and 25% of those aged 40 to 45.

RISK FACTORS

Genital or pelvic infections (venereal or sexually transmitted diseases)

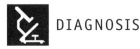 ## DIAGNOSIS

WHAT THE DOCTOR LOOKS FOR

A thorough history and physical examination should be performed on each partner.

TESTS AND PROCEDURES

- Blood tests
- Semen analysis, postcoital test
- The basal body temperature may be charted.
- Tissue from the uterus can be obtained by biopsy for laboratory analysis.
- The reproductive tract can be evaluated with a special radiology procedure called a "hysterosalpingogram" (HSG).
- The reproductive tract can be visually examined by laparoscopy.
- Many specialized tests are available, but only from fertility specialists in specialized facilities.

 ## TREATMENT

GENERAL MEASURES

- Infertility is managed in the outpatient setting.
- The cause of infertility should be identified and treated.
- Information about adoption may be provided when appropriate.
- Donor insemination may be considered.
- Surgery may be required.

ACTIVITY

- Men with low sperm counts should avoid hot tubs and saunas.
- If the sperm count is low sperm, intercourse should be timed to occur approximately every 36 hours during the fertile period. Delay of intercourse beyond 7 days also adversely affects semen quality.

 ## MEDICATIONS

COMMONLY PRESCRIBED DRUGS

- Clomiphene citrate
- Bromocriptine

CONTRAINDICATIONS

- Pituitary failure
- Ovarian cysts

PRECAUTIONS

Drugs have many precautions; read drug product information.

DRUG INTERACTIONS

Bromocriptine: alcohol, antihypertensives, tricyclic antidepressants, phenothiazine

OTHER DRUGS

- Human chorionic gonadotropin
- Menotropins; human menopausal gonadotropin (hMG)
- Gonadotropin-releasing hormone (GnRH) analogs
- Metformin (Glucophage)

 ## FOLLOW-UP

PATIENT MONITORING

See *Diagnosis*

PREVENTION

Prevention of sexually transmitted disease (STD) and pelvic inflammatory disease

COMPLICATIONS

Complications of pregnancy

WHAT TO EXPECT

- About half of couples conceive during the second year of unprotected intercourse.
- If the couple has been infertile for 4 or more years, the prognosis tends to be poor.

 ## MISCELLANEOUS

OTHERS

With aging, the effects of diseases (e.g., endometriosis) increase; cumulative exposure from environmental or occupational hazards can also play a role in fertility problems.

FURTHER INFORMATION

- RESOLVE, 5 Water St., Arlington, MA 02174
- Fertility Research Foundation, 1430 Second Avenue, Suite 103, New York, NY 10021, (212) 744-5500
- American College of Obstetricians & Gynecologists, 409 12th St, SW, Washington, DC 20024-2188, (800) 762-ACOG

Fertility Problems

Doctor
Office
Phone
Pager

Special notes to patient:

Fibrocystic Breast Disease

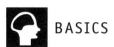 BASICS

DESCRIPTION

Fibrocystic breast disease, also called "benign breast disease," includes benign disorders (e.g., lumps and pain). The disease does not have a well-defined set of symptoms and has no clear cause. Benign lumps are usually smooth, regular, and somewhat mobile beneath the skin. Benign breast disease also includes nipple discharge, pain, inflammatory conditions, and growth disorders.

SIGNS AND SYMPTOMS

- May have no symptoms
- Breast pain
- Breast tenderness
- Pain subsides after menstrual cycle
- Smooth masses
- Tense masses
- Masses that change
- Masses in both breasts
- Breast engorgement
- Breast thickening
- Nipple discharge

CAUSES

- The cause of benign breast disease is unknown.
- Possible causes include hormone disorders, dietary fat intake.

SCOPE

It is estimated that at least 50% of women have benign breast symptoms during their lifetime.

MOST OFTEN AFFECTED

Symptoms tend to occur in menstruating women.

RISK FACTORS

- Unknown
- The effect of methylxanthine-containing substances (e.g., coffee, tea, cola, and chocolate) is uncertain.

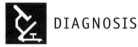 DIAGNOSIS

WHAT THE DOCTOR LOOKS FOR

The doctor will do a complete physical examination and identify the cause of symptoms.

TESTS AND PROCEDURES

- Blood tests
- Mammography
- Ultrasound can be used to assist in diagnosis.
- A sample of breast tissue can be obtained by biopsy for laboratory analysis.

 TREATMENT

GENERAL MEASURES

- Benign breast disease is managed in the outpatient setting.
- Biopsy or surgery may require hospitalization.
- Symptoms frequently resolve spontaneously.
- Cold compresses may be helpful.
- Use a well-fitting, supportive brassiere (worn night and day).
- Surgery may be required.

ACTIVITY

No restrictions. Avoid activities that can cause trauma to the breasts.

DIET

Avoid methylxanthines (coffee, tea, chocolate, caffeine-containing soda).

 MEDICATIONS

COMMONLY PRESCRIBED DRUGS

- Spironolactone (Aldactone), vitamin A, vitamin E, oral contraceptives
- Danazol (Danocrine), bromocriptine

CONTRAINDICATIONS

Read drug product information.

PRECAUTIONS

Read drug product information.

DRUG INTERACTIONS

Read drug product information.

 FOLLOW-UP

PATIENT MONITORING

- Patients may have an increased risk of cancer.
- See the doctor as often as necessary.

- Women should have a mammogram at 35 years of age, at least every 1 to 2 years after age 40, and yearly after age 50.
- When physical examination, mammography, and needle aspiration are used in combination, detection rates for breast cancer range from 93% to 100%.

PREVENTION

Avoiding caffeine may reduce breast pain.

COMPLICATIONS

- Physical examinations and mammograms may be difficult to interpret.
- Cancer

WHAT TO EXPECT

Benign breast disease is chronic, recurring, and intermittent.

 MISCELLANEOUS

PEDIATRIC

Biopsy in children should be avoided.

GERIATRIC

Not as common among the elderly.

FURTHER INFORMATION

- American College of Obstetricians & Gynecologists, 409 12th St., SW, Washington, DC 20024-2188, (800) 762-ACOG
- Booklet on Breast Self Examination from Primary care and Care and Cancer, 17 Prospect St., Huntington, NY 11743, (516) 424-8900
- National Cancer Institute, (800) 4-CANCER

Fibrocystic Breast Disease

Doctor
Office
Phone
Pager

Special notes to patient:

Food Allergy

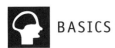 ## BASICS

DESCRIPTION
Food allergy is a hypersensitivity reaction caused by certain foods.

SIGNS AND SYMPTOMS
- Gastrointestinal: nausea, vomiting, diarrhea, abdominal pain, flatulence, bloating
- Dermatologic: hives, rash, swelling, dermatitis, pallor, flushing
- Respiratory: runny nose, asthma, cough, earache
- Neurologic: fatigue, fainting, headache
- Other symptoms: systemic reaction, growth retardation, bed-wetting

CAUSES
- Any food or ingested substance can cause allergic reactions. Most commonly implicated foods include cow's milk, egg whites, wheat, soy, peanut, fish, tree nuts (walnut and pecan), shellfish, melons, sesame seeds, sunflower seeds, and chocolate.
- Several food dyes and additives can cause allergic-like reactions.

SCOPE
- The incidence of food allergy ranges from 1% to 7% of the population.
- In children up to 4 years of age, the incidence is between 8% to 16%.
- Only about 3% to 4% of children above 4 years of age have persisting food allergy.

MOST OFTEN AFFECTED
- Food allergy can affect all ages, but is more common in infants and children.
- Males are affected twice as often as females.
- A family history can increase the risk of food allergy by 50%.

RISK FACTORS
- Allergies
- Family members with a history of food allergies

 ## DIAGNOSIS

WHAT THE DOCTOR LOOKS FOR
- The doctor will take a careful history and perform a thorough physical examination to rule out other causes of symptoms.
- Gastrointestinal, dermatologic, respiratory, neurologic, or other signs and symptoms can mimic a variety of diseases.

TESTS AND PROCEDURES
- Blood tests
- Allergy tests: prick test, challenge test
- A stool sample can be obtained for laboratory analysis.
- The digestive tract can be evaluated by an x-ray study.

 ## TREATMENT

GENERAL MEASURES
- Food allergies are usually managed in the outpatient setting.
- Avoiding the offending food is the most effective way to manage food allergy.
- Individuals with severe allergy should carry epinephrine for self-administration in the event that the offending food is ingested unknowingly and a severe reaction develops immediately.
- The success of immunotherapy and hyposensitization has not been proved.

ACTIVITY
No restrictions

DIET
As determined by tests

 ## MEDICATIONS

COMMONLY PRESCRIBED DRUGS
- Treatment of symptoms: antihistamine
- Cromolyn
- Ketotifen (not available in the United States)

CONTRAINDICATIONS
Read drug product information.

PRECAUTIONS
Read drug product information.

DRUG INTERACTIONS
Read drug product information.

 ## FOLLOW-UP

PATIENT MONITORING
See the doctor as often as needed.

PREVENTION
Avoid the offending food(s).

COMPLICATIONS
- Severe allergic reaction (anaphylaxis)
- Swelling
- Asthma
- Intestinal distress
- Patches of rash or dry skin

WHAT TO EXPECT
- Most infants will outgrow their food hypersensitivity by 2 to 4 years of age. It may be possible to reintroduce the offending food cautiously into the diet (particularly helpful when the food is one that is difficult to avoid).
- Adults with food hypersensitivity (particularly to milk, fish, shellfish, or nuts) tend to maintain their allergy for many years.

 ## MISCELLANEOUS

FURTHER INFORMATION
Patient support-Food Allergy Network, 4744 Holly Ave., Fairfax, VA 22030-5647, (703) 691-3179

Food Allergy

Doctor
Office
Phone
Pager

Special notes to patient:

_____
_____
_____
_____
_____
_____
_____
_____
_____
_____
_____
_____
_____
_____
_____
_____

Food Poisoning, Bacterial

 ## BASICS

DESCRIPTION
Bacterial food poisoning includes a variety of illnesses resulting from ingestion of food contaminated with disease-causing bacteria.

SCOPE
Although the true extent of food poisoning is unknown, an estimated 6.3 million cases occur per year in the United States. About 1 of 10 Americans suffer food-borne diarrhea annually.

MOST OFTEN AFFECTED
Food poisoning affects all ages, males and females with equal frequency.

SIGNS AND SYMPTOMS
- Food poisoning is suspected when multiple persons become ill after eating the same meal.
- Nausea, vomiting, cramps, diarrhea, fever 1 to 72 hours after meal
- Bloody diarrhea without fever 3 to 5 days after meal

CAUSES
Bacterial contamination

RISK FACTORS
- Ingestion of:
- Egg salad, cream-filled pastries, gravy
- Cereals, fried rice, dried foods, herbs
- Raw or under-cooked pork, poultry, beef, seafood, eggs, dairy products
- Raw vegetables, contaminated water

 ## DIAGNOSIS

WHAT THE DOCTOR LOOKS FOR
- The doctor takes a thorough history and conducts a physical examination to identify the cause of signs and symptoms.
- Identifying the source of contamination may involve detailed study.

TESTS AND PROCEDURES
- A stool sample can be obtained for laboratory analysis.
- Suspected food sources can be cultured.
- The intestinal tract can be examined by sigmoidoscopy.

 ## TREATMENT

GENERAL MEASURES
- Most cases of food poisoning are self-limiting and do not require therapy.
- Food poisoning is usually managed in the outpatient setting.
- Individuals with severe food poisoning may require hospitalization.
- Oral solutions for rehydration; intravenous (IV) fluids may be necessary for severe dehydration (particularly among the elderly).
- For infants, rehydration products (e.g., Pedialyte) provide adequate fluid and salt replacement. Do not use for more than 1 to 2 days without seeing the doctor again.

ACTIVITY
Bed rest for comfort, if needed during the acute phase

DIET
- Eliminate contaminated food.
- Bland diet during recovery
- Nothing by mouth if excessive vomiting or diarrhea

 ## MEDICATIONS

COMMONLY PRESCRIBED DRUGS
Antibiotics

CONTRAINDICATIONS
Read drug product information.

PRECAUTIONS
Read drug product information.

DRUG INTERACTIONS
Read drug product information.

 ## FOLLOW-UP

PATIENT MONITORING
See the doctor as often as necessary, based on symptoms and health status. Serious cases require hospitalization.

PREVENTION
- Do not eat raw seafood, meats, or poultry.
- Avoid unpasteurized dairy products.
- Thoroughly clean food preparation areas.
- Cool any prepared foods not immediately consumed.

COMPLICATIONS
- Cardiovascular collapse
- Irregular heart rhythm
- Severe infection
- Seizures or coma

WHAT TO EXPECT
In most cases, signs and symptoms resolve over a few days.

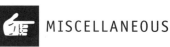 ## MISCELLANEOUS

PEDIATRIC
- Outbreaks of food poisoning can occur at daycare centers.
- Newborns and infants are a high risk for complications and death.

GERIATRIC
- Outbreaks of food poisoning can occur in nursing homes.
- Significant cause of death

PREGNANCY
Some infections can affect the newborn, with severe consequences.

Food Poisoning, Bacterial

Doctor
Office
Phone
Pager

Special notes to patient:

Frostbite

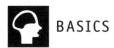 ## BASICS

DESCRIPTION
Frostbite is a complication of exposure to cold, resulting in diminished blood flow to the affected part (especially hands, face, or feet). Dehydration, tissue destruction, and ultimately cell death occur. In severe cases, deep tissue freezing can damage underlying blood vessels, muscles, and nerve tissue.

SIGNS AND SYMPTOMS
- Injured area first appears cold, hard, and white and has no sensation.
- After rewarming, the area is blotchy-red, swollen, and painful
- Loss of skin sensation
- Numbness
- Throbbing pain
- Tingling sensation
- Excessive sweating
- Joint pain
- Pallor
- Swelling
- Sensation of heat
- Blistering
- Blue discoloration
- Skin death
- Gangrene

CAUSES
- Prolonged exposure to cold
- Refreezing thawed extremities

SCOPE
- About 4,800 cases of frostbite occur annually in the United States.

MOST OFTEN AFFECTED
Frostbite affects all ages, males and females with equal frequency.

RISK FACTORS
- Impaired mental function
- Alcohol or drug abuse
- Mental illness
- Ambient temperature less than 0°F (−17.8°C)
- Smoking
- Elderly
- Circulatory disorders

 ## DIAGNOSIS

WHAT THE DOCTOR LOOKS FOR
The doctor will perform a physical examination and may use various imaging techniques to determine the extent and severity of frostbite.

TESTS AND PROCEDURES
- Blood tests
- Decreased hepatic function
- Electrocardiogram (ECG)
- Ultrasound can be used to assist in diagnosis.

 ## TREATMENT

GENERAL MEASURES
- Frostbite can be managed in the outpatient setting or may require hospitalization, depending on severity.
- Provide emergency first aid as needed, including rescue breathing and cardiopulmonary resuscitation (CPR).
- Prevent refreezing. It may be necessary to keep frostbitten part frozen until patient can be transported to a care facility.
- Rewarming must be done carefully and cautiously.
- Keep victim dry. If conscious, give warm fluids with high sugar content.
- Prevent damage to other body parts.

ACTIVITY
- As tolerated; protect injured body parts.
- Physical therapy should begin once healing progresses sufficiently.

DIET
- As tolerated
- Warm oral fluids

 ## MEDICATIONS

COMMONLY PRESCRIBED DRUGS
- Warm intravenous (IV) fluids
- Heated oxygen
- Levothyroxine, hydrocortisone
- Tetanus toxoid
- Pain relievers
- Antibiotics

CONTRAINDICATIONS
Read drug product information.

PRECAUTIONS
Read drug product information.

DRUG INTERACTIONS
Read drug product information.

OTHER DRUGS
Nifedipine, pentoxifylline

 ## FOLLOW-UP

PATIENT MONITORING
- The doctor will see the patient often during hospitalization.
- See the doctor as often as necessary during follow-up.

PREVENTION
- Dress in layers with appropriate cold weather gear.
- Cover exposed areas and extremities appropriately.
- Prepare properly for trips to cold climates.
- Avoid alcohol when out in the cold; alcohol interferes with the body's heat conservation mechanism.
- Recognize the early signs of cold exposure and take appropriate action.

COMPLICATIONS
- Metabolic disturbance
- Irregular heart rhythm
- Tissue loss, gangrene
- Death

WHAT TO EXPECT
- Loss of sensation and the formation of blisters.
- The affected areas will heal or mummify without surgery. The process can take 6 to 12 months. Person may be sensitive to cold and experience burning and tingling.

 ## MISCELLANEOUS

GERIATRIC
- Increased risk of death
- More sensitive to temperature extremes

Frostbite

Doctor
Office
Phone
Pager

Special notes to patient:

Gallstones

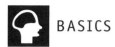
BASICS

DESCRIPTION
Gallstones, or cholelithiasis, is the formation of cholesterol- or pigment-containing stones in the gallbladder.

SIGNS AND SYMPTOMS
- Most people have no symptoms.
- About 5% to 10% of people with gallstones develop symptoms annually.
- Fewer than 50% of those with gallstones develop symptoms over their lifetime.
- Episodes of stomach pain, radiating to the back
- Nausea
- Vomiting
- Intolerance for fatty food (not proved)
- Indigestion

CAUSES
- Production of cholesterol-rich bile
- Changes in bile composition or flow
- Blood disorders
- Gallbladder infection

SCOPE
Gallstones affect 8% to 10% of the population in the United States.

MOST OFTEN AFFECTED
The incidence of gallstones increases with age, peaking in the 50s. Gallstones occur more frequently in American Indians and Hispanics and are twice as frequent in females as males.

RISK FACTORS
- Digestive disorders (short gut syndrome, inflammatory bowel disease)
- Multiple births
- Long-term total parenteral nutrition (TNP)
- Cirrhosis of the liver
- Blood disorders
- Prosthetic cardiac valves
- Rapid weight loss
- Childhood cancer
- Native-American descent
- Female gender

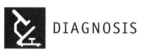
DIAGNOSIS

WHAT THE DOCTOR LOOKS FOR
- The doctor will perform a physical examination to identify the cause of symptoms.
- Causes of similar symptoms include hepatitis, pancreatitis, coronary artery disease, appendicitis, pneumonia, cancer, kidney stones, and numerous other conditions.

TESTS AND PROCEDURES
- A specialized imaging procedure, hepatobiliary radionuclide scan, can be done to assist in diagnosis.
- The gallbladder can be evaluated by a radiology procedure called "oral cholecystogram."
- Ultrasound or computed tomography (CT scan) can also be used.

TREATMENT

GENERAL MEASURES
- Gallstones can be medically managed in the outpatient setting.
- Surgical procedures for the treatment of gallstones require hospitalization.
- Only gallstones that cause symptoms are treated.
- Stones that do not cause symptoms are observed.
- Surgery may be open or minimally invasive.
- Direct contact dissolution may be an option.
- Extracorporeal shock wave lithotripsy (i.e., "stone busting," which is under study, but not approved by the US Food and Drug Administration)

DIET
Low-fat diet may be helpful.

MEDICATIONS

COMMONLY PRESCRIBED DRUGS
- Pain relievers for symptoms
- Ursodiol (ursodeoxycholic acid, Actigall)
- Chenodiol (Chenix)
- Methyl tert-butyl ether

CONTRAINDICATIONS
Known drug allergy

PRECAUTIONS
Can cause severe diarrhea

OTHER DRUGS
Nonsteroidal antiinflammatory drugs (NSAIDs)

FOLLOW-UP

PATIENT MONITORING
- See the doctor as often as necessary to evaluate health.
- Contact the doctor if stones start causing symptoms.

COMPLICATIONS
- Acute inflammation
- Common bile duct stones
- Intestinal disorders
- Liver disorders
- Gallbladder cancer

WHAT TO EXPECT
- Less than half of patients with gallstones develop symptoms.
- Cholecystectomy (removal of gallbladder): 0.5% to 5.0% death rate, 10% to 40% complication rate
- Of individuals with gallstones, 10% to 15% will also have stones in the bile duct.
- After cholecystostomy, stones may recur in bile duct.

MISCELLANEOUS

PEDIATRIC
- Gallstones are uncommon before 10 years of age.
- Associated with blood disorder

GERIATRIC
Incidence of gallstones increases with age.

FURTHER INFORMATION
National Digestive Diseases Information Clearinghouse, Box NDDIC, Bethesda, MD 20892, (301) 468-6344

Gallstones

Doctor
Office
Phone
Pager

Special notes to patient:

Gastritis

 ## BASICS

DESCRIPTION
Gastritis is an inflammation of the lining of the stomach.

SIGNS AND SYMPTOMS
- Epigastric distress, often aggravated by eating
- Loss of appetite
- Nausea, with or without vomiting
- Significant bleeding is unusual.
- Hiccups

CAUSES
- Alcohol
- Aspirin and other nonsteroidal antiinflammatory drugs (NSAIDs)
- Irritation from reflux
- Stress
- Radiation
- Infection
- Pernicious anemia
- Other stomach disorders

MOST OFTEN AFFECTED
Gastritis affects all ages, males and females in equal frequency.

RISK FACTORS
- Age more than 60 years
- Exposure to potentially noxious drugs or chemical agents
- Shock

 ## DIAGNOSIS

WHAT THE DOCTOR LOOKS FOR
- The doctor will perform a physical examination to identify the cause of symptoms.
- Other conditions with similar signs and symptoms include other gastrointestinal disorders, peptic ulcer disease, pancreatic disease, and stomach cancer.

TESTS AND PROCEDURES
- Special tests can be done to detect *Heliobacter pylori*, a bacterium that causes ulcers.
- The stomach can be inspected by gastroscopy.
- A sample of stomach tissue can be obtained by biopsy for laboratory analysis.

 ## TREATMENT

GENERAL MEASURES
- Gastritis is managed in the outpatient setting, except for severe hemorrhage.
- No specific therapy for gastritis (except treatment of *H. pylori* infection)
- Intravenous (IV) fluid and salts may be required if vomiting prevents food intake.
- Consider discontinuing NSAIDs or adding misoprostol.
- Discontinue smoking.

ACTIVITY
Usually no restriction

DIET
Restriction depends on severity of symptoms; avoid caffeine.

 ## MEDICATIONS

COMMONLY PRESCRIBED DRUGS
- Antacids
- Cimetidine (Tagamet), ranitidine (Zantac), famotidine (Pepcid), or nizatidine (Axid)
- Sucralfate (Carafate)
- Misoprostol (Cytotec)
- To eradicate *H. pylori*: bismuth (such as Pepto-Bismol), metronidazole, tetracycline, amoxicillin, omeprazole

CONTRAINDICATIONS
Drug allergy

PRECAUTIONS
- Bismuth causes black stools.
- Read drug product information.

DRUG INTERACTIONS
Read drug product information.

 ## FOLLOW-UP

PATIENT MONITORING
- The doctor may repeat gastroscopy after 6 weeks if gastritis has been severe or if no symptomatic response to treatment occurs.
- See the doctor as often as necessary.

PREVENTION
- Avoid known or potentially injurious drugs or chemical agents.
- Individuals susceptible to shock should receive preventive therapy.

COMPLICATIONS
Bleeding

WHAT TO EXPECT
- Most cases clear spontaneously when the cause has been identified and treated.
- Recurrence of *H. pylori* infection may require a repeated course of treatment.

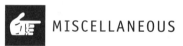 ## MISCELLANEOUS

PEDIATRIC
Gastritis rarely occurs in infants or children.

Gastritis

Doctor
Office
Phone
Pager

Special notes to patient:

Gastroesophageal Reflux Disease

 ## BASICS

DESCRIPTION

Gastroesophageal reflux disease (GERD) is the reflux of gastric contents into the esophagus, which causes irritation or inflammation of the esophagus.

SIGNS AND SYMPTOMS

- Heartburn
- Regurgitation
- Difficulty swallowing
- Chest pain
- Asthma
- Hoarseness, laryngitis, difficulty speaking
- Cough
- Sensation of a ball in the throat
- In infants: vomiting, failure to thrive, apnea

CAUSES

- Disorder of stomach muscle
- Pregnancy
- Scleroderma
- Other gastric disorders

SCOPE

- The incidence of reflux disorder is increasing; 65% of adults have experienced heartburn and 24% have had symptoms for more than 10 years.
- Heartburn is reported by 30% to 80% of pregnant women.

MOST OFTEN AFFECTED

Reflux disorder can affect all ages, males and females in equal frequency.

RISK FACTORS

- Certain foods: high-fat content foods, yellow onions, chocolate, peppermint, citrus fruits, spicy tomato drinks
- Hernia
- Cigarette smoking
- Excessive alcohol
- Coffee
- Certain medications
- Nasogastric tube
- Chest trauma
- In children: Down syndrome, mental retardation, cerebral palsy

 ## DIAGNOSIS

WHAT THE DOCTOR LOOKS FOR

- The doctor will perform a physical examination, particularly of the stomach and esophagus.
- Other conditions that may be responsible for the symptoms include infections, Crohn's disease, angina, cancer, and drug side effects.

TESTS AND PROCEDURES

- The pH (a measurement of acidity or alkalinity) of the upper digestive tract can be monitored.
- Other specialized testing can be done, including esophageal manometry, acid perfusion (Bernstein) test, and gastric analysis.
- Barium swallow or other radiologic procedures can be used to evaluate the upper digestive tract.
- Endoscopy (a procedure in which a tube with a camera on the end is inserted into the esophagus) can be done to examine the esophagus and stomach.
- A sample of esophageal or stomach tissue can be obtained by biopsy for laboratory analysis.

 ## TREATMENT

GENERAL MEASURES

- GERD is managed in the outpatient setting.
- Hospitalization may be required for surgery.
- Elevate head of bed and avoid lying down directly after meals.
- Avoid stooping, bending, tight-fitting garments.
- Avoid drugs that worsen the condition.
- Lose weight, if overweight.
- Avoid voluntary burping.
- Surgery may be necessary.

ACTIVITY

Full activity

DIET

Avoid chocolate, peppermint, onions, high-fat foods, alcohol, tobacco, coffee, and citrus juices.

 ## MEDICATIONS

COMMONLY PRESCRIBED DRUGS

- H^2 blockers: cimetidine (Tagamet), ranitidine (Zantac), famotidine (Pepcid), nizatidine (Axid)
- Severe disease: omeprazole (Prilosec), lansoprazole (Prevacid), rabeprazole (Aciphex), H^2 blockers

CONTRAINDICATIONS

Allergies to drugs used to treat the disorder

PRECAUTIONS

Drugs have many precautions; read drug product information.

DRUG INTERACTIONS

Drugs have many interactions; read drug product information.

OTHER DRUGS

- Antacids: alumina-magnesium (Gaviscon)
- Metoclopramide (Reglan)
- Bethanechol (Urecholine)

 ## FOLLOW-UP

PATIENT MONITORING

- See the doctor as often as necessary.
- Endoscopy may be repeated at 6 to 12 weeks if symptoms do not respond to treatment.
- Annual (or every other year) endoscopy to detect changes early

PREVENTION

- Long-term maintenance therapy, along with lifestyle and diet modification
- Scarring may require periodic procedures.
- Surgery should be considered for patients with severe disease.

Gastroesophageal Reflux Disease

Doctor
Office
Phone
Pager

Special notes to patient:

Gastroesophageal Reflux Disease

COMPLICATIONS

- Scarring
- Bleeding
- Esophageal disorders
- Lung, ear, nose, or throat disorders
- Chest pain
- Cancer

WHAT TO EXPECT

- Most of those with reflux disorders respond well to therapy.
- Symptoms and inflammation often return promptly when treatment is stopped.
- Relapse prevention therapy often requires that the full healing dose be maintained.
- Surgery produces excellent short-term results.

 MISCELLANEOUS

PEDIATRIC

- Reflux symptoms usually resolve by age 18 months.
- Vomiting, weight loss, and failure to thrive are more common than heartburn.
- Positional treatment: use an infant seat for 2 to 3 hours after meals; thicken feedings.
- Surgery for severe symptoms (apnea, choking, persistent vomiting) is successful in 85% to 95% of cases.

GERIATRIC

Complications are more likely among the elderly.

PREGNANCY

Heartburn is more common early in pregnancy.

- Tends to recur in later pregnancies
- Eat multiple small meals, avoid lying down for 2 to 3 hours after meals, elevate the head of the bed at night.
- Antacids or H_2 blockers are probably safe in the third trimester.

FURTHER INFORMATION

Digestive Diseases Clearinghouse, Suite 600, 1555 Wilson Blvd., Rosslyn, VA 22209, (212) 685-3440

Gastroesophageal Reflux Disease

	Doctor
	Office
	Phone
	Pager

Special notes to patient:

Genital Warts

 ## BASICS

DESCRIPTION

Genital warts, also called "venereal warts" or "condyloma acuminata," are soft, skin-colored, fleshy warts that are caused by the human papilloma virus (HPV). Warts appear in the vagina, on the cervix, around the external genitalia and rectum, and occasionally, in the throat. Warts can appear singly or in groups, small or large. The disease is highly contagious, and has an incubation period of 1 to 6 months.

SIGNS AND SYMPTOMS

- May be no symptoms
- Soft tumors
- Smooth to very rough surface
- Multiple finger-like projections
- Can be rough and cauliflower-like
- Penile lesions often smooth, in groups of three or four
- Itching
- Irritation
- Bleeding

CAUSES

Human papilloma viruses (HPV)

SCOPE

At least 10% to 20% of sexually active women may be infected with HPV.

MOST OFTEN AFFECTED

Individuals 15 to 30 years of age, males and females in equal frequency.

RISK FACTORS

- Young adult
- Sexually active
- Not using condoms
- Sexual activity at a young age
- Cigarette smoking
- Poor hygiene
- Pregnancy
- White
- History of genital warts

 ## DIAGNOSIS

WHAT THE DOCTOR LOOKS FOR

The doctor will perform a physical examination to identify the disorder and associated conditions.

TESTS AND PROCEDURES

- Blood tests
- A sample of tissue can be obtained by biopsy for laboratory analysis.
- Other specialized tests can be performed.
- The reproductive tract can be examined by endoscopy.

 ## TREATMENT

GENERAL MEASURES

- Genital warts are managed in the outpatient setting.
- Treatment is determined by location and size of warts.
- Small warts can be treated with topical applications.
- Cryotherapy
- Larger warts require laser treatment, electrocoagulation, or surgery.

ACTIVITY

No restrictions

DIET

No special diet

 ## MEDICATIONS

COMMONLY PRESCRIBED DRUGS

- Podophyllin in tincture of Benzoin
- Podofilox (Condylox)

CONTRAINDICATIONS

Podophyllin should not be used during pregnancy or on oral, cervical, urethral, or anal warts. It can be used on a small number of vaginal warts with careful drying after application.

PRECAUTIONS

Podophyllin: Wash treated areas 1 to 4 hours after application and use ointments to protect surrounding skin.

OTHER DRUGS

- Trichloroacetic acid (TCA)
- Fluorouracil

FOLLOW-UP

PATIENT MONITORING

- See the doctor every 2 weeks for treatment until warts clear
- For women, Pap test every year
- Sex partners should be monitored.

PREVENTION

- Use of condoms by infected men
- Use of condoms by male sexual partners of individuals treated for HPV infection
- Abstinence by women until treatment completed
- Circumcision may prevent recurrence in some men.

COMPLICATIONS

- Cervical dysplasia
- Cancer
- Male urethral obstruction

WHAT TO EXPECT

- Warts clear with treatment or spontaneously regress.
- Recurrence is common with all forms of therapy.
- Infection can persist indefinitely without symptoms.

 ## MISCELLANEOUS

OTHERS

Genital warts are increasing in an ever-younger population. A recent study of 487 college women showed an HPV infection rate of 48%.

PREGNANCY

Warts often grow larger in pregnancy and improve after delivery.
HPV can be transmitted to an infant at time of delivery and cause problems.

Genital Warts

Doctor
Office
Phone
Pager

Special notes to patient:

German Measles

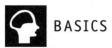 BASICS

DESCRIPTION

Rubella, or German measles, is a viral infection of children and adults that results in skin eruptions. Often, the infection does not produce symptoms; however, it can potentially cause fetal infection and birth defects in pregnant women.

SIGNS AND SYMPTOMS

- Enlarged glands
- Low-grade fever
- Skin eruptions
- Reddened eyes
- Acute rhinitis
- Malaise
- Headache
- Joint pain, especially in young women
- No symptoms (25% to 50%)
- Birth defects (congenital rubella)

CAUSES

Infection with the rubella virus

SCOPE

About 0.09 cases of rubella occur per 100,000 persons per year. Outbreaks occur in confined populations (e.g., prisons, schools).

MOST OFTEN AFFECTED

Children 5 to 9 years of age; males and females affected in equal proportion

RISK FACTORS

- Inadequate immunization
- Immune system disorders
- Immunosuppressive therapy
- Pregnancy
- Crowded living conditions
- School, daycare
- Late winter, spring seasons

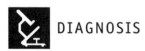 DIAGNOSIS

WHAT THE DOCTOR LOOKS FOR

- The doctor will perform a physical examination to identify the presence of rubella.
- Numerous other conditions that can cause similar signs and symptoms should be investigated.

TESTS AND PROCEDURES

- Blood tests
- Body fluids can be sampled for laboratory analysis.
- A sample of placenta can be obtained by biopsy to diagnose congenital rubella.

 TREATMENT

GENERAL MEASURES

- Rubella is managed in the outpatient setting.
- Most cases are mild and self-limited. Treatment is for symptomatic relief.

ACTIVITY

Contact isolation for 7 days after onset of rash; bed rest is not necessary.

DIET

No special diet

 MEDICATIONS

COMMONLY PRESCRIBED DRUGS

Acetaminophen for fever

OTHER DRUGS

None

 FOLLOW-UP

PATIENT MONITORING

See the doctor as often as necessary.

PREVENTION

Rubella vaccine

COMPLICATIONS

- Childhood rubella
  - Brain damage
  - Bleeding disorder
  - Testicular pain
  - Mild hepatitis
- Congenital rubella
  - Miscarriage
  - Stillbirth
  - Premature delivery
  - Progressive brain damage
  - Hormone disorders
- Rubella vaccine
  - Enlarged lymph glands
  - Fever
  - Rash
  - Joint pain (older girls or women)

WHAT TO EXPECT

- Childhood rubella
  - Fever, 1 to 2 days
  - Rash, 3 days
  - Runny nose, 5 days
  - Enlarged lymph nodes, 1 week
  - Joint pain (when present), 2 weeks
  - Complete and full recovery without complications is the rule.
- Congenital rubella
  - Varied and unpredictable spectrum of consequences
  - Prognosis is excellent when only minor defects are present.

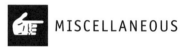 MISCELLANEOUS

PEDIATRIC

- Rubella is a milder disease in children than it is in adults.
- Adolescents and young adults currently account for about 60% of all new cases.

PREGNANCY

Women vaccinated against rubella are advised not to become pregnant for at least 3 months after receiving the vaccine. The vaccine can cross the placenta. However, no case of congenital rubella has ever occurred in newborns of women who were inadvertently vaccinated while pregnant.

German Measles

Doctor
Office
Phone
Pager

Special notes to patient:

Gingivitis

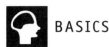 ## BASICS

DESCRIPTION
Gingivitis, an inflammation of the gums, is a significant oral infection.

SIGNS AND SYMPTOMS
- Bad breath (halitosis)
- Painless gum swelling
- Gum redness
- Change of normal gum contours
- Bleeding when flossing or brushing
- Swelling of gums between teeth
- Narrow band of bright red gum surrounding tooth

CAUSES
- Not contagious
- Inadequate plaque removal
- Blood disorders
- Oral contraceptive side effect
- Infection
- Allergic reaction
- Endocrine disturbances (e.g., pregnancy, menses)
- Chronic disease

SCOPE
Gingivitis affects 90% of the population in the United States.

MOST OFTEN AFFECTED
Primarily adults, males and females in equal proportions

RISK FACTORS
- Diabetes mellitus
- Poor dental hygiene
- Mouth breathing
- Faulty dental work
- Infection with human immunodeficiency virus (HIV)

 ## DIAGNOSIS

WHAT THE DOCTOR LOOKS FOR
- The doctor will perform a physical examination to evaluate the affected area and also identify any associated conditions (e.g., inflammation of the tongue [glossitis]).
- The cause of gingivitis should be identified and treated.

TESTS AND PROCEDURES
A sample of material from the affected area can be obtained for laboratory analysis.

 ## TREATMENT

GENERAL MEASURES
- Gingivitis is managed in the outpatient setting.
- Irritating factors should be eliminated (plaque, faulty dentures).
- Good oral hygiene
- Regular dental check-ups
- No smoking
- Warm saline rinses twice daily
- Preventive by dental hygienist

ACTIVITY
No restrictions

DIET
Assure that the diet contains adequate vitamins and minerals.

 ## MEDICATIONS

COMMONLY PRESCRIBED DRUGS
- Antibiotics: penicillin V, erythromycin
- Topical steroids: triamcinolone in Orabase

CONTRAINDICATIONS
Allergy to antibiotics

PRECAUTIONS
Erythromycin frequently causes significant gastrointestinal upset.

DRUG INTERACTIONS
Read drug product information.

OTHER DRUGS
Other antibiotics

 ## FOLLOW-UP

PATIENT MONITORING
See the doctor or dentist until gingivitis resolves.

PREVENTION
- Good oral hygiene, daily brushing and flossing
- Cleaning by a dentist or hygienist at least every 6 months

COMPLICATIONS
Severe periodontal disease

WHAT TO EXPECT
- The outcome is generally favorable; gingivitis responds well to appropriate treatment.
- May develop periodically again in the future or become chronic (long-lasting)

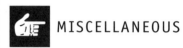 ## MISCELLANEOUS

PEDIATRIC
Mild cases of gingivitis are common in children and usually require no treatment.

GERIATRIC
Gingivitis is more frequent among the elderly, because of lifelong accumulation rather than increased susceptibility.

FURTHER INFORMATION
American Dental Association, 211 E. Chicago Avenue, Chicago, IL 60611, (800) 621-8099

Gingivitis

	Doctor
	Office
	Phone
	Pager

Special notes to patient:

Glaucoma

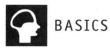 ## BASICS

DESCRIPTION

Glaucoma is generally defined as abnormally high pressure within the eye, which is caused by impaired circulation of fluid. Ultimately, excessive pressure damages the optic nerve and leads to loss of vision. Chronic open-angle glaucoma, the most common form of the disease, may cause no symptoms until it is well advanced. Primary angle-closure glaucoma is an eye emergency.

SIGNS AND SYMPTOMS

- Chronic open-angle glaucoma:
  - No symptoms until advanced disease
  - Gradual painless vision loss
- Primary angle-closure glaucoma
  - Pain or dull ache in or around one eye
  - Blurred vision
  - Symptoms occur when watching TV or movies in dark room, reading, or when fatigued.
  - Relieved by sleep or rest
  - Enlarged pupil
  - Excessive tearing
  - Halos around lights
  - Headache
  - Nausea and vomiting
  - Swelling of eyelid
  - Reddened eyes

SCOPE

Glaucoma affects approximately 4% of persons 40 years of age or older. More than 90% of those affected have chronic open-angle glaucoma.

MOST OFTEN AFFECTED

Glaucoma primarily affects those above 40 years of age, but can occur at any age. Males and females are affected with equal frequency. It is more frequent in African-Americans and Asians than in whites.

CAUSES

- Impaired flow of fluids within the eye
- Too much fluid within the eye (rare)

RISK FACTORS

- Family history
- Diabetes mellitus
- African-American ancestry

 ## DIAGNOSIS

WHAT THE DOCTOR LOOKS FOR

- The doctor will perform a physical examination to assess the extent and severity of signs and symptoms.
- Other conditions known to be associated with glaucoma (e.g., diabetes mellitus) should be identified and treated.

TESTS AND PROCEDURES

Vision tests can be performed, including the measurement of intraocular pressure (IOP) and evaluation of the visual field.

 ## TREATMENT

GENERAL MEASURES

- Glaucoma is managed in the outpatient setting.
- Treatment of glaucoma is directed at lowering IOP.
- Glaucoma cannot be cured.
- Usually medical therapy can lower the IOP sufficiently to prevent optic nerve damage and vision loss.
- Early detection and adequate treatment can prevent visual loss in virtually every case.
- When medical therapy fails, laser or conventional surgery is indicated.

ACTIVITY

For acute form, bedrest until attack subsides

DIET

No special diet

 ## MEDICATIONS

COMMONLY PRESCRIBED DRUGS

- Timolol, betaxolol, levobunolol, carteolol, metipranolol
- Epinephrine, dipivefrin, apraclonidine
- Dorzolamide
- Pilocarpine, carbamylcholine
- Physostigmine, demecarium bromide, echothiophate iodide, and isoflurophate
- Acetazolamide (Diamox), dichlorphenamide, methazolamide
- Primary angle-closure glaucoma:
  - Glycerin, isosorbide dinitrate, mannitol
  - Acetazolamide (Diamox), dorzolamide
  - Timolol (Timoptic), levobunolol (Betagan), betaxolol (Betoptic)
  - Pilocarpine Prednisolone acetate (Pred Forte)
  - Apraclonidine (Iopidine)

CONTRAINDICATIONS

Some drugs cannot be prescribed to individuals with asthma or allergies to sulfa drugs.

PRECAUTIONS

Drugs should be used with caution in people with cardiovascular disease, kidney stones, lung disease, diabetes mellitus, liver disease, or a history of allergy to sulfa drugs.

DRUG INTERACTIONS

Drugs have many interactions; read drug product information.

 ## FOLLOW-UP

PATIENT MONITORING

See the doctor every 3 to 4 months for the remainder of life.

COMPLICATIONS

Eye disorders, visual loss, blindness

WHAT TO EXPECT

- Treatment is required for the remainder of lifetime.
- The vision outcome is excellent unless the diagnosis is delayed until the disorder is far advanced.

 ## MISCELLANEOUS

FURTHER INFORMATION

- Foundation for Glaucoma Research, 490 Post Street, Suite 830, San Francisco, CA 94102, (415) 986-3162
- American Academy of Ophthalmology, 655 Beach Street, San Francisco, CA 94109, (415) 561-8500

Glaucoma

Doctor
Office
Phone
Pager

Special notes to patient:

Glomerulonephritis, Acute

 ## BASICS

DESCRIPTION

Glomerulonephritis is the inflammation of kidney structures in response to an infection. The kidney can be damaged as a result. This condition is most common in children. It is characterized by the abrupt appearance of blood in the urine, often accompanied by high blood pressure and swelling.

SIGNS AND SYMPTOMS

- Blood in urine
- Scant volume of urine
- Swelling, particularly of the face and eyes in the morning and feet and ankles in the afternoons and evenings
- High blood pressure
- Dark or tea-colored urine
- Fever (rare)
- Sore throat
- Respiratory infection
- Weight gain
- Abdominal pain
- Loss of appetite
- Back pain
- Pallor
- Impetigo

CAUSES

Viral or bacterial infection

SCOPE

About 20 cases of glomerulonephritis per 100,000 persons occur in the United States annually; occurs with impetigo in the late summer and with sore throat in the winter.

MOST OFTEN AFFECTED

- Of cases, 60% occur in children 2 to 12 years of age.
- Only 10% of cases occur in individuals above 40 years of age.
- More frequent in males than females

RISK FACTORS

- Of cases, 15% occur after infection with microbes known to cause the disease.
- Cycles of epidemics
- Cases without symptoms are 20 times more common.

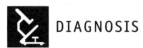 ## DIAGNOSIS

WHAT THE DOCTOR LOOKS FOR

- The doctor will perform a physical examination to assess the presence and severity of disease.
- Other diseases with similar symptoms include other kidney disorders and systemic lupus erythematosus.

TESTS AND PROCEDURES

- Blood tests
- Fluid from the throat can be sampled for laboratory analysis.
- Urinalysis and culture
- A sample of kidney tissue can be obtained by biopsy for laboratory analysis.

 ## TREATMENT

GENERAL MEASURES

- Acute glomerulonephritis is usually managed in the inpatient setting until the condition has improved.
- Most patients can be followed safely as outpatients.
- Decrease salt consumption until swelling and high blood pressure clear.
- Decrease fluids
- Control high blood pressure
- Dialysis may be necessary.

ACTIVITY

Full activity can be resumed after improvement. Blood may appear in urine after exercise for up to 2 years.

DIET

- No added salt until swelling and high blood pressure clear
- Restrict proteins
- Avoid high-potassium foods

 ## MEDICATIONS

COMMONLY PRESCRIBED DRUGS

- Sodium polystyrene sulfonate (Kayexalate), calcium gluconate, calcium carbonate (Turns)
- Oxygen
- Sodium bicarbonate
- Infection: penicillin, erythromycin
- Hypertension: furosemide, hydralazine (Apresoline), nifedipine

CONTRAINDICATIONS

Read drug product information.

PRECAUTIONS

Read drug product information.

DRUG INTERACTIONS

Read drug product information.

 ## FOLLOW-UP

PATIENT MONITORING

- See the doctor as often as necessary, depending on the severity of disease.
- Blood pressure measurement and urinalysis should be repeated at 2, 4, and 8 weeks and 4, 6, and 12 months.
- Periodic blood tests

PREVENTION

Infections should be treated aggressively.

COMPLICATIONS

- Eye disorders
- Brain disorders
- Severe kidney disease

WHAT TO EXPECT

- Acute glomerulonephritis is usually self-limiting, within 2 to 3 weeks.
- Immediate death rate is very low.
- Long-term outcome in children is excellent; almost all recover completely.
- May be a greater risk of death among adults or in those with preexisting kidney disease
- Symptoms can be worsened by an illness but rarely after 12 months.
- Urine may be darker after strenuous exercise.

 ## MISCELLANEOUS

PEDIATRIC

Acute glomerulonephritis is common among children 2 to 16 years of age.

FURTHER INFORMATION

National Kidney Foundation, 30 E. 33rd Street, Suite 1100, New York, NY 10016, (212) 8899910

Glomerulonephritis, Acute

Doctor
Office
Phone
Pager

Special notes to patient:

Gonorrhea

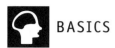
BASICS

DESCRIPTION

- Gonorrhea, or "clap," is a sexually transmitted disease affecting the reproductive and urinary system. Gonorrhea is caused by the bacterium *Neisseria gonorrhoeae*. Virtually any mucous membrane can be infected (i.e., urethra, vagina).
- In women, gonorrhea can affect the fallopian tubes and ovaries. Upper genital tract infection in women is referred to as "pelvic inflammatory disease" (PID).
- In men, the epididymis and testicle can become infected.
- *N. gonorrhoeae* can also infect the joints and cause arthritis.
- A person can have the disease without having symptoms.

SIGNS AND SYMPTOMS

- Adolescent and adult males:
  - Pus-like discharge from the urethra
  - Difficult or painful urination
  - Testicular pain
  - Scarring of the urethra
- Adolescent and adult females without PID:
  - Often no symptoms
  - Vaginal discharge
  - Painful or difficult urination
- Adolescent and adult females with PID:
  - Menstrual cramps
  - Lower abdominal pain and tenderness
  - Fever
  - Infertility
  - Chronic pelvic pain
- Either sex, if engaging in anal intercourse
  - Rectal discharge
  - Urgency to defecate
  - Rectal burning or itching
- Either sex, other syndromes:
  - Throat infection
  - Eye infection (rare)
  - Other: fever, chills, joint pain, painful skin lesions, heart disease, meningitis
- Infants and children
  - Eye infection
  - Pneumonia
  - Vaginal discharge
  - Rectal infection
  - Throat infection
  - Other forms of infection

SCOPE

Gonorrhea affects more than 200 per 100,000 people per year in the U.S.

MOST OFTEN AFFECTED

Individuals 15 to 29 years of age; males have symptoms more often than females.

CAUSES

Infection with *N. gonorrhoeae*

RISK FACTORS

- Sexual exposure to an infected individual without barrier protection (condom)
- Multiple sexual partners
- Infant: passage through the infected birth canal of the mother
- Children: sexual abuse by infected individual
- Autoinoculation (finger to eye)
- For PID: use of intrauterine devices

DIAGNOSIS

WHAT THE DOCTOR LOOKS FOR

The doctor will perform a physical examination to identify the presence of disease or other conditions with similar symptoms (e.g., urinary tract infection).

TESTS AND PROCEDURES

- A sample of fluid can be obtained for laboratory analysis.
- Blood or fluid withdrawn from joint can be cultured.
- Ultrasound or computed tomography (CT) scan can be done to assist with diagnosis.

TREATMENT

GENERAL MEASURES

- Uncomplicated cases of gonorrhea can be managed in the outpatient setting.
- Severe cases or infection of infant may require hospitalization.
- Notification and treatment of sexual contacts is required.
- Abstain from sexual activity until after follow-up examination.
- Tests for syphilis, human immunodeficiency virus (HIV)

ACTIVITY

Fully active for uncomplicated disease

DIET

No special diet

MEDICATIONS

COMMONLY PRESCRIBED DRUGS

- Antibiotics: ceftriaxone, cefixime, ofloxacin, ciprofloxacin, doxycycline, azithromycin penicillin, erythromycin, clindamycin, metronidazole
- Sexual contacts of persons with gonorrhea should be evaluated and treated.

CONTRAINDICATIONS

Some drugs are contraindicated in pregnancy.

PRECAUTIONS

Read drug product information.

DRUG INTERACTIONS

Read drug product information.

OTHER DRUGS

Other antibiotics

FOLLOW-UP

PATIENT MONITORING

Follow-up visits with the doctor may not be necessary if the recommended treatment regimen is followed, unless symptoms persist.

PREVENTION

- For recurrence: no sexual intercourse until culture results are known and partners are tested and treated.
- For prevention of initial infection: condoms offer partial protection

COMPLICATIONS

- Urethral scarring in men
- Infertility in women
- Corneal scarring after eye infections
- Joint disease
- Heart disease

WHAT TO EXPECT

A complete cure and a return to normal function can be expected with adequate, prompt therapy.

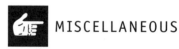

PREGNANCY

PID during pregnancy can lead to miscarriage or premature delivery.

Gonorrhea

Doctor
Office
Phone
Pager

Special notes to patient:

Gout

 ## BASICS

DESCRIPTION
Gout is an inflammation of joint, bones, and related structures by the formation of urate crystals.

SIGNS AND SYMPTOMS
- Rapid acute onset (within 24 hours) of severe pain, swelling, redness, and warmth in one or two joints
- Soft tissue redness, swelling, warmth
- Exquisite tenderness
- Nodules within the skin or bone
- Fever, chills
- Carpal tunnel syndrome
- Kidney stones

CAUSES
- High levels of uric acid in the bloodstream
- Dietary excess (e.g., anchovies, sardines, sweetbreads, kidney, liver, and meat extracts)
- Metabolic disorders
- Lead poisoning
- Kidney disease
- Blood disorders

SCOPE
Gout is rare among individuals under 18 years of age. Incidence increases with age.

MOST OFTEN AFFECTED
Gout primarily affects individuals 30 to 60 years of age, affecting males 20 times more often than females.

RISK FACTORS
- Consumption of alcohol
- Family history of gout
- Polynesian ancestry
- Medications
- Surgery or trauma
- Obesity
- High blood pressure
- Vascular disease
- Diabetes
- Kidney disease
- Hormone disorders
- Blood disorders
- Radiation treatment
- Down syndrome

 ## DIAGNOSIS

WHAT THE DOCTOR LOOKS FOR
- The doctor will perform a physical examination to assess the presence and severity of disease.
- Other conditions that can cause similar symptoms include arthritis and other joint or bone disorders.

TESTS AND PROCEDURES
- Blood tests
- Fluid or tissue from an affected joint can be withdrawn for laboratory analysis.
- X-ray study, bone scans

 ## TREATMENT

GENERAL MEASURES
- Gout is usually managed in the outpatient setting, except for severe joint infection or if treatment fails.
- Treatment is aimed at the underlying cause of gout.

ACTIVITY
Rest affected joints until acute phase is controlled.

DIET
Reduce consumption of fat, alcoholic beverages, sardines, anchovies, liver, and sweetbreads.

MEDICATIONS

COMMONLY PRESCRIBED DRUGS
Nonsteroidal antiinflammatory drugs (NSAIDs), probenecid, allopurinol

CONTRAINDICATIONS
Drugs have numerous contraindications; read drug product information.

PRECAUTIONS
- Probenecid and allopurinol may contribute to gout attacks.
- Reduce NSAID dosage if renal or liver disease is present.
- Allopurinol can cause skin rashes.

DRUG INTERACTIONS
Numerous drug interactions; read drug product information.

OTHER DRUGS
Colchicine, steroids, sulfinpyrazone, hormone (corticotropin)

 ## FOLLOW-UP

PATIENT MONITORING
- See the doctor as often as necessary to assess health and manage drug therapy.
- Blood tests may be repeated weekly or monthly.

PREVENTION
Avoid drugs, diets, and habits that make gout worse, if possible.

COMPLICATIONS
- Increased risk of infection
- Kidney stones or other kidney disease
- Nerve disease

WHAT TO EXPECT
- With early treatment, gout can be totally controlled.
- If attacks recur, medication may need adjustment.
- Acute attack can occur during the first 6 to 24 months of therapy.

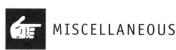 ## MISCELLANEOUS

GERIATRIC
Usually related to medications

PREGNANCY
Usual pregnancy precautions when taking medications

Gout

Doctor
Office
Phone
Pager

Special notes to patient:

Halitosis

 BASICS

DESCRIPTION

Halitosis is an unpleasant breath odor. Contrary to popular belief, gastrointestinal disorders do not generally cause halitosis; therefore, breath odor does not reflect the state of the digestive system or bowel function.

CAUSES

- Inhaled or ingested substances
- Gum or dental disease
- Fermentation of food in mouth
- Systemic disease (tonsillitis, pneumonia, lung abscess)
- Liver disease
- Diabetes
- Infection
- Cancer of the respiratory tract

 TREATMENT

GENERAL MEASURES

Specific causes of halitosis should be identified and treated.

Halitosis

Doctor
Office
Phone
Pager

Special notes to patient:

Headache, Cluster

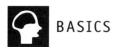 ## BASICS

DESCRIPTION
Cluster headaches are attacks of severe headache that are typically localized on one side around the eye or temple. They are associated with excessive tearing of the eye on the opposite side, runny nose, and nasal congestion. Attacks last from 30 minutes to 3 hours and occur one to six times per day.

SIGNS AND SYMPTOMS
- Sudden onset of severe headache
- Headache peaks within 15 minutes, lasts less than 3 hours
- Pain is one-sided and located around the eye, temple, or front part of the head; rare in other locations.
- Severe, piercing, exploding, penetrating (occasionally throbbing) pain
- Excessive tear production
- Reddened eyes
- Nasal stuffiness
- Runny nose
- Slow heart rate
- Nausea
- Perspiration
- Restlessness and agitation
- Attacks may occur at the same time of day for consecutive days; often, attacks occur within 90 minutes of falling to sleep.

CAUSES
Unknown

SCOPE
Cluster headaches affect 0.5% to 1% of adults in the United States.

MOST OFTEN AFFECTED
The average age of onset is 30 years in men, later in women. Cluster headaches occur six times more frequently in men than women.

RISK FACTORS
- Male gender
- Age greater than 30 years
- Small amounts of alcohol or nitroglycerine
- May be related to previous head trauma or surgery

WHAT THE DOCTOR LOOKS FOR
- The doctor will perform a physical examination to identify the presence and severity of cluster headaches.
- Other disorders that cause similar symptoms include nerve disorders, migraine, blood vessel conditions, and other diseases.
- The doctor will look for conditions known to be associated with cluster headaches (e.g., heart disease).

TESTS AND PROCEDURES
Laboratory tests and x-ray studies are of limited value in the diagnosis of cluster headaches.

 ## TREATMENT

GENERAL MEASURES
- Cluster headaches are managed in the outpatient setting, except for those patients who are at risk of suicide.
- During cluster period, avoid alcohol, bright lights and glare, excessive emotion, and stress, as these may precipitate attacks.
- Avoid narcotic pain killers.
- Tobacco use may make treatment less effective.
- Surgery may be an option for some patients.

ACTIVITY
- Avoid self-injury during bouts of excruciating pain.
- Vigorous physical activity at first symptom may stop attack in some people.

DIET
- During cluster phase, alcohol, even in small amounts, frequently precipitates attacks.
- Rarely, specific foods may trigger attacks.

 ## MEDICATIONS

COMMONLY PRESCRIBED DRUGS
- Acute attack: oxygen, sumatriptan (Imitrex), dihydroergotamine mesylate (DHE 45)
- Prevention: verapamil, lithium carbonate (Eskalith), methysergide (Sansert), ergotamine, prednisone

CONTRAINDICATIONS
Read drug product information.

PRECAUTIONS
Read drug product information.

DRUG INTERACTIONS
Read drug product information.

OTHER DRUGS
- Lidocaine, phenylephrine
- Indomethacin, nifedipine, nimodipine

 ## FOLLOW-UP

PATIENT MONITORING
- See the doctor as often as necessary for monitoring of health and drug therapy.
- Anticipate cluster bouts and start preventive treatment early.

PREVENTION
- Alcohol, nitroglycerine, and some foods can induce cluster attack.
- Disturbances in sleep cycle can induce attacks.
- Strong emotions, anger, and excessive physical activity can induce attacks.
- Tobacco can slow response to medication.
- Narcotics can transform episodes of cluster to chronic cluster.

COMPLICATIONS
- Self-injury during attack
- Side effects of medication, including unmasking of coronary heart disease
- Potential for drug abuse

WHAT TO EXPECT
- Attacks of cluster headaches tend to recur.
- Prolonged periods of remission occur between clusters.
- Episodic clusters may evolve into chronic cluster and occasionally, vice versa.

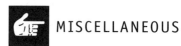 ## MISCELLANEOUS

PEDIATRIC
Cluster headaches are rare among children.

OTHERS
With age, cluster headaches are more likely to begin in women, often around the menopausal years.

PREGNANCY
Cluster headaches are rare in pregnancy.

Headache, Cluster

	Doctor
	Office
	Phone
	Pager

Special notes to patient:

Headache, Tension

 ## BASICS

DESCRIPTION

- Tension headaches are divided into two types:
  - Episodic: Usually linked to a stressful event; is of moderate intensity and self-limited; and usually responds to nonprescription remedies.
  - Chronic: Often occurs daily; located on both sides of the head, usually around the back or front part of the head; and is associated with muscles of the neck and scalp.

SIGNS AND SYMPTOMS

- Headache on both sides of the head
- Located in the front or back of the head, or generalized
- Dull, pressing, or band-like discomfort
- The intensity of pain varies throughout the day.
- Often present on waking or soon after
- For 75% of patients, chronic headaches occur for more than 5 years
- Insomnia
- Teeth grinding
- Not aggravated by physical activity
- Difficulty concentrating
- Muscular tightness or stiffness in neck and front or back of the head

CAUSES

- Poor posture
- Stress, anxiety
- Depression
- Osteoarthritis of neck
- Blood vessel disorder

SCOPE

Tension headaches are common in the United States.

MOST OFTEN AFFECTED

- Of tension headaches, 60% begin after age 20 (unusual for tension headaches to begin after age 50).
- Tension headaches affect females more frequently than males.
- Of sufferers, 40% have a family history of headache.

RISK FACTORS

Obstructive sleep apnea

 ## MEDICATIONS

Excessive caffeine

 ## DIAGNOSIS

WHAT THE DOCTOR LOOKS FOR

- The doctor will perform a physical examination to identify the type and severity of headache.
- Other disorders that can cause similar symptoms include bone conditions, dependency on caffeine or analgesics, depression, head injury, and other medical conditions.

TESTS AND PROCEDURES

- Blood tests
- X-ray study can be done of the neck.
- Computed tomography (CT) scan or magnetic resonance imaging (MRI) can be done to assist in diagnosis.

 ## TREATMENT

GENERAL MEASURES

- Tension headaches are managed in the outpatient setting.
- Relief measures: relaxation techniques; rest in quiet, dark room with cold washcloth over eyes; hot bath or shower; massaging back of neck and temples
- Biofeedback training offers an alternative that is often helpful.
- Change lifestyle to minimize stress; counseling may help.

ACTIVITY

Physical fitness and range of motion and strengthening exercises for the neck are encouraged.

DIET

- No proven link exists between diet and tension headache.

 ## MEDICATIONS

COMMONLY PRESCRIBED DRUGS

- Acute attack: nonsteroidal antiinflammatory drugs (NSAIDs):
  - Naproxen sodium (Naprosyn, Aleve)
  - Fenoprofen calcium (Nalfon)
  - Ibuprofen (Motrin, Advil)
  - Ketoprofen (Orudis)
- Prophylaxis for chronic tension headache: antidepressants
  - Amitriptyline (Elavil)
  - Desipramine (Norpramin)
  - Imipramine (Tofranil)
  - Nortriptyline (Pamelor)

CONTRAINDICATIONS

- NSAIDs and antidepressants are generally not suitable for children.
- Antidepressants should not be used with monoamine oxidase (MAO) inhibitors.

PRECAUTIONS

- Do not use antidepressants in presence of acute heart attack.
- Avoid dependence on nonprescription, caffeine-containing preparations.
- NSAIDs should be used with caution in individuals with a history of peptic ulcer disease.

DRUG INTERACTIONS

Antidepressants interact with alcohol.

OTHER DRUGS

- Propranolol (Inderal LA), nadolol (Corgard), atenolol (Tenormin)
- Isometheptene-dichloralphenazone-acetaminophen (Midrin)
- Other NSAIDs

 ## FOLLOW-UP

PATIENT MONITORING

See the doctor as often as necessary.

PREVENTION

- Physical therapy
- Biofeedback and relaxation
- Neck traction
- Injection of trigger points

COMPLICATIONS

- Risk of addiction or reliance on pain relievers
- Gastrointestinal bleeding from NSAID use
- Risk of epilepsy in individuals who experience tension headaches is fourfold that of the general population.

WHAT TO EXPECT

- Tension headaches usually follow a chronic course when life stress is not changed.
- Most cases are intermittent and should not interfere with work or normal life span.

Headache, Tension

	Doctor
	Office
	Phone
	Pager

Special notes to patient:

Headache, Tension

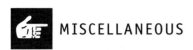 **MISCELLANEOUS**

PEDIATRIC
Only 15% will have onset at age younger than 10 years.

GERIATRIC
Onset of new headache in the elderly is cause for careful study.

OTHERS
It is unusual for tension headaches to begin after age 50.

FURTHER INFORMATION
National Headache Foundation, 5252 N. Western Ave., Chicago, IL 60625, (800) 843-2256

Headache, Tension

Doctor
Office
Phone
Pager

Special notes to patient:

Head Lice

 ## BASICS

DESCRIPTION

Lice, or pediculosis, is an infestation by parasites that feed on human blood. A mature female louse lays eggs, or nits, which appear as small white spots cemented to the base of hair. Lice can infest head, body, or pubic hair.

SIGNS AND SYMPTOMS

- Head lice (pediculosis capitis):
  - Found most often on the back of the head and neck and behind the ears
  - Nits are white spots on the hair shaft that cannot be moved.
  - Itching
  - Prickling sensation of the scalp
  - Eyelashes may be involved
- Body lice (pediculosis corporis):
  - Affects individuals with poor hygiene
  - Adult lice live and lay their nits in the seams of clothing.
  - Most common symptom is itching that leads to scratching and infection.
  - Uninfected bites appear as red spots.
- Pubic lice (*Phthirus pubis*):
  - Itching of groin and rectal area
  - May have no symptoms during 30-day incubation period
  - Delay in treatment may lead to development of widespread groin inflammation and infection.
  - Pubic hair is the most common site.
  - Lice can spread to hair around rectum, abdomen, armpit, chest, beard, eyebrows, and eyelashes.
  - Infested adult patients can spread lice to eyelashes of children.

CAUSES

Lice are transmitted by close personal contact and contact with objects such as combs, hats, clothing, and bed linen.

SCOPE

Head lice affects 10% to 40% of students in schools where accurate surveys have been conducted.

MOST OFTEN AFFECTED

- Most common in adults: pubic lice
- Most common in children: head lice
- More common in females than males

RISK FACTORS

- Body lice: inability to change and launder clothing, overcrowded sleeping quarters
- Pubic lice: sexual contact with an infected person

 ## DIAGNOSIS

WHAT THE DOCTOR LOOKS FOR

The doctor will perform a physical examination to identify lice and nits.

 ## TREATMENT

GENERAL MEASURES

- After treatment with shampoo or lotion, nits remain in scalp or pubic hair.
- Nits are best removed with a very fine comb (nit comb). Removal may be made easier by soaking the hair in a solution of equal parts water and white vinegar and wrapping wet scalp in a towel for at least 15 minutes.
- Repeat treatment periodically as needed for stubborn nits.
- All family contacts possibly infested with head lice should be treated at the same time.

ACTIVITY

No restrictions

DIET

No special diet

 ## MEDICATIONS

COMMONLY PRESCRIBED DRUGS

- Lindane (Kwell)
- Pyrethrins-piperonyl butoxide (Rid)
- Permethrin (Nix)
- Eyelash infestation: careful manual removal of lice and nits or application of petroleum jelly (Vaseline) three or four times a day for 8 to 10 days

CONTRAINDICATIONS

Avoid lindane in infants and pregnant women.

PRECAUTIONS

- Medication should never be used to treat eyelash infections.
- Accidental ingestion and gross overuse of lindane may be associated with central nervous system toxicity.

OTHER DRUGS

Malathion (Ovide)

 ## FOLLOW-UP

PATIENT MONITORING

As needed

PREVENTION

- Changing and laundering clothing eliminates risk of head lice.
- Careful follow-up in schools by public health nurses may help prevent recurrence and spread of head lice.
- Washing combs, brushes, hats, coats, collars, sheets, pillow cases, and so on will help to prevent reinfestation.

COMPLICATIONS

Persistent itching can be caused by too frequent use of medication.

WHAT TO EXPECT

- With appropriate treatment, the cure rate is more than 90%.
- Recurrence is common, mainly from reinfection and failure to comply with treatment.

 ## MISCELLANEOUS

FURTHER INFORMATION

Mayo Foundation for Medical Education and Research, Section of Patient and Health Education, Sieber Subway, Rochester, MN 55905, (507) 284-8140

Head Lice

Doctor
Office
Phone
Pager

Special notes to patient:

Heart Attack

 ## BASICS

DESCRIPTION

Heart attack, or acute myocardial infarction (AMI), is the rapid development of heart muscle death resulting from a sustained and complete reduction of blood flow. The blockage is caused by a blood clot generated by an atherosclerotic plaque on the lining of the artery. The consequences of heart attack depend on the size and location of the blockage and how quickly blood flow can be restored.

SIGNS AND SYMPTOMS

- Pain in the arm, back, jaw, upper abdomen, neck, chest
- Heaviness, viselike tightness of the chest
- Anxiety
- Lightheadedness, pallor, weakness, fainting
- Nausea, vomiting, profuse sweating
- Cough, difficulty breathing, wheezing
- Irregular heart rhythms

CAUSES

- Blockage of heart artery by blood clot
- Coronary artery disorders
- Oxygen imbalance
- Cocaine use

SCOPE

About 600 heart attacks occur per 100,000 persons per year in the United States.

MOST OFTEN AFFECTED

Individuals above 40 years of age; more common in males until age 70, when frequency among females becomes equal

RISK FACTORS

- High levels of cholesterol in the bloodstream
- History of early heart disease in family
- Smoking
- Diabetes mellitus
- High blood pressure
- Sedentary life style
- Aging
- Hostile, high-strung, frustrated personality
- High levels of fats and triglycerides in bloodstream

 ## DIAGNOSIS

WHAT THE DOCTOR LOOKS FOR

- The doctor will perform a physical examination to identify that a heart attack has occurred.
- Conditions that can cause similar signs and symptoms include aortic aneurysm, lung disorders, pancreatitis, spasm of the esophagus, and other heart conditions.
- The degree of heart impairment will be assessed.

TESTS AND PROCEDURES

- Blood tests
- Chest x-ray study
- Electrocardiography (ECG) and echocardiography can be done.
- Special radiology procedures, radionuclide studies, can be done to assist in diagnosis.
- Blood vessels of the heart can be assessed by an imaging procedure (angiography).

 ## TREATMENT

GENERAL MEASURES

- Heart attack requires hospitalization.
- Call 911 for help; do not drive to hospital.
- Provide emergency first aid as needed, including rescue breathing and cardiopulmonary resuscitation (CPR).
- In the hospital, goals are pain relief, treatment of electrical and mechanical complications, and limiting damage to heart muscle.
- Emergency percutaneous transluminal angioplasty (PTCA), or balloon angioplasty, may be done.

ACTIVITY

- Bed rest for first 24 hours
- Medically supervised rehabilitation plan

DIET

Nothing by mouth until stable; later, low-fat, low-salt diet

 ## MEDICATIONS

COMMONLY PRESCRIBED DRUGS

- Acute phase:
  - Alteplase [tissue plasminogen activator (TPA), Activase]
  - Heparin
  - Aspirin
  - Nitrates
  - Lidocaine
  - Oxazepam, Lorazepam
  - Morphine
  - Metoprolol (Lopressor)
  - Oxygen
  - Stool softeners: milk of magnesia, docusate sodium (dioctyl sodium sulfosuccinate)
- Recovery phase:
  - Beta-blockers
  - Nitrates
  - Angiotensin-converting enzyme (ACE) inhibitors

CONTRAINDICATIONS

Read drug product information.

PRECAUTIONS

Read drug product information.

DRUG INTERACTIONS

Read drug product information.

OTHER DRUGS

- Streptokinase
- Atenolol

 ## FOLLOW-UP

PATIENT MONITORING

See the doctor as often as needed.

PREVENTION

- Avoid risk factors
- Recognize the signs and symptoms of heart attack and take prompt action.
- Aspirin (81 mg/day) may be helpful in preventing heart attacks. See your doctor before taking daily aspirin.

Heart Attack

Doctor
Office
Phone
Pager

Special notes to patient:

Heart Attack

COMPLICATIONS

- Heart failure
- Shock
- Heart rupture
- Structural heart damage
- Clot formation in heart or lungs
- Inflammation of heart
- Irregular heart rhythm
- Cardiac arrest
- Death

WHAT TO EXPECT

- Overall mortality rate of heart attack is 10% during the hospital phase, with an additional 10% mortality rate during the year after. More than 60% of the deaths occur within 1 hour of the onset of the heart attack.
- Outcome can be good with prompt diagnosis and proper treatment.

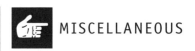 MISCELLANEOUS

GERIATRIC

Complications are more frequent among the elderly.

FURTHER INFORMATION

American Heart Association, 7320 Greenville Avenue, Dallas, TX 75231, (214) 373-6300

Heart Attack

Doctor
Office
Phone
Pager

Special notes to patient:

Heat Exhaustion and Heat Stroke

 ## BASICS

DESCRIPTION

- Heat exhaustion and heat stroke are severe illnesses caused by dehydration, loss of salts, and failure of the body's temperature regulation mechanisms.
- Heat exhaustion is an acute heat injury caused by dehydration.
- Heat stroke is an extreme injury with failure of temperature regulation that profoundly affects the central nervous system.

SIGNS AND SYMPTOMS

- Heat exhaustion:
  - Fatigue and lethargy
  - Weakness
  - Dizziness
  - Nausea, vomiting
  - Muscle ache, soreness
  - Headache
  - Profuse sweating
  - Rapid heart rate
  - Low blood pressure
  - Lack of coordination
  - Agitation
  - Intense thirst
  - Rapid breathing
  - Tingling sensation
  - Core temperature elevated but below 103°F (39.4°C)
- Heat stroke:
  - Exhaustion
  - Confusion, disorientation
  - Coma
  - Hot, flushed, dry skin
  - Core temperature above 105°F (40.5°C)

CAUSES

Failure of heat-dissipating mechanisms or an overwhelming heat stress leading to a rise in core body temperature, dehydration, and salt depletion.

SCOPE

Varies depending on preexisting conditions and environmental factors

MOST OFTEN AFFECTED

Heat injuries are more likely to occur in children and the elderly. Males and females are affected with equal frequency.

RISK FACTORS

- Poor adaptation to heat
- Poor physical conditioning
- Salt or water depletion
- Obesity
- Fever
- Gastrointestinal illness
- Chronic illnesses: diabetes, high blood pressure, heart disease
- Alcohol or drug abuse
- High heat and humidity, poor air circulation in environment
- Heavy, restrictive clothing

 ## DIAGNOSIS

WHAT THE DOCTOR LOOKS FOR

- The doctor will perform a complete physical examination to assess the extent of heat injury.
- Other possible causes of symptoms should be identified and treated.

TESTS AND PROCEDURES

- Blood tests
- Urinalysis
- The rectal temperature may be monitored.

 ## TREATMENT

GENERAL MEASURES

- Heat injuries are emergencies that are best managed in a hospital.
- Remove person to a cooler location.
- Provide emergency first aid as needed [rescue breathing, cardiopulmonary resuscitation (CPR)].
- Rapid cooling: remove clothing, wet patient down, apply ice packs.
- Intravenous (IV) replacement of fluids and salts

ACTIVITY

Rest with legs elevated

DIET

- Cool or cold clear liquids only (noncarbonated)
- Avoid caffeine.
- Unrestricted salt

 ## MEDICATIONS

COMMONLY PRESCRIBED DRUGS

IV saline (salt water) fluids

FOLLOW-UP

PATIENT MONITORING

- The doctor will see the patient often, if hospitalization is required.
- For minor cases of heat injury, no follow-up may be needed.
- See the doctor as often as necessary.

PREVENTION

- Avoid dehydration with proper fluids during activity or exercise: 8 oz of fluid for every 15 minutes of moderate exercise.
- Allow acclimatization to hot weather through proper conditioning and activity modification.
- Dress appropriately with loose-fitting, open-weave, light-colored clothing.
- Maintain as much skin exposure as possible in hot, humid conditions, while using proper sun block protection.
- Recognize the signs and symptoms of heat stress and act accordingly.

COMPLICATIONS

- Major organ system failure
- Irregular heart rhythms or heart attack
- Pulmonary conditions
- Coma, seizures
- Acute kidney failure
- Bleeding disorders
- Liver disease

WHAT TO EXPECT

- Recovery is good when mental function is not altered. Recovery occurs within 24 to 48 hours in most cases.
- The death rate for heat stroke (10% to 80%) is directly related to the duration and intensity of injury, as well as to the speed and effectiveness of treatment.

 ## MISCELLANEOUS

PEDIATRIC

Children are susceptible to heat injury.

GERIATRIC

The elderly are susceptible to heat injury.

PREGNANCY

Pregnant women may be more susceptible to dehydration.

Heat Exhaustion and Heat Stroke

Doctor
Office
Phone
Pager

Special notes to patient:

Hemorrhoids

 ## BASICS

DESCRIPTION

Hemorrhoids, or piles, are varicose or enlarged veins of the rectum. They can occur internally or externally. Hemorrhoids can be acute (of short duration), chronic (long-lasting), or relapsing.

SIGNS AND SYMPTOMS

- Rectal bleeding
- Anal protrusion
- Anal pain
- Itching
- Constipation
- Straining with defecation
- Bowel incontinence
- Blood or mucus in stool
- Sensation of incomplete emptying of the bowel
- Anal fissure
- Anal infection
- Anal ulceration

CAUSES

Dilated veins of rectum

SCOPE

Common

MOST OFTEN AFFECTED

Hemorrhoids primarily affect adults, although they can occur at any age. Males and females are affected with equal frequency.

RISK FACTORS

- Pregnancy
- Colon cancer
- Liver disease
- Constipation
- Occupations that require prolonged sitting
- Loss of muscle tone in old age, rectal surgery, episiotomy, anal intercourse
- Obesity

 ## DIAGNOSIS

WHAT THE DOCTOR LOOKS FOR

The doctor will perform a physical examination to identify the presence of hemorrhoids.

TESTS AND PROCEDURES

The colon can be examined by anoscopy or sigmoidoscopy.

 ## TREATMENT

GENERAL MEASURES

- Hemorrhoids are managed in the outpatient setting, except when surgery is required.
- Mild symptoms or prevention:
  - Avoid prolonged sitting on toilet
  - Avoid straining
  - Avoid constipation by using stool softeners
  - Use soap and water for clean-up after stool
- For pain: sitz baths with soapy water or Epson salts
- Surgery may be needed for persistent and severe disease.
- Other treatments include incision of hemorrhoid, rubber band ligation, injection therapy, cryosurgery, and laser surgery.

ACTIVITY

- No restrictions
- Physical fitness is encouraged.
- Avoid prolonged sitting and straining on the toilet.

DIET

High-fiber diet

 ## MEDICATIONS

COMMONLY PRESCRIBED DRUGS

- Prevention:
  - Fiber supplements
  - Stool softeners
- Pain:
  - Analgesic sprays or ointments: benzocaine (Hurricane), dibucaine (Nupercainal)
- Itching
  - Hydrocortisone ointment (Anusol-HC; Cortifoam)
- Bleeding:
  - Astringent suppositories (Preparation H)
  - Hydrocortisone ointment (Anusol; Cortifoam)

CONTRAINDICATIONS

Read drug product information.

PRECAUTIONS

Read drug product information.

DRUG INTERACTIONS

Read drug product information.

 ## FOLLOW-UP

PATIENT MONITORING

See the doctor as often as needed, depending on treatment.

PREVENTION

- Avoid constipation
- Lose weight, if overweight
- Avoid prolonged sitting on the toilet.
- Avoid prolonged sitting, especially at work; get up and move around periodically.

COMPLICATIONS

- Thrombosis
- Infection
- Ulcers
- Anemia (rare)
- Incontinence

WHAT TO EXPECT

- Spontaneous improvement
- Recurrence

MISCELLANEOUS

PEDIATRIC

Hemorrhoids are uncommon in infants and children. Occasionally, hemorrhoids result from chronic constipation, fecal impaction, and straining at stool. Surgery is rarely required.

GERIATRIC

Hemorrhoids are common in the elderly, along with rectal prolapse.

PREGNANCY

Hemorrhoids are common in pregnancy, and they usually resolve after pregnancy. No treatment is required unless they are extremely painful.

Hemorrhoids

Doctor
Office
Phone
Pager

Special notes to patient:

Hepatitis, Viral

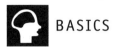 ## BASICS

DESCRIPTION
Viral hepatitis is a group of viral infections involving the liver.

SCOPE
- Hepatitis A virus (HAV): 50% of people above 49 years of age have been exposed; HAV is found in 25% of cases of acute hepatitis.
- Hepatitis B virus (HBV): About 200,000 persons are infected annually; more than 500,000 persons are carriers of HBV.
- Hepatitis C virus (HCV): HCV is becoming the most common cause of acute and chronic viral hepatitis; 150,000 persons are infected annually.

MOST OFTEN AFFECTED
Hepatitis occurs in all age groups. It is rare in infants, and susceptibility increases with age. Males are affected more often than females.

SIGNS AND SYMPTOMS
- Fever
- Malaise, fatigue
- Nausea
- Loss of appetite
- Jaundice
- Dark urine
- Abdominal pains
- Headache
- Vomiting

CAUSES
- Viral infection
- Multiple, different viruses can cause infection.
- Maximal infectivity occurs 2 weeks before the appearance of jaundice.
- Transmitted sexually, by blood or its products, or during pregnancy

RISK FACTORS
- Healthcare workers or other occupational risks
- Dialysis
- Recipients of blood, blood products
- Intravenous (IV) drug users; individuals with tattoos
- Sexually active homosexual males
- Household exposure
- Unprotected sex
- Needle stick
- Organ transplantation

 ## DIAGNOSIS

WHAT THE DOCTOR LOOKS FOR
- The doctor will perform a physical examination to identify the signs and symptoms of viral hepatitis.
- Other causes of similar symptoms include Infectious mononucleosis, drug or alcohol abuse, and other liver disorders.

TESTS AND PROCEDURES
- Blood tests
- Tests can be done to identify virus.
- A sample of liver tissue can be obtained for laboratory analysis.
- Ultrasound can be used to assist with diagnosis.

 ## TREATMENT

GENERAL MEASURES
- Viral hepatitis is usually managed on an outpatient basis.
- Hospitalization may be required.
- Segregation is advised for food handlers or healthcare workers.
- Acute cases must be reported to public health department.
- Liver transplantation may be necessary.

ACTIVITY
As tolerated

DIET
Adequate calories; balanced nutrition

 ## MEDICATIONS

COMMONLY PRESCRIBED DRUGS
- Interferon, ribavirin (Virazole)
- Amantadine (Symmetrel)
- Steroids

CONTRAINDICATIONS
Read drug product information.

PRECAUTIONS
- Bleeding disorders, immune system disorders, seizures, pregnancy, fertile age group, lactation.
- Read drug product information.

DRUG INTERACTIONS
Read drug product information.

OTHER DRUGS

 ## FOLLOW-UP

PATIENT MONITORING
- See the doctor as often as necessary.
- Blood tests will be periodically repeated.
- Biopsy of liver may need to be repeated in chronic cases.
- Monitoring for metabolic complications

PREVENTION
- Use safe sex practices.
- Do not share needles.
- Practice good sanitation habits.
- It is currently recommended that all individuals receive vaccination against HBV.
- Vaccination against HAV is recommended for some individuals, including travelers, sewage workers, military personnel, daycare staff and children, homosexual men, and food handlers.

COMPLICATIONS
Severe liver disease, cancer, or failure

WHAT TO EXPECT
- The outcome varies, depending on the virus causing hepatitis.
- Severity of liver disease is a good indicator of outcome.
- Can progress to chronic disease

 ## MISCELLANEOUS

OTHERS
Alcohol abuse is a major factor for chronic liver disease.

PREGNANCY
Hepatitis virus can be transmitted to babies. Pregnant women should be screened for HBV.

Hepatitis, Viral

Doctor
Office
Phone
Pager

Special notes to patient:

Herpes Simplex

 ## BASICS

DESCRIPTION
Herpes simplex is a viral disease that usually causes painful blisters in clusters on the skin, cornea, or mucous membranes. Herpes simplex can occur in other, more serious forms. Newborns or individuals with immune system disorders are at greater risk of complications or death.

SIGNS AND SYMPTOMS
- Blisters: usually cluster and open as painful ulcerated lesions, often with a reddened base
- Variations include:
  - Infection on a finger: intense itching and pain, followed by blisters that can merge; accompanied by swelling, reddening, and pain; heals over 2 to 3 weeks
  - Fever; sore, swollen, and reddened throat; small blisters on throat and mouth, rapidly increasing to involve roof of mouth, cheek, tongue, and often lips and cheeks; resolves in 10 to 14 days
  - Genital herpes: see *Herpes, Genital*
  - Infection of eye or lid; lasts 2 to 3 weeks
  - Diffuse rash-like eruption
  - Newborn infection; life-threatening and usually acquired by vaginal birth of infected mother
- Recurring diseases include:
  - Recurrent lesions on lips; usually less than one recurrence per 6 months, but 5% to 25% may have more than one attack per month; may be precipitated by sunlight, fever, trauma, menstruation, stress; pain, burning, itching can last 6 to 48 hours before blisters appear, often at edge of lip; will ulcerate and crust within 48 hours; heals within 8 to 10 days
  - Eye infection: may affect cornea, eye lid, or whites of eye; ulcers, vision loss; may cause permanent visual loss
  - Genital herpes: see *Herpes, Genital*

CAUSES
Infection with herpes simplex virus

SCOPE
- Herpes infection is widespread; up to 20% of adults may be contagious.
- From 30% to 100% of population subgroups have been exposed to herpes simplex virus.

MOST OFTEN AFFECTED
Herpes affects all ages, males and females in equal proportion.

RISK FACTORS
- Immune system disorders
- Newborns: if exposed to infected mother during birth canal or if exposed in nursery
- Prior herpes infection
- Sexual intercourse with infected person
- Occupational exposure (healthcare worker)

 ## DIAGNOSIS

WHAT THE DOCTOR LOOKS FOR
- The doctor will complete a physical examination to look for the signs of herpes infection.
- Other conditions that may appear similar include impetigo and numerous other skin diseases.

TESTS AND PROCEDURES
- Fluid from a blister can be sampled for laboratory analysis.
- A sample of skin can be obtained by biopsy.
- Tests for other sexually transmitted diseases can be performed.

 ## TREATMENT

GENERAL MEASURES
- Herpes is managed on an outpatient basis.
- Intermittent, cool, moist dressings
- Genital herpes: Painful urination may be helped by pouring a cup of warm water over the genitals while urinating, or sitting in a warm bath to urinate.

ACTIVITY
No restrictions

DIET
Avoid acidic foods if mouth is involved.

 ## MEDICATIONS

COMMONLY PRESCRIBED DRUGS
- Acyclovir (Zovirax)
- Valacyclovir (Valtrex)
- Famciclovir (Famvir)
- Penciclovir (Denavir)

CONTRAINDICATIONS
Allergy to or intolerance of drug

PRECAUTIONS
Numerous precautions; read drug product information.

DRUG INTERACTIONS
Read drug product information.

OTHER DRUGS
- Foscarnet
- Other topical medications: Acyclovir, vidarabine (Vira-A), idoxuridine and trifluorothymidine

 ## FOLLOW-UP

PATIENT MONITORING
See the doctor as often as necessary.

PREVENTION
- Avoid contact with newborns or individuals with immune system disorders.
- Wash hands often.
- For genital herpes: Avoid sexual contact while disease is active; condoms can reduce the risk of transmission but are not perfect; maintain mutually monogamous sexual relations.

COMPLICATIONS
- Brain infection or inflammation
- Pneumonia
- Blood poisoning

WHAT TO EXPECT
- Good for treatment of recurrent episodes
- Expect frequent recurrences.

 ## MISCELLANEOUS

GERIATRIC
Decreased immune response of old age can increase risk of herpes.

PREGNANCY
Cesarean section may be required, if lesions are active during labor.

Herpes Simplex

Doctor
Office
Phone
Pager

Special notes to patient:

Herpes, Genital

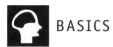 ## BASICS

DESCRIPTION
Genital herpes is caused by herpes simplex virus infection of the genital organs.

SIGNS AND SYMPTOMS
- Of individuals infected with herpes simplex, 60% to 70% show no symptoms.
- Fever
- Headache
- Malaise
- Muscle ache and pain
- Burning genital pain
- Painful urination
- Pain during intercourse
- Numbness or tingling of the lower back
- Swollen glands in groin
- Urinary retention
- Blisters: Blisters appear on a swollen, reddened base; they ulcerate, crust over, and heal within 21 days. Blisters persist longer on dry skin.
- Recurrent genital herpes: Symptoms (burning, numbness, tingling of skin) can occur at the site of old lesion about 24 hours before the eruption of new blisters.

SCOPE
Up to one third of the population in the United States is infected with herpes; 300,000 to 700,000 new cases occur annually.

MOST OFTEN AFFECTED
Individuals 18 to 40 years of age, females more frequently than males

RISK FACTORS
- Sexual activity
- Clothing, wet towels (rare)
- Triggers (recurrent)
  - Genital trauma
  - Menstrual period
  - Infection
  - Emotional stress
  - Sunlight

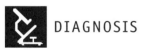 ## DIAGNOSIS

WHAT THE DOCTOR LOOKS FOR
- The doctor will perform a physical examination to identify the presence of genital herpes.
- The doctor will also look for conditions known to be associated with genital herpes, including other sexually transmitted diseases.

TESTS AND PROCEDURES
- Blood tests
- A sample of blister fluid can be obtained for laboratory analysis.
- Pap smear

 ## TREATMENT

GENERAL MEASURES
- Genital herpes is managed in the outpatient setting.
- Most care of genital herpes is self-care.
- Cool compresses, ice packs to perineum, sitz baths
- Local perineal hygiene
- Analgesics: nonsteroidal antiinflammatory drugs (NSAIDs)
- Topical anesthetics: lidocaine

ACTIVITY
- Avoid intercourse in the presence of genital lesions.
- Appropriate rest, if systemic symptoms are present

DIET
No special diet

 ## MEDICATIONS

COMMONLY PRESCRIBED DRUGS
Acyclovir (Zovirax)

CONTRAINDICATIONS
Allergy to acyclovir

PRECAUTIONS
Acyclovir is not approved for routine use in pregnancy; drug is excreted in breast milk.

DRUG INTERACTIONS
Drugs have many interactions; read drug product information.

OTHER DRUGS
- Acyclovir topical ointment: less effective
- Foscarnet
- Vidarabine
- Famciclovir (Famvir)
- Valacyclovir (Valtrex)

 ## FOLLOW-UP

PATIENT MONITORING
- Acute episode: See the doctor if complications develop.
- Latent infection: annual Pap smear

PREVENTION
- Use condoms and spermicide during sexual intercourse.
- Avoid multiple sexual partners.
- Avoid stress, when possible.

COMPLICATIONS
- Vaginal discharge
- Bacterial infection
- Urinary retention
- Meningitis
- Transmission to baby
- Increased risk for human immunodeficiency virus (HIV) infection

WHAT TO EXPECT
- Resolution of signs and symptoms in 14 to 21 days; recurring episodes heal in 7 to 10 days
- Blisters recur in more than 50% of infected individuals; individuals with immune system disorders average three to four episodes per year.

MISCELLANEOUS

PEDIATRIC
Genital herpes in a child may be a sign of sexual abuse.

PREGNANCY
- First episode of genital herpes infection during pregnancy is associated with an increased rate of miscarriage and preterm labor.
- Greatest risk for neonatal infection occurs at time of delivery.
- Cesarean section may be required.
- Acyclovir therapy can be considered for women with genital herpes who are beyond 36 weeks of their pregnancy.

FURTHER INFORMATION
Herpes Resource Center ASHA/HRC, P.O. Box 13827, Research Triangle Park, North Carolina 27709-9940, HRC Hotline (919) 361-8488; web page http://sunsite.unc.edu./ASHA/

Herpes, Genital

Doctor
Office
Phone
Pager

Special notes to patient:

Hirsutism

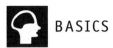 BASICS

DESCRIPTION

- Hirsutism is excessive hair growth because of increased male hormones.
- Often accompanied by menstrual irregularities
- Virilization involves extreme masculinization effects (e.g., deep voice, enlarged clitoris, balding).

SIGNS AND SYMPTOMS

- Hair thickens and darkens in "male" pattern (i.e., beard, moustache, chest hair).
- Usually accompanied by irregular menstruation and absence of ovulation
- Usually accompanied by acne
- May be accompanied by infertility
- Onset is usually gradual.

CAUSES

- Hormone disorder
- Ovarian disease
- Ovarian cancer

SCOPE

Hirsutism affects about 8% of adult women.

MOST OFTEN AFFECTED

Females, after puberty

RISK FACTORS

- Family history of hirsutism
- Absence of ovulation

 DIAGNOSIS

WHAT THE DOCTOR LOOKS FOR

- The doctor will perform a thorough physical examination to evaluate hirsutism and identify the cause.
- Other conditions known to be associated with hirsutism should be identified and treated (e.g., acne).

TESTS AND PROCEDURES

- A number of blood tests can be performed to assist with diagnosis.
- Computed tomography (CT) scan or ultrasound can be used to assess the reproductive tract.
- A sample of uterine tissue can be obtained by biopsy for laboratory analysis.
- Other specialized diagnostic testing can be done.

GENERAL MEASURES

- Hirsutism is managed in the outpatient setting.
- Cosmetic measures include plucking, bleaching, shaving, electrolysis, and cover-up cosmetics.
- Treatment is slow and often lifelong.
- Ovulation may need to be induced if pregnancy is desired.
- Use contraception as needed.
- Maintain ideal weight.
- Treat accompanying acne.

ACTIVITY

No special activity

DIET

No special diet

 MEDICATIONS

COMMONLY PRESCRIBED DRUGS

Oral contraceptives: estrogen, progesterone, medroxyprogesterone (Depo-Provera)
Dexamethasone

CONTRAINDICATIONS

Avoid medications in pregnancy.

OTHER DRUGS

Antiandrogenic drugs: spironolactone, cyproterone, flutamide, ketoconazole, leuprolide (Lupron), danazol, metformin

 FOLLOW-UP

PATIENT MONITORING

See the doctor as often as needed to monitor drug therapy.

PREVENTION

- Tumor must be ruled out.
- As hormone balance improves, fertility may increase; use contraception as needed.
- Avoid quackery and unlicensed electrolysis.

COMPLICATIONS

- Uterine bleeding and anemia
- Hormone excess can affect lipids, cardiac disease risk, and bone density.
- Poor self-image, shame

WHAT TO EXPECT

- Treatment takes 6 to 24 months and can be lifelong.
- Excellent outcome with long-term therapy for halting further hair growth
- Moderate to poor outcome for reversing current hair growth

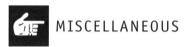 MISCELLANEOUS

GERIATRIC

Can occur after menopause

PREGNANCY

Hirsutism may be accompanied by infertility.

Hirsutism

Doctor
Office
Phone
Pager

Special notes to patient:

HIV Infection and AIDS

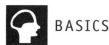 BASICS

DESCRIPTION

The human immunodeficiency virus (HIV) infects immune system cells, causing cell death and a decline in immune function. As a result, a person infected with HIV eventually develops acquired immunodeficiency syndrome (AIDS), which includes opportunistic infections, cancer, and neurologic lesions. HIV appears to have direct effects on the central nervous system, the gastrointestinal tract, and other systems.

SIGNS AND SYMPTOMS

- Chronic infection with variable course (50% of persons develop AIDS within 10 years)
- Acute infection: fever, rash, muscle aches, and malaise; this self-limited syndrome occurs about 6 to 8 weeks after infection
- Following infection is a variable period of time without symptoms.
- Lymph node enlargement persisting longer than 3 months
- Other diseases:
  - ▸ Constitutional: fever lasting more than 1 month, weight loss, persistent diarrhea, skin rash, severe chronic fatigue
  - ▸ Neurologic disease: dementia, nerve disorders
  - ▸ AIDS-defining opportunistic infections: *Pneumocystis carinii* pneumonia (PCP); toxoplasmosis, candidiasis, tuberculosis, other infections
  - ▸ Cancers: Kaposi's sarcoma, non-Hodgkin's lymphoma, other cancers

CAUSES

Human immunodeficiency virus (HIV)

SCOPE

More than 500,000 current cases of AIDS and more than 300,000 deaths have occured in the United States.

MOST OFTEN AFFECTED

Young adults 25 to 44 years of age; men are affected more frequently than women.

RISK FACTORS

- Sexual activity: Homosexual men are at greatest risk, but all sexually active people are at risk, depending on the risk factors of, and number of sexual partners.
- Intravenous (IV) drug use (sharing of contaminated needles)
- Recipients of blood products
- Hemophiliacs who have received pooled plasma products are at high risk.
- Children of HIV-infected women
- Healthcare workers' greatest risk is needle stick.

 DIAGNOSIS

WHAT THE DOCTOR LOOKS FOR

- The doctor will perform a physical examination to identify any of the conditions associated with HIV infection or AIDS.
- The doctor should screen for HIV infection in cases of prolonged illness without a ready explanation.

TESTS AND PROCEDURES

- Blood tests. CD4 cells (the cells infected and destroyed by HIV) are counted; CD4 cell count gives an indication of the severity of HIV infection.
- Any number of radiology procedures or special tests can be done to assist in diagnosis, depending on the nature of opportunistic infections or other conditions.

 TREATMENT

GENERAL MEASURES

- HIV infection is managed by a primary care provider in an outpatient setting.
- Infectious disease or HIV specialist may be involved in acute episodes.
- Depending on CD4 cell counts, individuals with HIV infection may receive antiviral therapy or preventive treatment for PCP, toxoplasmosis, or *Mycobacterium avium complex*.

ACTIVITY

Regular exercise is encouraged. Many community HIV groups have organized "wellness" activities.

DIET

- Good nutrition is encouraged.
- Avoid raw eggs, unpasteurized milk, and other potentially contaminated foods.
- Vitamin supplements may be required.

 MEDICATIONS

COMMONLY PRESCRIBED DRUGS

- Didanosine (ddI, Videx), lamivudine (3TC, Epivir), stavudine (d4T, Zerit), zalcitabine (ddC, Hivid), zidovudine (AZT, Retrovir), Abacavir (ABC, Ziagen)
- Indinavir (Crixivan), ritonavir (Norvir), saquinavir (Fortovase), amprenavir (Agenerase)
- Nevirapine (Viramune), efavirenz (Sustiva), delaviridine (Rescriptor)

CONTRAINDICATIONS

Significant drug interactions; read drug product information.

PRECAUTIONS

Antiretroviral drugs have significant toxicities; read drug product information.

DRUG INTERACTIONS

Drugs have potentially life-threatening interactions; read drug product information.

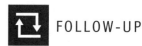 FOLLOW-UP

PATIENT MONITORING

- See the doctor as frequently as needed, based on the person's health, psychological status, and the need to monitor drug therapy.
- Blood tests every 3 to 6 months.

PREVENTION

- Avoid unscreened blood products.
- Avoid unprotected sexual intercourse.
- Use condoms.
- Avoid injection drug abuse.
- Avoid contact with body fluids of HIV-infected individuals.

COMPLICATIONS

- Immune system deficiency
- Opportunistic infections
- Neuropsychiatric symptoms
- HIV-associated cancers

HIV Infection and AIDS

	Doctor
	Office
	Phone
	Pager

Special notes to patient:

HIV Infection and AIDS

WHAT TO EXPECT

- When HIV infection leads to AIDS, life expectancy is 2 to 3 years.
- AIDS-defining opportunistic infections usually do not develop until CD4 counts are less than 200.
- CD4 counts decline at a rate of 50 to 80 per year, with more rapid decline as counts drop below 200.

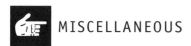# MISCELLANEOUS

PEDIATRIC

Progresses more rapidly in infants

GERIATRIC

Progresses more rapidly in individuals above 50 years of age

PREGNANCY

The risk of bacterial pneumonia may be increased during pregnancy, and the risk of premature birth is also increased in HIV-infected women. Zidovudine (AZT) has been shown to decrease the risk of HIV transmission to infants.

FURTHER INFORMATION

- National AIDS Hotline (800) 342-2437 [Spanish (800) 342-7432]
- National Institute of Health AIDS Clinical Trials Group (800) 874-2572; Information on AIDS/HIV clinical trials
- American Foundation for AIDS Research: (212) 719-0033; new treatments and research

HIV Infection and AIDS

	Doctor
	Office
	Phone
	Pager

Special notes to patient:

Hodgkin's Disease

 ## BASICS

DESCRIPTION
Hodgkin's disease is a cancer of the lymph system.

SIGNS AND SYMPTOMS
- Painless, enlarged lymph nodes
- Fever
- Night sweats
- Weight loss
- Fatigue
- Loss of appetite
- Unexplained itching

CAUSES
Unknown

SCOPE
About 7,900 new cases of Hodgkin's disease occur annually in the United States.

MOST OFTEN AFFECTED
Hodgkin's disease peaks at age 20 and 70 years. It is more common in males than females, and it may be inherited.

RISK FACTORS
Immune system disorder

 ## DIAGNOSIS

WHAT THE DOCTOR LOOKS FOR
- The doctor will perform a physical examination to identify the signs and symptoms of Hodgkin's disease.
- Other similar-appearing conditions include other types of cancer, sarcoidosis, or drug reaction.

TESTS AND PROCEDURES
- Blood tests
- Chest x-ray study
- Computed tomography (CT) scan of the chest, abdomen, and pelvis may be done.
- Specialized radiology procedures can be done, including lymphangiogram, gallium scan, and bone scan.
- Ultrasound can be used to assist in diagnosis.
- A sample of liver or lymph tissue can be obtained for laboratory analysis.
- A sample of bone marrow can be obtained for laboratory analysis.
- Exploratory surgery may be necessary to assess the extent of disease.

 ## TREATMENT

GENERAL MEASURES
- Hodgkin's disease can be managed in the inpatient or outpatient setting.
- Hospitalization may be required.
- The disease will be "staged" to define its nature.
- Treatment is aimed at cure with minimal toxicity.
- Treatment can be radiation, chemotherapy, or a combination.
- Bone marrow transplantation may be required.

ACTIVITY
As tolerated

DIET
No restrictions

 ## MEDICATIONS

COMMONLY PRESCRIBED DRUGS
- MOPP chemotherapy
  - Mechlorethamine (Mustargen)
  - Vincristine (Oncovin)
  - Procarbazine
  - Prednisone
- "ABVD" chemotherapy
  - Doxorubicin (Adriamycin)
  - Bleomycin
  - Vinblastine
  - Dacarbazine

CONTRAINDICATIONS
Read drug product information.

PRECAUTIONS
Read drug product information.

DRUG INTERACTIONS
Read drug product information.

 ## FOLLOW-UP

PATIENT MONITORING
See the doctor as often as necessary for health status monitoring.

COMPLICATIONS
- Secondary cancers
- Sterility
- Hypothyroidism
- Bone marrow suppression
- Infections
- Anemia
- Bleeding disorders
- Heart disease
- Lung disease

WHAT TO EXPECT
Hodgkin's disease has a 75% overall survival rate.

 ## MISCELLANEOUS

PREGNANCY
- If fertility is maintained after treatment, pregnancy can be normal.
- Pregnancy is not known to have a negative impact on the course of Hodgkin's disease.
- Hodgkin's disease is not known to adversely affect the pregnancy or fetus if treatment can be postponed until delivery.
- Disease can progress during pregnancy if treatment is delayed.

FURTHER INFORMATION
Leukemia Society of America, 733 3rd Avenue, New York, NY 10017, (212) 573-8484

Hodgkin's Disease

Doctor
Office
Phone
Pager

Special notes to patient:

Huntington's Chorea

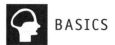 ## BASICS

DESCRIPTION

Huntington's chorea is an inherited disease characterized by dementia and spasmodic muscle movement. It has a gradual onset and slow progression. Symptoms usually do not develop until after 30 years of age. By the time the disease is diagnosed, the patient has usually had children and passed the disease to another generation.

SIGNS AND SYMPTOMS

- Spasmodic, involuntary movement of the limb and facial muscles
- Difficulty swallowing
- Difficulty speaking
- Impaired memory, judgment
- Intellectual decline
- Emotional disturbances, mood swings
- Depression
- Anxiety
- Mania
- Delusions
- Agitation, aggression
- Urinary incontinence
- Bowel incontinence
- Weight loss
- Difficulty walking
- Unsteadiness
- Hyperkinesia
- Abnormal eye movements
- Facial twitching
- Apathy, withdrawal
- Dementia
- Rigidity
- Hallucinations
- Delusions
- Paranoia
- Impulsiveness

CAUSES

Hereditary genetic defect

SCOPE

Approximately four to eight cases of Huntington's chorea per 100,000 people occur in the United States annually.

MOST OFTEN AFFECTED

Individuals 16 to 75 years of age, males and females in equal frequency

RISK FACTORS

Family history

 ## DIAGNOSIS

WHAT THE DOCTOR LOOKS FOR

- The doctor will perform a physical examination to identify the signs and symptoms of Huntington's chorea.
- The doctor may take a detailed family medical history.

TESTS AND PROCEDURES

- Blood tests
- Genetic tests
- Special imaging procedures can be used to assist in diagnosis, including computed tomography (CT) scan, magnetic resonance imaging (MRI), or positron emission tomography (PET).

 ## TREATMENT

GENERAL MEASURES

- Huntington's chorea is managed in the outpatient setting.
- Genetic counseling should be considered.
- Electroconvulsive therapy (ECT) can be considered for drug-resistant depression.
- Speech and occupational therapy may be of benefit.

ACTIVITY

Full activity as long as possible

DIET

No special diet, but soft diet with liquid supplements may be needed.

 ## MEDICATIONS

COMMONLY PRESCRIBED DRUGS

Haloperidol (Haldol)

CONTRAINDICATIONS

Read drug product information.

PRECAUTIONS

Can cause reactions; read drug product information.

DRUG INTERACTIONS

Read drug product information.

OTHER DRUGS

- Reserpine
- Tetrabenazine
- Tricyclic antidepressants
- Antipsychotics

 ## FOLLOW-UP

PATIENT MONITORING

See the doctor as often as necessary.

PREVENTION

Genetic counseling

COMPLICATIONS

- Choking
- Brain injury
- Spasmodic muscle movement
- Personality changes
- Dementia
- Death
- Suicide

WHAT TO EXPECT

The outcome is poor; disease leads to progressive impairment and is fatal within 20 years.

 ## MISCELLANEOUS

PEDIATRIC

Usually does not occur until after puberty

GERIATRIC

Usually fatal before reaching old age

FURTHER INFORMATION

Newsletter and printed information available from: Huntington's Disease Society of America, 140 W. 22nd St., 6th Fl., New York, NY 10011-2420, (212) 242-1968; fax (212) 243-2443

Huntington's Chorea

Doctor
Office
Phone
Pager

Special notes to patient:

Hypertension, Essential

BASICS

DESCRIPTION

Essential hypertension is the sustained elevation of blood pressure (systolic blood pressure 140 millimeters of mercury [mm Hg] or greater, diastolic blood pressure of 90 mm Hg or greater, or both). Hypertension is a strong risk factor for cardiovascular disease. Essential hypertension is also known as benign, idiopathic, familial, genetic, or chronic hypertension. It is sometimes referred to simply as "high blood pressure."

SIGNS AND SYMPTOMS

- Hypertension typically causes no symptoms, except in extreme cases or after related cardiovascular complications.
- Hypertension can cause headaches, especially at higher blood pressures. Headaches are commonly felt in the back of the head and are present on awakening.
- Retina damage caused by hypertension may be observed by the doctor.

CAUSES

- More than 90% of hypertension has no identified cause. This type of hypertension is called "essential" or "primary hypertension."
- Secondary causes of hypertension include:
  - Kidney disease
  - Hormonal disorders
  - Blood vessel conditions
  - Chemical: drugs, industrial substances

SCOPE

Hypertension affects 50 million Americans, or about 20% of the adult population.

MOST OFTEN AFFECTED

Essential hypertension usually occurs in individuals in their 20s and 30s. It is more common in men than women. Blood pressure tends to run higher in males. Most importantly, men have a significantly higher risk of cardiovascular disease at any given blood pressure. Blood pressure levels appear to run in families, but no clear genetic pattern has been identified.

RISK FACTORS

- Family history of hypertension or cardiovascular disease
- Obesity
- Alcohol consumption
- Excess dietary sodium
- Stress
- Physical inactivity

WHAT PHYSICIAN LOOKS FOR

The doctor will take a complete history and thoroughly examine the patient to assess physical condition. The examination should include evaluation of the heart and pulses, the abdomen, and the eyes. A diagnosis of hypertension is made if the average of at least three properly performed blood pressure measurements exceeds 90 mm Hg diastolic or 160 mm Hg systolic. The doctor will look for potential cardiovascular, cerebrovascular, and renal disease as well as diabetes.

TESTS AND PROCEDURES

- Blood workup includes a complete blood count and chemistry tests.
- Complete urinalysis (sometimes reveals proteinuria)
- Chest x-ray study
- Tests can be performed to assess the kidney (e.g., an intravenous pyelogram [IVP] or a renal arteriogram).
- Special urine tests may be ordered.
- Special imaging can be done to assess blood vessels.
- The kidney can be biopsied if disease is suspected.
- An electrocardiogram (ECG) can be done to evaluate the heart.

TREATMENT

GENERAL MEASURES

- Hypertension is generally treated on an outpatient basis.
- The goal of treatment is to achieve a blood pressure diastolic less than 90 mm Hg and systolic less than 160 mm Hg.
- Treatment should be individualized, based on risk factors.
- Obese persons may significantly lower blood pressure by reducing weight.
- Smoking cessation is an important part of a cardiovascular risk reduction program.
- Biofeedback and relaxation exercises may reduce blood pressures.

ACTIVITY

Normal activity with an appropriate aerobic fitness program

DIET

- A reduced-salt diet may benefit some patients.
- Alcohol consumption should be reduced to less than 1 oz/day.
- Decrease saturated fats and increase monounsaturated fats in the diet.
- Potassium and calcium supplements may be helpful.

MEDICATIONS

COMMONLY PRESCRIBED DRUGS

- First-line choices of drugs include the following categories and their representatives:
  - Diuretics (hydrochlorothiazide, chlorthalidone, indapamide)
  - Alpha-adrenergic agents (prazosin, terazosin, doxazosin)
  - Angiotensin-converting enzyme (ACE) inhibitors (captopril, enalapril, fosinopril, lisinopril, ramipril, quinapril, benazepril)
  - Angiotensin II receptor blocker (losartan)
  - Calcium channel blockers (diltiazem, felodipine, isradipine, nicardipine, nifedipine, nitrendipine, verapamil, amlodipine)
  - Beta-blockers (acebutolol, atenolol, metoprolol, nadolol, penbutolol, pindolol, propranolol, timolol, betaxolol, bisoprolol)

CONTRAINDICATIONS

- Diuretics may worsen gout and diabetes.
- Beta-blockers may be contraindicated in reactive airway disease (asthma), heart failure, heart block, diabetes, and peripheral vascular disease.
- Diltiazem or verapamil should be used cautiously with heart failure or block.

PRECAUTIONS

See product information.

DRUG INTERACTIONS

See product information.

OTHER DRUGS

- Other drugs may be used in combination with those listed above:
  - Centrally acting adrenergic inhibitors (clonidine, guanabenz, guanfacine, methyldopa)
  - Peripherally acting adrenergic inhibitors (guanadrel, guanethidine, reserpine labetalol)
  - Vasodilators (hydralazine, minoxidil)
  - Loop diuretics (furosemide, bumetanide, ethacrynic)
  - Potassium-sparing diuretics (amiloride, spironolactone triamterene)
  - Valsartan, irbesartan, candesartan, telmisartan

Hypertension, Essential

Doctor
Office
Phone
Pager

Special notes to patient:

Hypertension, Essential

 FOLLOW-UP

PATIENT MONITORING

- See the doctor at least every 3 to 6 months.
- The effectiveness of treatment should be evaluated.
- Quality of life issues should be considered, including sexual function.

PREVENTION

- Be aware of risks of cardiovascular disease.
- Make healthful changes to diet and lifestyle.
- Maintain an appropriate level of physical activity.
- Reduce or manage stress, and stop smoking.
- Limit consumption of alcoholic beverages.
- Comply with drug regimens and other treatment.
- Hypertension usually causes no symptoms and requires a lifetime of treatment even if you are feeling well.

COMPLICATIONS

- Congestive heart failure
- Myocardial infarction (heart attack)
- Stroke
- Hypertensive heart disease
- Kidney disease
- Eye disease

WHAT TO EXPECT

The outcome of hypertension is good, if adequately controlled.

 MISCELLANEOUS

PEDIATRIC

- Blood pressure should be measured during routine examinations.
- Hypertension can accompany a wide variety of acute and chronic illnesses among children.

GERIATRIC

Isolated systolic hypertension is more common among the elderly. Therapy is effective, although adverse reactions to medications are more frequent.

PREGNANCY

Elevated blood pressure during pregnancy can be either chronic hypertension or preeclampsia. Some medications can adversely affect the fetus.

Hypertension, Essential

Doctor
Office
Phone
Pager

Special notes to patient:

Hyperthyroidism

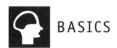 ## BASICS

DESCRIPTION

Hyperthyroidism is caused by the excess production of thyroid hormone. Types of hyperthyroidism include Grave's disease and goiter.

SIGNS AND SYMPTOMS

- In adults:
  - Nervousness
  - Increased sweating
  - Heat intolerance
  - Palpitations and rapid heart rate
  - Difficulty breathing
  - Fatigue and weakness
  - Weight loss
  - Increased appetite
  - Protruding eyes
  - Goiter
  - Tremor
  - Warm and moist skin
  - Mood swings
- In children:
  - Growth abnormalities
  - Eye abnormalities

SCOPE

Hyperthyroidism affects 1 of 1,000 women and 1 of 3,000 men.

MOST OFTEN AFFECTED

Hyperthyroidism can affect any age. It peaks in individuals 20 to 30 years of age. It is more common in females than males.

CAUSES

- Autoimmune disease
- Iodine disturbance
- Unknown

RISK FACTORS

- Positive family history
- Female gender
- Other autoimmune disorders
- Iodide replacement after iodide deprivation

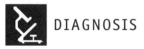 ## DIAGNOSIS

WHAT THE DOCTOR LOOKS FOR

- The doctor will perform a thorough physical examination to identify the presence of hyperthyroidism.
- Other conditions that can cause similar signs and symptoms include anxiety, cancer, diabetes, and other disorders.

TESTS AND PROCEDURES

- Blood tests
- A special radiology procedure called a "thyroid scan" can be done to assist in diagnosis.

 ## TREATMENT

GENERAL MEASURES

- Hyperthyroidism is managed in the outpatient setting, except for treatment of thyroid storm, a life-threatening condition that can cause heart failure, fever, and mania.
- Treatment consists of antithyroid drugs, therapeutic iodine.
- Surgery may be required (rare).

ACTIVITY

Modified according to severity of disease

DIET

Sufficient calories to prevent weight loss

 ## MEDICATIONS

COMMONLY PRESCRIBED DRUGS

- Propylthiouracil (PTU)
- Methimazole (Tapazole)
- Radioiodine therapy: sodium iodine131 (Iodotope I-131).
- Beta-blocker: propranolol (Inderal)

CONTRAINDICATIONS

- Radioiodine therapy: pregnancy and nursing
- Propranolol: congestive heart failure, asthma, chronic bronchitis, pregnancy, hypoglycemia

PRECAUTIONS

- Can cause dermatitis or liver damage
- Radioiodine therapy often causes permanent hypothyroidism and can cause birth defects if given during pregnancy.

DRUG INTERACTIONS

Oral blood-thinners (anticoagulants)

OTHER DRUGS

Ipodate sodium (Oragrafin)

 ## FOLLOW-UP

PATIENT MONITORING

- See the doctor as often as necessary.
- Repeat blood tests twice a year
- After radioiodine therapy, blood tests at 6 weeks, 12 weeks, 6 months, and annually thereafter

COMPLICATIONS

- Hypoparathyroidism
- Hypothyroidism
- Visual loss or double vision
- Cardiac failure in the elderly with underlying heart disease
- Muscle wasting

WHAT TO EXPECT

With precise diagnosis and adequate treatment, the outcome of treatment is good.

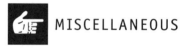 ## MISCELLANEOUS

GERIATRIC

- Characteristic symptoms and signs may be absent in elderly.
- Harder to diagnose
- Cardiac failure more likely

PREGNANCY

- Symptoms can be confusing.
- Radioiodine therapy is absolutely contraindicated.

Hyperthyroidism

Doctor
Office
Phone
Pager

Special notes to patient:

Hypothermia

 ## BASICS

DESCRIPTION

Hypothermia occurs when the core body temperature falls below 95°F (35°C). It can take several hours or several days to develop. As the body temperature falls, all organ systems are affected. Blood flow to the brain decreases and the metabolic rate declines rapidly. Patients who have been immersed for as long as 45 minutes in very cold water and appear to be dead have been resuscitated.

SIGNS AND SYMPTOMS

- Mild (93.2°F to 95°F; 34°C to 35°C):
  - Lethargy
  - Mild confusion
  - Shivering
  - Loss of fine motor coordination
  - Increased pulse and blood pressure
- Moderate (86°F to 93.2°F; 30° to 34°C):
  - Delirium
  - Slow heart rate
  - Low blood pressure
  - Slow breathing rate
  - Bluish discoloration around lips, eyes, and nail beds
  - Irregular heart rhythm
  - Semicoma and coma
  - Muscular rigidity
  - Generalized swelling
- Severe (< 86°F; 30°C):
  - Very cold skin
  - Rigidity
  - No breathing
  - No pulse
  - Unresponsive
  - Fixed pupils

CAUSES

- Decreased heat production
- Increased heat loss
- Impaired temperature regulation

SCOPE

Unknown

MOST OFTEN AFFECTED

Very young and the elderly; males affected slightly more than females

RISK FACTORS

- Malnutrition
- Cold water immersion
- Homelessness
- Outdoor workers
- Trauma victims
- Alcohol or drug consumption
- Mental illness
- Drug intoxication
- Hormone disorders
- Central nervous system disorders
- Severe infection
- Cardiovascular disease
- Pneumonia
- Liver failure
- Kidney failure
- Extensive skin disease
- Excessive fluid loss
- Hypothermia

 ## DIAGNOSIS

WHAT THE DOCTOR LOOKS FOR

- The doctor will perform a physical examination, including measuring core body temperature.
- Other conditions known to be associated with hypothermia should be investigated, including trauma, stroke, and intoxication.

TESTS AND PROCEDURES

- Arterial blood can be drawn for analysis.
- A number of blood tests can be performed to assist in diagnosis.
- Blood can be cultured for microbiologic analysis.
- Electrocardiogram (ECG)
- X-ray study of the neck, chest, and abdomen can be done.

 ## TREATMENT

GENERAL MEASURES

- Hypothermia is usually managed at a hospital emergency department or intensive care unit.
- Provide emergency first aid as needed, including rescue breathing and cardiopulmonary resuscitation (CPR).
- Remove wet garments.
- Protect against heat loss and wind chill.
- Maintain horizontal position.
- Move victim to a warm location as quickly as possible; alert 911.

ACTIVITY

Bed rest

DIET

Warm fluids only, if alert and able to swallow. Avoid fluids containing caffeine (coffee, hot chocolate).

 ## MEDICATIONS

COMMONLY PRESCRIBED DRUGS

- Antibiotics
- Resuscitation: bretylium, magnesium sulfate, sodium bicarbonate, dextrose intravenous (IV) solution
- Thiamine
- Naloxone
- Levothyroxine

 ## FOLLOW-UP

PATIENT MONITORING

The doctor and other healthcare providers will see the patient often during hospitalization. See the doctor as often as necessary following acute episode for treatment of the underlying cause of hypothermia.

PREVENTION

- Wear appropriate clothing for cold weather, with particular attention to head, feet, and hand coverings.
- If walking or climbing in cold climate, carry survival bags lined with "space" blankets for use if stranded or injured.
- Avoid alcohol, especially if anticipating exposure to cold weather.
- Pay attention to early symptoms and take proper action (e.g., drinking warm fluids, moving indoors).
- Keep the home adequately heated.

Hypothermia

_____ Doctor
_____ Office
_____ Phone
_____ Pager

Special notes to patient:

Hypothermia

COMPLICATIONS

- Irregular heart rhythms
- Shock
- Pneumonia
- Fluid in lungs
- Pancreatitis
- Peritonitis
- Gastrointestinal bleeding
- Kidney damage
- Bleeding disorder
- Metabolic disorder
- Gangrene of extremities

WHAT TO EXPECT

- Death from hypothermia is declining because of faster recognition and better care.
- Death rate depends on the severity of underlying cause of hypothermia.
- In previously healthy individuals, recovery is usually complete.
- Death rate in healthy patients is less 5%.
- Death rate in patients with other medical illness is more than 50%.

 MISCELLANEOUS

PEDIATRIC

- Infants are at increased risk of hypothermia because of their limited ability to produce heat when placed in a cold environment.
- A child's body temperature drops faster than an adult's when immersed in cold water.

GERIATRIC

- Older adults have a lower metabolic rate and it is more difficult for them to maintain normal body temperature when environmental temperature drops below 64.4°F (18°C).
- Aging also impairs the ability to detect temperature changes.
- This population also has increased incidence of diseases that decrease heat production or impair temperature regulation.

Hypothermia

_____ Doctor
_____ Office
_____ Phone
_____ Pager

Special notes to patient:

Hypothyroidism, Adult

 ## BASICS

DESCRIPTION

Hypothyroidism, or myxedema, is a condition resulting from the decreased action of thyroid hormone in the body.

SIGNS AND SYMPTOMS

- Onset may be insidious, subtle
- Weakness, fatigue, lethargy
- Cold intolerance
- Diminished memory
- Hearing impairment
- Constipation
- Muscle cramps
- Joint pain
- Loss of sensation, tingling feeling
- Modest weight gain
- Decreased sweating
- Heavy menstrual flow
- Depression
- Carpal tunnel syndrome
- Dry, coarse skin
- Dull facial expression
- Coarsening or huskiness of voice
- Puffiness around eyes
- Swelling of hands and feet
- Slow heart rate
- Low body temperature
- Reduced body and scalp hair
- Enlarged tongue

CAUSES

- Iodine therapy or thyroid surgery
- Thyroid disorders

SCOPE

- Hypothyroidism affects up to 5 to 10 per 1,000 persons in the United States.
- Affects 6% to 10% of women and 2% to 3% of men above 65 years of age

MOST OFTEN AFFECTED

Individuals above 40 years of age; 5 to 10 times more common in females than males

RISK FACTORS

- Risk increases with increasing age.
- Autoimmune diseases

 ## DIAGNOSIS

WHAT THE DOCTOR LOOKS FOR

- The doctor will perform a thorough physical examination to identify the signs and symptoms of hypothyroidism.
- Conditions that can cause similar signs and symptoms include heart failure, kidney disease, depression, and other disorders.
- Other conditions known to be associated with hypothyroidism should be investigated (e.g., diabetes mellitus and other hormone disorders).

TESTS AND PROCEDURES

Blood tests

 ## TREATMENT

GENERAL MEASURES

- Hypothyroidism is managed in the outpatient setting, except for complicating emergencies (coma, hypothermia).
- The goals of treatment are to restore and maintain a normal thyroid state.

ACTIVITY

As tolerated

DIET

- High-bulk diet may be helpful to avoid constipation.
- Low-fat diet for obese patients

 ## MEDICATIONS

COMMONLY PRESCRIBED DRUGS

Levothyroxine (Synthroid, Levothroid)

CONTRAINDICATIONS

Read drug product information.

PRECAUTIONS

Read drug product information.

DRUG INTERACTIONS

- Oral anticoagulants
- Insulin
- Oral hypoglycemics
- Estrogen
- Oral contraceptives
- Cholestyramine
- Ferrous sulfate

 ## FOLLOW-UP

PATIENT MONITORING

- See the doctor every 6 weeks until condition is stabilized, then every 6 months.
- Contact the doctor to report any signs of infection or heart problems.

COMPLICATIONS

- Congestive heart failure
- Coma
- Increased susceptibility to infection
- Colon disorder
- Organic psychosis with paranoia
- Adrenal crisis
- Infertility
- Hypersensitivity to opiates
- Bone softening

WHAT TO EXPECT

- With early treatment, striking transformations in improved appearance and mental function. Return to normal state is the rule.
- Relapses will occur if treatment is interrupted.
- If untreated, may progress to myxedema coma

 ## MISCELLANEOUS

GERIATRIC

Characteristic signs and symptoms are different or absent in the elderly. Hypothyroidism is common in the elderly.

Hypothyroidism, Adult

Doctor
Office
Phone
Pager

Special notes to patient:

Immunizations

BASICS

DESCRIPTION

Immunizations, also called "vaccinations," are substances that prevent specific diseases.

TREATMENT

GENERAL MEASURES

- Discuss the consequences of specific diseases and risks of immunizations with your doctors.
- Minor redness, swelling, or soreness at the site of injections can be expected; ice packs and acetaminophen may help relieve discomfort.
- Acetaminophen may relieve fever caused by immunizations.
- Adverse effects should be promptly reported to the doctor.

ACTIVITY

No restrictions after immunization

DIET

No specific restrictions after immunization

MEDICATIONS

COMMONLY PRESCRIBED DRUGS

- Recommendations for vaccinations are as follows:
- Hepatitis B:
  - Infants
  - Healthcare workers
  - Laboratory personnel who might be exposed to the virus
  - Intravenous drug users
  - Male homosexuals
  - Persons with a sexually transmitted disease
- Pneumococcal:
  - All persons above 65 years of age
  - Individuals with chronic disease, diabetes mellitus, or infected with the human immunodeficiency virus (HIV)
- Influenza:
  - All persons above 50 years of age
  - Healthcare workers
  - Individuals with chronic disease, diabetes mellitus, or infected with HIV
- Diphtheria, tetanus, pertussis (DTP):
  - All children starting at age 2 months
  - May be given up to the 7th birthday
- Tetanus and diphtheria:
  - All persons 7 years of age or older, every 10 years
- Measles, mumps and rubella (MMR):
  - Children at 12 to 15 months, and again at 4 to 6 or 11 to 12 years of age
  - Adults (especially medical personnel and daycare workers) without prior immunization or uncertain immunizations born after 1957
  - International travelers
  - College students
- Varicella (chickenpox):
  - Children at 2 to 18 months of age
  - Children 18 months to 12 years who have not already had chickenpox
  - Healthcare workers who have not already had chickenpox
  - Others who have not already had chickenpox
- Polio:
  - All children starting at 2 months of age
  - Adults traveling to areas where polio is prevalent
- *Hemophilus influenzae* type B:
  - All children starting at 2 months of age
- Hepatitis A:
  - Travelers to high-risk countries
  - Patients with chronic liver disease
  - Members of high-risk communities and ethnic groups
  - Homosexual males
  - Street-drug users
  - Laboratory personnel who might be exposed

CONTRAINDICATIONS

Vaccination may be contraindicated by allergies, pregnancy, active tuberculosis, and immune deficiency.

PRECAUTIONS

- Precautions should be taken with DTP if an individual has suspected neurologic disease or has had an adverse event (fever, seizure, spell of inconsolable crying) after a previous DPT vaccination.
- The following are NOT contraindications and DTP may be given if present:
  - Family history of convulsions
  - Family history of sudden infant death syndrome (SIDS)
  - Family history of adverse event following DTP
  - Temperature of 105°F or less following a prior DTP

POSSIBLE DRUG INTERACTIONS

Avoid aspirin and other salicylates for 6 weeks before varicella vaccination.

OTHER DRUGS

None

FOLLOW-UP

PATIENT MONITORING

None routinely needed

POSSIBLE COMPLICATIONS

- Fever, malaise, and minor local reactions (redness, pain) are the most common results of immunization.
- Vaccines rarely cause allergic reaction, high fever, or seizures.
- Some debatable evidence suggests that DTP may cause encephalopathy on rare occasions.

WHAT TO EXPECT

The outcome after vaccination is usually good. Most people who receive immunization develop protective antibodies.

MISCELLANEOUS

PEDIATRIC

Most vaccines are given to children before they enter school. DTP immunization of the preterm infant should not be delayed unless specific contraindications exist.

GERIATRIC

Pneumococcal, influenza, and tetanus are needed in older age groups.

PREGNANCY

MMR and varicella should not be routinely given to women who are pregnant or who are planning pregnancy in the next 3 months (MMR) or next 1 month (varicella).

Immunizations

Doctor
Office
Phone
Pager

Special notes to patient:

Impetigo

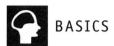 ## BASICS

DESCRIPTION

Impetigo is a superficial infection of the skin that produces fluid-filled blisters. Impetigo typically begins as a reddened, tender pimple that rapidly progresses into a blister before forming a shallow ulcer covered by a yellowish crust.

SIGNS AND SYMPTOMS

- Begins as a tender red bump or pimple in the skin
- Can develop slowly or spread rapidly
- Develops into fluid-filled blisters
- When blisters break, produces a weeping, shallow red ulcer that becomes covered with a honey-colored crust
- Most often occurs on the face around the mouth and nose or at a site of trauma
- Can form "satellite lesions" at multiple areas of the body

CAUSES

- Bacterial infection
- Can be transmitted by direct contact or by insect bite
- Can be the result of contamination at site of trauma

SCOPE

Unknown

MOST AFFECTED

Impetigo primarily affects children 2 to 5 years of age, males and females in equal proportion.

RISK FACTORS

- Warm, humid environment
- Tropical or subtropical climate
- Summer or fall season
- Minor trauma, insect bites, and so on
- Poor hygiene, epidemics during war, and so forth
- Person-to-person spread within families
- Poor health with anemia and malnutrition
- Complication of head lice, scabies, chickenpox, eczema
- Contact dermatitis

 ## DIAGNOSIS

WHAT THE DOCTOR LOOKS FOR

The doctor will rule out other causes of similar conditions (e.g., chickenpox, herpes, insect bites, and burns).

TESTS AND PROCEDURES

- No blood tests are usually required.
- A small amount of the lesion contents can be sampled after removal of the crust to test for the presence of bacteria.

 ## TREATMENT

GENERAL MEASURES

- Impetigo is managed on an outpatient basis.
- Remove crusts from lesions and gently wash two to three times a day.
- Can be associated with malnutrition and anemia, crowded living conditions, poor hygiene, and neglected minor trauma; these factors should also be addressed during treatment, if present.
- Good hygiene habits are important to prevent possible spread.

ACTIVITY

No restrictions

DIET

No special diet

 ## MEDICATIONS

COMMONLY PRESCRIBED DRUGS

Antibiotics for 7 to 10 days: erythromycin base, mupirocin (Bactroban) topical ointment, dicloxacillin.

CONTRAINDICATIONS

Some antibiotics should not be given to people with known allergies.

PRECAUTIONS

Refer to product information.

POSSIBLE DRUG INTERACTIONS

- Erythromycin interacts with theophyllines, astemizole, Fexofenadine (Allegra), and other drugs.
- Refer to product information.

OTHER DRUGS

- First generation cephalosporins: cephalexin, cefaclor, cephradine, cefadroxil
- Amoxicillin-clavulanate acid
- Vancomycin
- Clindamycin
- Ciprofloxacin plus rifampin (rifampicin)
- Clarithromycin

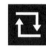 ## FOLLOW-UP

PATIENT MONITORING

If the lesions do not clear within 7 to 10 days, they should be cultured for microbiologic evaluation.

PREVENTION

Close attention to good hygiene habits, particularly handwashing, is important to prevent the spread of impetigo within families.

COMPLICATIONS

- Infection can persist, or become worse.
- In rare cases, bacterial infection can affect the kidney or cause blood poisoning.

WHAT TO EXPECT

With treatment, impetigo usually completely resolves within 7 to 10 days.

PEDIATRIC

Impetigo can occur in newborns by contamination in the nursery.

Impetigo

Doctor
Office
Phone
Pager

Special notes to patient:

Impotence

 ## BASICS

DESCRIPTION
Erectile problems (dysfunction), or impotence, is the dissatisfaction with size, rigidity, or duration of erection. Includes problems of arousal, desire, orgasm, sensation, and relationships. Temporary periods of impotence occur in about half of adult males and are not abnormal.

SIGNS AND SYMPTOMS
- Reduction of erectile size and rigidity
- Inability to maintain or achieve an erection
- Reduced body hair
- Breast growth
- Testicular atrophy or absence
- Deformed penis
- Vascular disease
- Nerve disease

CAUSES
- Endocrine
- Neurologic
- Vascular
- Medication
- Psychological
- Structural

SCOPE
About 10% of men have erectile dysfunction, but the true incidence is probably higher.

MOST OFTEN AFFECTED
Men 40 years of age and older

RISK FACTORS
- Pelvic surgery
- Medication
- Disorders listed in Causes

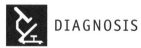 ## DIAGNOSIS

WHAT THE DOCTOR LOOKS FOR
The doctor will perform a complete physical examination to identify causes of erectile dysfunction (e.g., hormone, neurologic, vascular, and psychological disorders or drug side effects).

TESTS AND PROCEDURES
- Blood tests
- Special nerve tests may be performed.
- Tests can be performed to assess penile blood flow.
- Ultrasound can be used to assist in diagnosis.

 ## TREATMENT

GENERAL MEASURES
- Erectile dysfunction is managed by a primary care provider in an outpatient setting.
- Therapy includes vacuum erectile devices, sensate focus therapy, injection therapy, and penile implants.
- Reduce performance pressure.
- Psychiatrists, psychologists, sex therapists, vascular surgeons, urologists, endocrinologists, neurologists, plastic surgeons, and so on can be consulted for cases that do not improve with therapy.

ACTIVITY
No restrictions

DIET
Control diabetes if present.

 ## MEDICATIONS

COMMONLY PRESCRIBED DRUGS
- Testosterone cypionate
- Bromocriptine
- Penile injection of phentolamine and papaverine
- Alprostadil (Caverject)
- Sildenafil (Viagra)

CONTRAINDICATIONS
- Injections are contraindicated for men with bleeding disorders, sickle cell disease or trait, or penile deformities.
- Avoid drug allergies.

PRECAUTIONS
Injection therapy can cause persistent erection, scarring, low blood pressure, or nausea.

OTHER DRUGS
Use vacuum erection device before injections.

 ## FOLLOW-UP

PATIENT MONITORING
- See the doctor as often as needed.
- Therapy may include sex partner.

PREVENTION
Sex therapist or marriage counselor may help to speed recovery and prevent future problems.

WHAT TO EXPECT
- Because the cause of erectile dysfunction is unspecified for most men, vacuum erection device, injection therapy, and penile implants have improved the outlook greatly.
- Vacuum erection device fails in about 20% of cases.
- Many men stop injection therapy.
- Of men with penile implants, 10% to 30% do not use them.
- About 15% of men improve spontaneously.

GERIATRIC
Aging alone is not a cause of erectile dysfunction.

Impotence

	Doctor
	Office
	Phone
	Pager

Special notes to patient:

Influenza

BASICS

DESCRIPTION
Influenza is an acute, usually self-limited illness caused by the influenza virus. Also called the "flu" or "grip," it is marked by fever and inflammation of the nose, throat, eyes, and respiratory tract. Outbreaks occur almost every winter with varying degrees of severity.

SIGNS AND SYMPTOMS
- Sudden onset of:
- High fever
- Muscle aches, sometimes severe and lasting for days
- Sore throat
- Nonproductive cough
- Headache
- Swollen neck lymph nodes
- Chills
- Nasal congestion
- Malaise
- Runny nose
- Sneezing

CAUSES
Influenza virus is transmitted from person to person, usually by an airborne route.

SCOPE
Each year, 250,000 to 500,000 new cases of influenza occur. Attack rates in healthy children are 10% to 40% each year.

MOST OFTEN AFFECTED
Influenza most often affects young children (3 months to 16 years of age) and young adults (16 to 40 years of age). Males and females affected with equal frequency. Deaths are highest among the elderly (>75 years of age) and those with other medical illnesses, such as lung disease.

RISK FACTORS
- People at increased risk for contracting influenza include:
  - Patients in semiclosed environments (e.g., nursing homes)
  - Students, prisoners
  - People living in crowded, close environments during times of epidemics
- Medical conditions that increase the risks of complications arising from influenza include:
  - Chronic lung diseases
  - Heart disease
  - Metabolic diseases
  - Blood disorders
  - Cancer
  - Pregnancy in the third trimester
  - Infants and the elderly
  - Suppression of the immune system

DIAGNOSIS

WHAT THE DOCTOR LOOKS FOR
- The doctor will look for other causes of similar signs and symptoms, (e.g., the common cold, bronchitis, pneumonia, tonsillitis, and other viral infections).
- During the physical examination, the doctor will consider infectious illnesses that are currently spreading throughout the local community.

TESTS AND PROCEDURES
- Blood tests
- The nose or throat can be cultured for microbiologic analysis.
- Chest x-ray study

TREATMENT

GENERAL MEASURES
- Influenza is managed on an outpatient basis, except for treatment of severe complications or treatment of persons in high-risk groups.
- Treatment of symptoms: saline nasal spray, gargling
- Cool-mist, ultrasonic humidifier to increase moisture of breathed air.
- Hospitalized patients may require oxygen or ventilatory support.
- Smoking should be avoided.

ACTIVITY
Physical activity as tolerated

DIET
Fluid intake should be increased

MEDICATIONS

COMMONLY PRESCRIBED DRUGS
- Rimantadine is effective against influenza A. Rimantadine is now preferred over amantadine because it has fewer side effects.
  - Effective if given within the first 48 hours of onset of symptoms.
  - Rimantadine is not approved for influenza in children.
- Oseltamivir (Tamiflu)
- Zanamivir (Relenza)
- Oseltamivir and zanamivir are effective for influenza types A and B. Shortens duration by 1 day.
- Antifever drugs:
  - Acetaminophen. This drug should be used to control fever in children.
  - Aspirin should not be given to children under 16 years of age because of the risk of Reye's syndrome
- Antibiotics, in cases of a bacterial infection

CONTRAINDICATIONS
Nursing mothers; pregnancy unless benefits outweigh risks

PRECAUTIONS
- Amantadine and rimantadine:
  - Can cause mild side effects, including lightheadedness, insomnia, and anxiety, which are related to the dose and resolve when the drug is stopped. Drugs can impair the ability to perform hazardous activities or to drive a motor vehicle. Amantadine causes more side effects than rimantadine.
  - Can affect underlying seizure disorders and worsen epilepsy
  - Can cause psychosis in some people
  - Patients with congestive heart failure who take amantadine should be observed closely for deterioration.
  - Patients above 65 years of age or with kidney impairment should receive a lower dose

SIGNIFICANT POSSIBLE INTERACTIONS
Read drug product information.

OTHER DRUGS
- Ribavirin is reported to be effective against influenza types A and B.
- Ibuprofen or other nonsteroidal antiinflammatory drugs (NSAIDs) can be used for relief of symptoms.

FOLLOW-UP

PATIENT MONITORING
- In mild cases, usually no follow-up is required.
- Moderate or severe cases should be followed until symptoms resolve and any complications are treated effectively.

PREVENTION
The incubation period of influenza is 1 to 4 days. Infected persons are most contagious during period of peak symptoms.

Influenza

Doctor
Office
Phone
Pager

Special notes to patient:

Influenza

- Influenza vaccine
  - Recommended for all adults 65 years of age and older
  - Recommended for individuals at high risk with heart, lung, metabolic or kidney diseases; diabetes; suppression of the immune system (e.g., HIV-infected individuals); alcoholism; long-term aspirin therapy.
  - Recommended for healthcare providers, home care providers, staff and residents of nursing homes and other chronic care facilities, homeless persons, public safety workers, and those in close contact with high-risk individuals.
  - Should be administered in the fall before the influenza season
  - Some side effects possible (e.g., fever and mild, local reaction at vaccination site).
- Amantadine and rimantadine:
  - May be used for prevention in high-risk groups during epidemics of influenza A. It should not be considered a substitute for vaccination unless vaccine is contraindicated.
  - Take for duration of outbreak, if no vaccine given. Discontinue after 14 days, if used in addition to vaccine.

WHAT TO EXPECT

Recovery from influenza is favorable

COMPLICATIONS

- Middle-ear infection
- Pneumonia
- Reye's syndrome
- Acute sinusitis
- Croup
- Apnea in neonates
- Bronchitis
- Death

PEDIATRIC

Reye's syndrome is a rare and severe complication associated with aspirin use. Do not give aspirin to children with influenza; use acetaminophen.

GERIATRIC

- The elderly are more likely to have complications.
- Immunization is recommended for all individuals 50 years of age and older.

PREGNANCY

- Women with medical problems that place them at risk for complications of influenza should receive influenza vaccine regardless of trimester.
- Women who are in the third trimester of pregnancy during influenza season should consider being vaccinated.
- Amantadine should not be given to pregnant women.

Influenza

Doctor
Office
Phone
Pager

Special notes to patient:

Inner Ear Infection

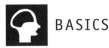 BASICS

DESCRIPTION
Inner ear infection, called "labyrinthitis," is an inflammation of the vestibular system of the inner ear. It has many possible causes. The most constant and pervasive symptom is vertigo.

SIGNS AND SYMPTOMS
- Vertigo
- Dizziness
- Hearing loss
- Nausea and vomiting
- Ringing in ear (tinnitus)
- Perspiration
- Increased salivation
- Generalized malaise

CAUSES
- Physiologic: mismatch of sensory systems, such as a stop after whirling turns, heights, motion sickness
- Disorder of inner ear, nerve, or brain
- Infections
- Tumors
- Blood vessel disorders
- Drug side effects
- Head injury

SCOPE
Unknown

MOST OFTEN AFFECTED
All ages beyond infancy, males and females in equal proportion

RISK FACTORS
- Trauma
- Stress
- Drug use
- Virus infection
- Cardiovascular disease

 DIAGNOSIS

WHAT THE DOCTOR LOOKS FOR
- The doctor will perform a physical examination to identify the signs and symptoms of labyrinthitis.
- Other conditions that can cause similar signs and symptoms include Meniere's syndrome, head injury, bacterial infection, cancer, and multiple sclerosis.

TESTS AND PROCEDURES
- Special diagnostic tests may be performed (e.g., electronystagmography, caloric test, doll's eye test).
- Computed tomography (CT) scan or magnetic resonance imaging (MRI) can be used to assist in diagnosis.

 TREATMENT

GENERAL MEASURES
- Labyrinthitis is managed in the outpatient setting.
- When possible, treatment is directed at the underlying disorder causing labyrinthitis.
- Treatment of symptoms accompanies specific treatment.

ACTIVITY
Lie still with eyes closed in darkened room during acute attacks. Otherwise, activity as tolerated.

DIET
Reduced-sodium diet

 MEDICATIONS

COMMONLY PRESCRIBED DRUGS
- Promethazine (Phenergan)
- Diazepam
- Prochlorperazine suppositories
- Meclizine
- Scopolamine, transdermal

CONTRAINDICATIONS
Read drug product information.

PRECAUTIONS
All the listed medications have significant adverse reactions. Use with caution. Avoid scopolamine in the elderly. Read drug product information.

SIGNIFICANT POSSIBLE INTERACTIONS
Read drug product information

 FOLLOW-UP

PATIENT MONITORING
See the doctor as often as needed.

PREVENTION
No preventive measures

COMPLICATIONS
Permanent hearing loss

WHAT TO EXPECT
The outcome depends on cause. Labyrinthitis often clears completely.

PEDIATRIC
Labyrinthitis is unusual in children.

GERIATRIC
- Labyrinthitis is common in the elderly.
- Avoid scopolamine or use with extreme caution in this age group.

PREGNANCY
Avoid medications.

Inner Ear Infection

Doctor
Office
Phone
Pager

Special notes to patient:

Insect Bites and Stings

BASICS

DESCRIPTION

Insects can bite or sting and inject poison, invade tissue, and transmit disease. This discussion here is limited to the irritative, poisonous, and allergic effects of insects.

- Harmful insects of the United States include:
  - Bees: bumblebees, sweat bees, honeybees
  - Wasps: hornets, wasps
  - Ants: fire ants, harvester ants
  - Brown recluse spider
  - Black widow spider
  - Hobo spiders
  - Scorpions
  - Mosquitoes
  - Flies: deer, horse, black, stable, and biting midges
  - Lice: body, head, pubic
  - Bugs: kissing, bed, wheel
  - Fleas: human, cat, dog
  - Mites: itch mite (scabies), red bugs (chiggers)
  - Ticks
  - Caterpillars: Puss, browntail, buck
  - Centipedes
- Typical reactions include:
  - Local tissue irritation, inflammation, and destruction
  - Systemic (whole body) effects related to bite or sting toxin
  - Allergic reactions: immediate or delayed

SIGNS AND SYMPTOMS

- Local reactions:
  - Redness at site of bite or sting
  - Pain
  - Heat
  - Swelling
  - Itching
  - Blisters
  - Formation of ulcers
  - Weeping from site of bite or sting
- Toxic reactions:
  - Nausea
  - Vomiting
  - Headache
  - Fever
  - Diarrhea
  - Lightheadedness, fainting
  - Drowsiness
  - Muscle spasms
  - Swelling
  - Convulsions
- Systemic reactions: allergic
  - Itching eyes
  - Facial flushing
  - Hives
  - Dry cough
  - Chest/throat constriction
  - Difficulty breathing
  - Noisy breathing
  - Bluish discoloration around eyes, mouth, and nail beds (cyanosis)
  - Abdominal cramps
  - Nausea, vomiting
  - Vertigo
  - Chills, fever
  - Shock
  - Loss of consciousness
  - Involuntary bowel or bladder action
  - Frothy saliva
  - Respiratory failure
  - Cardiovascular collapse
  - Death
- Delayed reaction:
  - Serum sickness-like reactions
  - Fever
  - Malaise
  - Headache
  - Rash
  - Swollen hands
  - Aching of joints
- Unusual reactions:
  - Brain damage
  - Inflammation of nerves or blood vessels
  - Kidney failure
  - Extreme fear, anxiety

CAUSES

- Local tissue inflammation and destruction from poison
- Allergic reaction from previous sensitization
- Toxic reaction from large dose of poison

SCOPE

Insect bites and stings are widespread throughout the United States, with seasonal and regional variations.

MOST OFTEN AFFECTED

All age groups are affected, males and females in equal proportions.

RISK FACTORS

- Living environment
- Climate
- Season
- Clothing
- Lack of protective measures
- Perfumes, colognes
- Previous sensitization to insect toxin
- Increased risk in young and elderly individuals

DIAGNOSIS

WHAT THE DOCTOR LOOKS FOR

- Local reaction: punctures, foreign bodies, infection, inflammation, lesions, or eruptions of the skin
- Toxic reaction: chemical exposure, drug abuse, plants
- Allergic reaction: medications, illicit drugs, foods, topical products, environmental, plants, chemicals

TESTS AND PROCEDURES

- Any number of blood tests can be ordered by the doctor
- The insect causing sting or bite may be identified if available

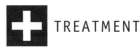

TREATMENT

GENERAL MEASURES

- The insect bite or sting victim can be treated as an outpatient or inpatient, depending on individual response to injury.
- Victims are hospitalized for severe reactions that threaten breathing or for shock, bronchospasm, severe swelling, or pain.
- First aid measures: activate emergency medical services in severe reactions.
- If the amount of venom or toxin is large (e.g., a swarm of bees) or victim has a history of allergic reaction, seek emergency care immediately.
- If victim carries epinephrine (a drug used to manage severe allergic reactions to insect bites or stings), use it.
- If available, over-the-counter antihistamines can also help alleviate allergic reactions.
- Local effects (depending on severity)
  - Remove stinger (scrape it out with a credit card or other flat, thin object—do not squeeze with tweezer).
  - Cleanse wound.
  - Apply cold packs to bite or sting site (alternate 10 minutes on/10 minutes off).
  - Elevate and rest affected part.
- Systemic effects (depending on severity and type of reaction)
  - Oxygen, if needed for respiratory distress
  - Rescue breathing may be needed.
  - Victim may be hospitalized and observed for 24 to 48 hours.
- Surgical repair may be required for severe spider-bite lesions.

ACTIVITY

Rest to limit spread of poison.

DIET

No special diet; nothing by mouth if severe systemic reaction

Insect Bites and Stings

	Doctor
	Office
	Phone
	Pager

Special notes to patient:

Insect Bites and Stings

 ## MEDICATIONS

COMMONLY PRESCRIBED DRUGS

- Local effects (depending on severity)
  - Analgesics: acetaminophen, ibuprofen
  - Antihistamines: diphenhydramine (Benadryl) (25–50 mg) four times a day
  - Steroids, topical or oral: prednisone (20–40 mg/day)
  - Antibiotics
- Systemic effects (depending on severity and type of reaction)
- Epinephrine
  - Diphenhydramine for rash, wheezing, swelling
  - Aminophylline, if needed for bronchospasm
  - Intravenous (IV) fluids if needed for shock
  - Hydrocortisone, if needed for severe hives or spider bite
  - Tetanus prophylaxis and antibiotics, if indicated
  - Diazepam (Valium)
  - Morphine or meperidine (Demerol) if needed for pain
- Antivenoms (e.g., black widow spider, scorpion) may be used in certain cases, based on availability and identification of organism.

CONTRAINDICATIONS
Read drug product information.

PRECAUTIONS
Treatment should not be delayed if the reaction is severe.

DRUG INTERACTIONS
Read drug product information.

OTHER DRUGS
Other antihistamines (e.g., loratadine and fexofenadine)

 ## FOLLOW-UP

PATIENT MONITORING
See primary care provider after caring for a significant wound.

PREVENTION
- Known hypersensitive persons should avoid reexposure.
- Future exposures could cause a more severe allergic response.
- An epinephrine injection may be prescribed for emergency use.
- Individuals with known sensitivity should wear medical identification (bracelet, tag) or carry a card.
- Persons who experience severe allergic reactions may consider desensitization with immunotherapy.

COMPLICATIONS
- Infection
  - Bacterial
  - Diseases associated with tick, fly, and mosquito bites: Lyme disease, rickettsial disease (Rocky Mountain spotted fever), arboviral encephalitis, malaria, leishmaniasis, trypanosomiasis
- Scarring
- Drug reactions
- Multisystem failure
- Death

WHAT TO EXPECT
- Minor reactions: excellent recovery
- Severe reactions: excellent recovery with prompt appropriate treatment

PEDIATRIC
More at risk

GERIATRIC
More at risk

PREGNANCY
Not a contraindication to treatment

Insect Bites and Stings

Doctor
Office
Phone
Pager

Special notes to patient:

Insomnia

 ## BASICS

DESCRIPTION
Insomnia is difficulty falling asleep or maintaining sleep, intermittent wakefulness, early morning awakening, or a combination. May be:

- Transient, caused by a life crisis, medical illness, grief, or change in environment
- Chronic, associated with medical and psychiatric conditions or drug use

SIGNS AND SYMPTOMS
- Perceived reduction in sleeping time
- Initial insomnia: difficulty falling asleep at the usual time
- Middle insomnia: wakefulness during the usual sleep cycle, "tossing and turning"
- Terminal insomnia: early awakening
- Daytime fatigue, sleepiness, and napping
- Anxiety in anticipation of sleep

CAUSES
- Medical illnesses: arthritis, gastroesophageal reflux disease, duodenal ulcer, Alzheimer's disease, restless leg syndrome, sleep apnea, lung disease, painful conditions (e.g., muscle cramps)
- Psychiatric illnesses: depression, anxiety, schizophrenia, manic disorders
- Drug-induced insomnia: alcohol, caffeine, nicotine
- Nonprescription drugs: diet aids, decongestants, cough preparations
- Prescribed drugs: steroids, theophylline, phenytoin (Dilantin), levodopa (Sinemet, Dopar)
- Jet lag (transient)
- Heavy smoking

SCOPE
Insomnia affects an estimated 30% of the adult population. It is one of the most common complaints in primary care practice.

MOST OFTEN AFFECTED
Insomnia can affect all age groups but is more common in the elderly. Males and females are affected equally.

RISK FACTORS
- Chronic illnesses
- Age above 50 years
- Multiple drug use
- Obesity

 ## DIAGNOSIS

WHAT THE DOCTOR LOOKS FOR
- The doctor will evaluate for known causes of insomnia.
- Some patients may have obstructive sleep apnea (snoring) that requires treatment.
- Patient may be evaluated for drug or alcohol dependence.
- Patient may be evaluated for depression or anxiety.

TESTS AND PROCEDURES
A sleep study (polysomnography) can be done to evaluate the patient.

 ## TREATMENT

GENERAL MEASURES
- Insomnia is usually managed in the outpatient setting.
- Sleep study may involve an overnight stay in a hospital.
- Transient insomnia
  - Lasts less than 3 to 4 weeks
  - Reassurance and supportive counseling may be helpful.
- Chronic insomnia
  - The underlying cause should be identified and addressed: pain, drugs, depression
  - Avoid alcohol after 5 PM or within 6 hours of retiring because it has a stimulant effect.
  - Person with insomnia should avoid daytime napping and should develop bedtime rituals conducive to sleep.
  - A thorough review of habits, drug intake, diet, and exercise pattern may reveal correctable causes of insomnia.
  - Drugs should be prescribed only if the above strategies fail.

ACTIVITY
No restriction on physical activity. A daily exercise routine is helpful. Avoid exercise close to bedtime.

DIET
Avoid caffeine. Avoid heavy, late-night snacks. Sometimes a light snack before bedtime may help. Avoid alcohol after 5 PM or within 6 hours of retiring. In some people, alcohol acts as a stimulant.

 ## MEDICATIONS

COMMONLY PRESCRIBED DRUGS
- Analgesics, as indicated for pain
- Benzodiazepines for insomnia: flurazepam (Dalmane), temazepam (Restoril), triazolam (Halcion)
- Tricyclic antidepressants: amitriptyline (Elavil)
- Nonbenzodiazepine agent: zolpidem (Ambien), zaleplon (Sonata)

CONTRAINDICATIONS
- Pregnancy and lactation
- Severe mental illness
- Acute narrow-angle glaucoma
- Significant liver disease
- Depressed patient who may be suicidal

PRECAUTIONS
- Benzodiazepines can cause agitated states in some people.
- Flurazepam can impair coordination and judgment.
- Triazolam has been associated with anterograde amnesia.
- Withdrawal psychosis and seizures can occur in some patients after abrupt cessation of insomnia drugs.
- Sedatives can cause "rebound insomnia."
- Sedatives can cause physical or psychological dependence.
- Amitriptyline can cause constipation and dizziness on standing.
- Zolpidem should be used with the same precautions as other sedative drugs. Most common reported side effects are drowsiness, dizziness, headache, and nausea.

DRUG INTERACTIONS
- Alcohol can magnify the sedative effects of the benzodiazepines.
- Blood levels of digoxin can be increased.
- Effect of levodopa may be reduced.

OTHER DRUGS
- Diphenhydramine (Benadryl) has been used to induce sleep in the elderly, but it can also cause confusion and "hangover."
- Chloral hydrate (Noctec) is favored by some physicians because it does not cause tolerance or withdrawal.

Insomnia

	Doctor
	Office
	Phone
	Pager

Special notes to patient:

Insomnia

- Melatonin, a pineal hormone, is marketed as a dietary supplement. It is increasingly being used as a self-medication for insomnia, but is not approved by the U.S. Food and Drug Administration. Appears to be useful for jet lag. Has mild hypnotic effect. No adverse effects have been reported, but controlled studies are lacking.
- L-Tryptophan, formerly widely used, is no longer available as a single ingredient in the United States.

 FOLLOW-UP

- Follow-up is based on the needs of the individual patient.
- The need for benzodiazepines should be reassessed periodically.
- A referral to psychosocial counseling can be made, if appropriate.

PREVENTION

Avoid all known causes of insomnia (e.g., caffeine, smoking), when possible.

COMPLICATIONS

- Transient insomnia can become chronic.
- Increased daytime sleepiness

WHAT TO EXPECT

Insomnia should resolve with time. The treatment of underlying symptoms is helpful.

GERIATRIC

- Benzodiazepines or other sedative-hypnotics should be prescribed with caution to elderly persons.
- Sleep habits normally change with age.

PREGNANCY

Transient insomnia can occur during pregnancy because of the discomfort of sleeping positions.

Insomnia

Doctor
Office
Phone
Pager

Special notes to patient:

Iron Deficiency Anemia

 ## BASICS

DESCRIPTION

Iron deficiency anemia is anemia caused by decreased stores of iron in the body. Other forms of anemia are related to the poor absorption or utilization of iron. The onset of iron deficiency anemia may be acute with rapid blood loss, or chronic with poor diet or slow blood loss. Iron deficiency is the most common cause of anemia in the United States.

SIGNS AND SYMPTOMS

- Initially, no symptoms
- Dry, peeling lips
- Shortness of breath
- Fatigue, listlessness
- Rapid heart rate, palpitations
- Headache
- Irritability, inability to concentrate
- Pain or tingling sensation in extremities
- Pallor
- Susceptibility to infection
- Brittle, spoon-shaped, nails

CAUSES

- Blood loss (e.g., menstruation, gastrointestinal bleeding)
- Poor iron intake
- Poor iron absorption
- Increased demand for iron (e.g., infancy, adolescence, pregnancy)
- Hookworms
- Stomach cancer

SCOPE

About 10% to 30% of the adult population have iron deficiency anemia.

MOST OFTEN AFFECTED

Iron deficiency anemia affects all ages. It is more common in females than males.

RISK FACTORS

See *Causes*

 ## DIAGNOSIS

WHAT THE DOCTOR LOOKS FOR

- The doctor will rule out anemia caused by poor iron metabolism or other causes.
- The doctor will evaluate for the presence of stomach cancer, especially in the elderly.
- Potential sources of bleeding will be investigated and ruled out.

TESTS AND PROCEDURES

- Blood tests to measure cells, hemoglobin, and iron compounds
- Bone marrow can be sampled for analysis to assist in diagnosis.
- Special tests can be done to identify other causes of iron loss (e.g., stool guaiac testing, endoscopy, and blood-clotting studies).
- Endoscopy (insertion of a tube with a small camera at its end into the esophagus) of the gastrointestinal tract can be done to identify hidden sources of bleeding.

 ## TREATMENT

GENERAL MEASURES

- Iron deficiency anemia is usually treated on an outpatient basis.
- The doctor should search for a cause of bleeding and treat it.

ACTIVITY

Patients with heart disease should reduce their physical activity.

DIET

- Adults should limit milk to 1 pint a day.
- Consume adequate protein- and iron-containing foods (e.g., meat, beans, and leafy green vegetables).
- Increase dietary fiber to decrease likelihood of constipation during iron replacement therapy.
- Do not ingest milk, other dairy products, antacids, or tetracycline within 2 hours of iron dosage.

 ## MEDICATIONS

COMMONLY PRESCRIBED DRUGS

Ferrous sulfate (iron). Dose can be reduced to ease gastrointestinal effects, which affect 15% of patients on standard iron therapy.

CONTRAINDICATIONS

Do not take iron while also taking antacids or tetracycline.

PRECAUTIONS

- Iron preparations cause black bowel movements.
- Iron overdose is highly toxic. Tablets should be kept out of the reach of small children.

DRUG INTERACTIONS

- Allopurinol
- Antacids
- Penicillamine
- Tetracycline
- Vitamin E

 ## FOLLOW-UP

PATIENT MONITORING

See the doctor regularly after blood tests return to normal to detect any return of anemia.

PREVENTION

- Good nutrition with adequate iron intake
- Gynecologic or other problems causing excess blood loss should be treated.

COMPLICATIONS

Hidden sources of bleeding (e.g., a malignancy) may not be identified.

WHAT TO EXPECT

Iron deficiency anemia is curable with iron therapy if the underlying cause can be identified and treated.

PEDIATRIC

Frequent problem in infants whose major source of nutrition is cow's milk

GERIATRIC

Accounts for 60% of anemias in people above 65 years of age

PREGNANCY

Common during pregnancy unless iron supplements are included in the diet

FURTHER INFORMATION

National Heart, Lung & Blood Institute, Communications & Public Information Branch, National Institutes of Health, Building 31, Room 41-21, 9000 Rockville Pike, Bethesda, MD 20892, (301) 251-1222

Iron Deficiency Anemia

Doctor
Office
Phone
Pager

Special notes to patient:

Irritable Bowel Syndrome

 ## BASICS

DESCRIPTION

Irritable bowel syndrome, also called "spastic" or "irritable colon," is a set of signs and symptoms of altered bowel habits, abdominal pain, and gaseousness in the absence of other disease.

SIGNS AND SYMPTOMS

- Most patients have all signs and symptoms, but not with every episode.
- Abdominal pain, usually lower quadrant, is relieved by defecation.
- Mucus in stools
- Constipation
- Diarrhea
- Distention
- Upper abdominal discomfort after eating
- Straining for normal consistency stools
- Urgency of defecation
- Feelings of incomplete evacuation
- Hard, round stool
- Nausea, vomiting (rarely)

CAUSES

The cause of irritable bowel syndrome is unknown.

SCOPE

- The incidence of irritable bowel syndrome in the United States is unknown, but it is second to upper respiratory infection as the cause for lost workdays.
- At least 15% of the population (uncommon in children and early teens) is affected.

MOST OFTEN AFFECTED

- Irritable bowel syndrome is rare in the late teens; it more commonly affects those in their late 20s.
- In a person above 40 years of age, the symptoms are likely caused by a different disease.
- Females are affected twice as often as males in the United States, whereas irritable bowel syndrome is more common in males than females in other parts of the world.

RISK FACTORS

- Other members of the family with the same or similar gastrointestinal disorder
- History of childhood sexual abuse
- Sexual or domestic abuse in women

 ## DIAGNOSIS

WHAT THE DOCTOR LOOKS FOR

The doctor will look for other causes of similar signs and symptoms (e.g., inflammatory bowel syndromes, lactose intolerance, infections).

TESTS AND PROCEDURES

- Laboratory tests can be ordered as needed to rule out other diseases and conditions.
- Imaging of the gastrointestinal tract can be done.
- Sigmoidoscopy can be done to visually inspect the large intestine.

 ## TREATMENT

GENERAL MEASURES

- Irritable bowel syndrome is managed on an outpatient basis.
- Heat to the abdomen may help relieve discomfort.
- Biofeedback or other techniques may help reduce stress.
- Problem stimulants should be avoided.

ACTIVITY

As normal

DIET

- Increase fiber.
- Avoid large meals; spicy, fried, fatty foods; and milk products.

 ## MEDICATIONS

COMMONLY PRESCRIBED DRUGS

- Bulk-producing agents: psyllium-containing products (Metamucil)
- Constipating agents (if diarrhea is significant): loperamide (Imodium), iphenoxylate-atropine (Lomotil)
- Antispasmodics/anticholinergics: dicyclomine (Bentyl) or lactase (LactAid)
- Anticholinergics/sedatives: chlordiazepoxide-clidinium (Librax), phenobarbital-hyoscyamine-atropine-hyoscine (Donnatal), amitriptyline HCL (Elavil)
- Antiflatulents: simethicone (Mylicon)
- For milk intolerance: lactase capsules or tablets

CONTRAINDICATIONS

Read drug product information.

PRECAUTIONS

Read drug product information.

DRUG INTERACTIONS

Read drug product information.

 ## FOLLOW-UP

PATIENT MONITORING

See the doctor as needed for symptoms.

PREVENTION

See *Diet*

WHAT TO EXPECT

- Irritable bowel syndrome does not progress to cancer or inflammatory disease.
- Acute episodes may recur throughout life, particularly when an individual is under stress. The frequency of episodes decreases with increasing age.

PREGNANCY

Some experts suggest that irritable bowel syndrome worsens during pregnancy. However, irritable bowel syndrome in the mother causes no increased risks to fetus or mother.

Irritable Bowel Syndrome

Doctor

Office

Phone

Pager

Special notes to patient:

Jaundice

 BASICS

DESCRIPTION

Jaundice is a term that describes the accumulation of bile pigment in the skin, mucous membranes, and eyes that causes a yellowish appearance.

CAUSES

- Jaundice is usually caused by blood disorders, heart or liver disease, viral infection, alcohol or drug use, stones in the bile ducts, or cancer of the pancreas or liver.
- A form of jaundice can be caused by pregnancy.
- Jaundice is common in newborns and usually resolves quickly with no long-term effects.

 TREATMENT

Because jaundice is a symptom rather than a disease in itself, treatment is directed at the underlying cause.

Jaundice

Doctor
Office
Phone
Pager

Special notes to patient:

Jet Lag

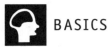 **BASICS**

DESCRIPTION

Jet lag, also called "circadian dysrhythmia," is a syndrome resulting from travel between different time zones. North-to-south travel does not cause jet lag. A person experiences jet lag when his or her body is out of sync with the local time (e.g., the clock shows that it is lunchtime, but the body says it is the middle of the night). The severity of jet lag depends on the number of time zones crossed and the direction of travel. Most people find traveling eastward and adapting to a shorter day more difficult than traveling westward and adapting to a longer day.

SIGNS AND SYMPTOMS

Extreme fatigue, sleep disturbances, loss of concentration, malaise, disorientation, sluggishness, gastrointestinal upset, and loss of appetite

CAUSES

Jet lag is a disturbance of the body's physiologic processes that control sleep and wakefulness, as well as alertness, hunger, digestion, temperature, and hormones.

 TREATMENT

- No clear evidence indicates the effectiveness of elaborate preventive self-remedies to avoid jet lag.
- The doctor may prescribe a short-acting sedative (e.g., lorazepam) for sleep during travel.
- Travelers should plan their destination activities to accommodate local time differences.
- The hormone melatonin shows promise as a jet lag remedy.

Jet Lag

Doctor
Office
Phone
Pager

Special notes to patient:

Kaposi's Sarcoma

 ## BASICS

DESCRIPTION

Kaposi's sarcoma (KS) is a form of skin cancer characterized by vascular tumors of skin and viscera. Several different forms of KS are seen, including a classic indolent (slow-growing) type and a form associated with acquired immune deficiency syndrome (AIDS) and other immune system disorders.

SIGNS AND SYMPTOMS

- Multiple purplish tumors on the skin
- Lesions can be tender or itchy.
- Skin tumors can appear on the face, arms, legs, or trunk.
- Lesions may also be in the mouth or other mucous membranes or on internal organs or lymph nodes.

CAUSES

It is believed that transmission of an as yet unidentified agent leads to the formation of KS. A herpes-related virus can cause KS.

SCOPE

The indolent form of KS is rare in the United States. It is common among persons with AIDS or immune deficiency.

MOST OFTEN AFFECTED

Kaposi's sarcoma affects individuals between 16 and 75 years of age. It tends to occur more often in males than females.

RISK FACTORS

- Infection with the human immunodeficiency virus (HIV)
- Treatment with immunosuppressant medications
- Transplantation and chemotherapy

 ## DIAGNOSIS

WHAT THE DOCTOR LOOKS FOR

The doctor looks for other possible causes of similar lesions of the skin (e.g., abnormal blood vessel growth).

TESTS

- A computed tomography (CT) scan of the chest and abdomen can be done to assess internal organs.
- A biopsy of a sarcoma or lymph node can be obtained to assist in diagnosis.
- Lesions can be examined by bronchoscopy, if the airway is affected.

 ## TREATMENT

GENERAL MEASURES

- KS is usually managed on an outpatient basis.
- If immunosuppressant medications have caused KS, dosages can be modified.
- If KS is related to HIV, drug therapy can be initiated.
- Treatment is otherwise determined by the extent of the disease.
- Lesions can be surgically removed, typically on an outpatient basis.
- Other treatments include radiation therapy, chemotherapy, immunotherapy, and antiviral therapy.
- The person with KS should be observed for a return of lesions or other change in condition.

ACTIVITY

Remain active as long as possible.

DIET

No special diet

 ## MEDICATIONS

COMMONLY PRESCRIBED DRUGS

- Chemotherapy agents: doxorubicin, bleomycin, vinblastine, vincristine
- Antiviral: interferon

CONTRAINDICATIONS

Read drug product information.

PRECAUTIONS

Read drug product information. Chemotherapy can suppress the function of bone marrow.

POSSIBLE DRUG INTERACTIONS

Read drug product information.

OTHER DRUGS

Uncontrolled studies indicate that some individuals respond to antiherpes medications.

 ## FOLLOW-UP

PATIENT MONITORING

Among those with HIV, other opportunistic infections must be aggressively treated.

PREVENTION

Safe sex practices reduce the risk of HIV transmission.

COMPLICATIONS

An aggressive form of KS affects at least one third of those infected with HIV.

WHAT TO EXPECT

- Better treatments may result in improved HIV-related KS survival.
- Individuals with the indolent form of KS typically survive for 10 years after diagnosis.

 ## MISCELLANEOUS

GERIATRIC

Indolent form most often occurs among elderly men.

Kaposi's Sarcoma

Doctor
Office
Phone
Pager

Special notes to patient:

Kidney Stones

 ## BASICS

DESCRIPTION
Kidney stones, also called "urolithiasis" or "renal colic," are the formation of hard mineral deposits called "calculi" within the urinary system.

SIGNS AND SYMPTOMS
- Usually sudden onset
- Severe agonizing pain, which can be felt from the rib cage to the groin, depending on the location of stone
- Patient is unable to obtain relief from discomfort.
- Nausea with or without vomiting
- Sweating
- Rapid heartbeat
- Abdominal distension
- Tenderness to deep abdominal examination
- Frequent, urgent, or difficult urination
- Fever
- Blood or pus in the urine
- May be asymptomatic if stone stays within kidney

CAUSES
Kidney stones are caused by a wide range of factors related to the body's water and mineral balance.

SCOPE
About 2% to 5% of the population in the United States can expect to have kidney stones, which affect 70 to 210 per 100,000 of the population in their lifetime.

MOST OFTEN AFFECTED
Kidney stones affect people ranging from 20 to 60 years of age. Incidence peaks at 20 to 30 years of age. Males are affected four times more often than females. The tendency to develop kidney stones seems to run in families.

RISK FACTORS
- Family history
- Hot climate
- Work in hot environment
- Inadequate fluid intake
- Diet high in minerals and vitamins
- Cancer
- Gout
- Use of diuretics (water pills)
- Bowel or kidney disease

 ## DIAGNOSIS

WHAT THE DOCTOR LOOKS FOR
The doctor looks for other medical disorders (e.g., kidney disease, diabetes, infection, intestinal conditions, or gynecologic problems).

TESTS AND PROCEDURES
- Urinalysis and culture
- Blood tests for electrolytes, chemistry, and hormones
- Stone can be analyzed to determine its chemical composition
- Urinary system can be assessed by x-ray study or ultrasound
- A special procedure called "intravenous pyelogram" (IVP) can be performed to evaluate the urinary system.

 ## TREATMENT

GENERAL MEASURES
- Most stones pass within 24 hours.
- About 80% of individuals with kidney stones are managed as outpatients.
- About 20% require hospitalization and treatment by a specialist.
- The doctor should provide reassurance to the patient.
- Patient should strain urine to recover stone for analysis.
- It is important to maintain adequate fluid intake.
- Doctor should make sure pain is controlled appropriately.
- Patient with intractable pain, urinary tract obstruction, large stones, infection, or other complicated conditions may be seen by a specialist.
- Surgical measures include:
  - Extracorporeal shock wave lithotripsy, which uses sound waves to shatter kidney stones
  - Urethroscopy, in which a stone is crushed and removed through an instrument inserted into the bladder
  - Minimally invasive techniques
  - Open surgery, which is performed on less than 5% of patients

ACTIVITY
Bedrest during acute phase if necessary. No restrictions after stone passes.

DIET
- Normal diet
- Drink 8 oz. water every 1 hour while awake and, if possible, every 2 hours during sleep hours.
- If stones consist of uric acid, eat less protein and take sodium bicarbonate to alkalinize urine.

MEDICATIONS

COMMONLY PRESCRIBED DRUGS
- Acute therapy
  - Pain control: meperidine (Demerol) or morphine or buprenorphine (Buprenex)
  - 3-day supply pain control: oxycodone-acetaminophen (Percocet), pentazocine (Talwin), hydrocodone-acetaminophen (Vicodin)
  - Uric acid stones: potassium citrate (Urocit-K)
  - Cystine stones: penicillamine (Cuprimine, Depen)
  - Infected stones: antibiotics
- Maintenance therapy:
  - Hypercalciuria: sodium cellulose phosphate, hydrochlorothiazide (HCTZ), K-citrate
  - Uric acid: allopurinol (Zyloprim), K-citrate
  - Cystine: K-citrate, penicillamine

CONTRAINDICATIONS
Penicillamine should not be given to those who are pregnant or have renal failure, aplastic anemia, or known allergic reactions.

PRECAUTIONS
Penicillamine requires regular blood tests and urinalysis.

DRUG INTERACTIONS
Read drug product information.

 ## FOLLOW-UP

PATIENT MONITORING
- Strain urine until stone passes or 72 hours after symptoms cease.
- Repeat urinalysis every 2 to 3 days.
- Repeat urinary system x-ray studies if no stone is passed.
- Stone should be analyzed when passed.

Kidney Stones

Doctor
Office
Phone
Pager

Special notes to patient:

Kidney Stones

- X-ray study should be repeated at 3 to 6 months and at 1 year. If no new stone develops, no further follow-up is needed.
- Further urinalysis and blood tests may be required for recurring kidney stones.

PREVENTION

Maintain adequate water intake to produce more than 2 L/day of urine, including one trip to the bathroom at night. Keep dietary calcium below 1 g/day.

COMPLICATIONS

- Kidney damage
- Infection

WHAT TO EXPECT

- In about 80% of cases, stones pass within 48 to 72 hours with outpatient therapy.
- About 60% of persons have no recurrence of kidney stones at 10 years.

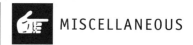

MISCELLANEOUS

PEDIATRIC

May be caused by inherited disorders

PREGNANCY

Pregnant women with kidney stones should be seen by a urologist.

Kidney Stones

Doctor
Office
Phone
Pager

Special notes to patient:

Laryngitis

 ## BASICS

DESCRIPTION

Laryngitis is an inflammation of the lining of the larynx. It is most common during late fall, winter, and early spring. In predisposed individuals, it can also occur intermittently during period of vocal misuse or abuse. It can be acute (brief) or chronic (long-lasting).

SIGNS AND SYMPTOMS

- Hoarseness
- Abnormal sounding voice
- Inability to speak
- Throat tickling
- Feeling of rawness in throat
- Constant urge to clear the throat
- Fever
- Malaise
- Painful or difficult swallowing
- Throat pain
- Cough
- Enlarged lymph glands in neck

CAUSES

- Infections: viral or bacterial
- Excessive use of voice
- Inhaling irritating substances
- Aspiration of caustic chemical
- Aging
- Damage during surgery
- Esophageal reflux

SCOPE

Laryngitis is common.

PREDOMINANT AGE

Laryngitis affects all ages, males and females equally.

RISK FACTORS

- Upper respiratory tract infection
- Bronchitis
- Pneumonia
- Influenza (flu)
- Pertussis (whooping cough)
- Measles
- Allergy
- Chronic rhinitis
- Chronic sinusitis
- Voice abuse
- Reflux of gastric contents
- Smoking
- Alcohol abuse
- Constant exposure to dust or other irritants

 ## DIAGNOSIS

WHAT THE DOCTOR LOOKS FOR

- The doctor will evaluate the patient for the presence of laryngitis.
- Other conditions that can cause similar signs and symptoms include croup, measles, diphtheria, vocal cord nodules, and throat cancer.

TESTS AND PROCEDURES

- Blood tests
- A sample of fluid from the throat can be obtained for laboratory analysis.
- The throat can be examined by laryngoscopy.
- A sample of tissue can be obtained by biopsy to assist in diagnosis.

 ## TREATMENT

GENERAL MEASURES

- Laryngitis is usually managed in the outpatient setting.
- Acute laryngitis:
  - Usually a self-limited illness and not severe
  - Vocal conservation without excessive voice use
  - Steam inhalations or cool-mist humidifier
  - Increase fluid intake
  - Pain relievers
  - Avoid smoking (or secondhand smoke) during acute phase
- Chronic:
  - Symptomatic treatment as above
  - Voice therapy
  - Stop smoking
  - Reduce alcohol intake
  - Occupational change or modification, if needed
  - For reflux laryngitis: elevate head of bed, other antireflux management
- Surgery may be necessary.

ACTIVITY

Rest until fever subsides, then no restrictions.

DIET

No special diet

 ## MEDICATIONS

None usually required

COMMONLY PRESCRIBED DRUGS (IF NEEDED)

- Pain relievers
- Antifever drugs
- Cough suppressants
- Penicillin, erythromycin

CONTRAINDICATIONS

Read drug product information.

PRECAUTIONS

Read drug product information.

DRUG INTERACTIONS

Read drug product information.

 ## FOLLOW-UP

PATIENT MONITORING

No follow-up is usually needed.

PREVENTION

- Avoid overuse of voice.
- Prompt treatment of respiratory infections
- Flu vaccine for individuals at high risk

COMPLICATIONS

Chronic hoarseness

WHAT TO EXPECT

Complete clearing of the inflammation without long-term effects

 ## MISCELLANEOUS

PEDIATRIC

Laryngitis is common in children.

GERIATRIC

The elderly may have more severe symptoms and healing may be slower.

PREGNANCY

Use antibiotics with caution.

Laryngitis

Doctor
Office
Phone
Pager

Special notes to patient:

Lazy Eye

 ## BASICS

DESCRIPTION

Amblyopia, also called "lazy eye," is a reduction in visual acuity in one eye that, in the absence of other disease, cannot be corrected by eyeglasses or contact lenses.

SIGNS AND SYMPTOMS

Decreased visual acuity in one eye

CAUSES

Multiple causes

SCOPE

Amblyopia affects about 2.5% of the population in the United States.

MOST OFTEN AFFECTED

Amblyopia may be present from birth or can occur at any age. Males and females are affected equally. An increased incidence is seen in children with one parent who has a history of amblyopia.

RISK FACTORS

None known

 ## DIAGNOSIS

WHAT THE DOCTOR LOOKS FOR

- A thorough eye examination should be performed.
- Other causes of visual acuity loss in one eye should be considered.

TESTS AND PROCEDURES

Examination by an ophthalmologist can include slit lamp and funduscopic examination of eye structures.

 ## TREATMENT

GENERAL MEASURES

- All children should have complete visual examinations before starting school.
- Children from families with a history of amblyopia or strabismus should have special examinations by an ophthalmologist.
- Correction of the underlying disorder should begin at the earliest opportunity.
- Glasses, patching, or both of the stronger eye may be helpful in encouraging visual development.
- Amblyopia never corrects itself spontaneously and always requires treatment.
- Children do not outgrow amblyopia.
- Surgical correction of an abnormal eye position may be required.

ACTIVITY

No restrictions

DIET

No special diet

 ## FOLLOW-UP

PATIENT MONITORING

See the doctor as often as needed, until the problem is resolved.

PREVENTION

None

COMPLICATIONS

Permanent and profound visual loss can develop if proper therapy is not begun early.

WHAT TO EXPECT

- In most cases, and with dearly diagnosis, amblyopia is a treatable condition.
- Patching therapy, eyeglasses, and surgical correction of abnormal eye positions can result in nearly normal vision, when performed early.
- Visual development occurs during the first several years of life; amblyopia therapy can be effective until approximately age 12 years.

 ## MISCELLANEOUS

PEDIATRIC

Commonly seen in young children

GERIATRIC

When seen among the elderly population, the diagnosis usually has been made early in childhood.

Lazy Eye

Doctor
Office
Phone
Pager

Special notes to patient:

Lead Poisoning

 ## BASICS

DESCRIPTION
Lead poisoning is a toxic condition that results from exposure to lead, an element having no known function in the human body.

SIGNS AND SYMPTOMS
- Often no symptoms
- Mild to moderate toxicity:
  - Can cause muscle or joint pain, loss of sensation, fatigue, irritability, lethargy, abdominal discomfort, difficulty concentrating, headache, tremor, vomiting, weight loss
- Severe toxicity:
  - Causes loss of appetite, metallic taste in mouth, constipation, severe abdominal cramps
  - Peripheral neuritis
  - Seizures; coma; and long-term effects including brain damage, retarded mental development, hyperactivity
  - Chronic exposure to lead can cause renal failure.

CAUSES
Inhalation of lead dust or fumes or ingestion of lead

SCOPE
Of preschoolers in the United States, 17% have lead poisoning. Sporadic cases have been reported in adults.

MOST OFTEN AFFECTED
- Children 1 to 5 years of age; adult workers in industries that use lead
- Males and females are affected equally.

RISK FACTORS
- Children who eat nonfood items (e.g., dirt)
- Children with iron deficiency anemia
- Resident or frequent visitor in deteriorating, pre-1960 housing with lead paint surfaces
- Children with seizures
- Children with hyperkinetic or autistic behavior
- Sibling or playmate with lead poisoning
- Dust from clothing of lead worker
- Lead dissolved in water from lead or lead-soldered plumbing
- Lead-glazed ceramics, especially with acidic food or drink
- Food stored in inverted plastic bread bags printed with colored ink
- Colored comics
- Soil near lead industries and roads
- Folk remedies
- Hobbies
- Occupational exposure
- Dietary: zinc or calcium deficiency

 ## DIAGNOSIS

WHAT THE DOCTOR LOOKS FOR
The doctor will perform a physical examination to identify the signs and symptoms of lead poisoning.

TESTS AND PROCEDURES
- Blood tests
- X-ray study of the abdomen or long bones

 ## TREATMENT

GENERAL MEASURES
- Lead poisoning is often managed in the outpatient setting.
- Hospitalization may be required for chelation therapy.
- Local health department may be notified.

ACTIVITY
Avoid activity at any site of potential lead contamination.

DIET
- If symptomatic, avoid excessive fluids.
- Consume adequate calcium and iron.
- Eat a low-fat diet to reduce lead absorption and retention.

 ## MEDICATIONS

COMMONLY PRESCRIBED DRUGS
- Oral chelation: succimer (Chemet)
- Intravenous (IV) chelation: dimercaprol (British anti-Lewisite, BAL), Ca EDTA edetate calcium disodium

CONTRAINDICATIONS
BAL should not be given to persons allergic to peanuts, because the drug solution contains peanut oil.

PRECAUTIONS
Chelation drugs have many precautions; read drug product information.

DRUG INTERACTIONS
Vitamins should not be given concurrently with oral chelation.

OTHER DRUGS
Penicillamine (d-penicillamine, Depen, Cuprimine)

 ## FOLLOW-UP

PATIENT MONITORING
- See the doctor after 7 to 10 days of treatment and then once or twice a month.
- Testing should be repeated periodically (e.g., every 3 months).

PREVENTION
- Identify potential sources of lead and decrease lead exposure. Wet mopping and dusting with a high-phosphate solution (e.g., powdered automatic dishwasher detergent, $\frac{1}{4}$ cup per gallon of water) will help control lead-bearing dust.
- If the source is in the home (e.g., lead paint), the patient must reside elsewhere until lead removal is completed.

Lead Poisoning

_____ Doctor
_____ Office
_____ Phone
_____ Pager

Special notes to patient:

Lead Poisoning

COMPLICATIONS
- Toxicity can be long lasting or permanent.
- Long-term lead exposure can cause chronic renal failure and gout.

WHAT TO EXPECT
- Symptomatic lead poisoning without brain damage generally improves with chelation therapy, but subtle effects may be long-lasting or permanent.
- If brain damage occurs, permanent effects (e.g., mental retardation, seizure disorder, blindness, paralysis) are seen in 25% to 50% of patients.

MISCELLANEOUS

PEDIATRIC
- Increasing evidence exists that low lead level exposure can be toxic to children.
- Children are at increased risk because of incomplete development of the brain.
- Common childhood behaviors such as frequent hand-to-mouth activity and pica (ingestion of nonfood products) greatly increase the risk of ingesting lead.

PREGNANCY
- Lead exposure in pregnancy is associated with reduced birthweight and premature birth.
- Lead causes birth defects in animals.

FURTHER INFORMATION
- The Inside Story: A Guide to Indoor Air Quality, EPA/400/1-88/004. EPA and Consumer Product Safety Commission, 1988. Lead and Your Drinking Water. EPA, 1988, OPA-87-006
- Because there is too much lead in your child's body . . . , Bock Pharmacal Co., (800) 727-2625

Lead Poisoning

Doctor
Office
Phone
Pager

Special notes to patient:

Leukemia, Acute Lymphoblastic in Adults (ALL)

 ## BASICS

DESCRIPTION

Acute lymphoblastic leukemia (ALL) is a cancerous proliferation and accumulation of immature white blood cells.

SIGNS AND SYMPTOMS

- Anemia: fatigue, shortness of breath, lightheadedness, chest pain, headache
- Insufficient platelets: pinpoint red spots, bruising, nosebleed, retinal bleeding
- Insufficient white blood cells: fever, infection
- Lymphatic disorder: enlarged glands, enlarged spleen or liver, bone pain
- Immune system suppression
- Metabolic disturbances: kidney failure
- Central nervous system: confusion, nerve disorder

CAUSES

Unknown. Epstein-Barr virus is suspected.

SCOPE

About 1,000 adult cases of ALL occur annually in the United States.

MOST OFTEN AFFECTED

Patient age averages 35 to 40 years, but incidence increases with age. Males are affected slightly more often than females.

RISK FACTORS

- Age above 60 years
- Exposure to agents such as benzene or radiation
- May follow aplastic anemia

 ## DIAGNOSIS

WHAT THE DOCTOR LOOKS FOR

The doctor will perform a physical examination to identify the presence of ALL. Other diseases can cause similar signs and symptoms, including other forms of leukemia or other cancers, immune system disorders, and noncancerous conditions.

TESTS AND PROCEDURES

- Blood tests.
- A sample of bone marrow can be obtained for laboratory analysis.
- Special genetic testing can be done.
- Chest x-ray study, ultrasound
- A sample of lymph node tissue can be obtained by biopsy for laboratory analysis.
- A sample of spinal fluid can be obtained by lumbar puncture (spinal tap).

 ## TREATMENT

GENERAL MEASURES

- Treatment of patients with ALL requires hospitalization for chemotherapy. Management after therapy is on an outpatient basis.
- Access to the resources and expertise of a major oncology center is important for appropriate support.
- The person with ALL must be isolated from infection.
- Surgery and/or bone marrow transplantation may be required.

ACTIVITY

Physical activity as tolerated

DIET

- Nutritional support
- Avoid alcohol

 ## MEDICATIONS

COMMONLY PRESCRIBED DRUGS (IF NEEDED)

- Optimal therapy is not yet known. Although all treatment regimens are still experimental, they are clearly effective for some patients.
- Drugs include cyclophosphamide, daunorubicin, vincristine, asparaginase, filgrastim (L-asparaginase), prednisone, methotrexate, hydrocortisone, mercaptopurine (6-mercaptopurine), cytarabine, doxorubicin, dexamethasone, thioguanine (6-thioguanine), and cytarabine.

OTHER DRUGS

Other experimental drugs

 ## FOLLOW-UP

PATIENT MONITORING

See the doctor daily or weekly during chemotherapy, monthly during maintenance therapy, and every 3 months thereafter.

COMPLICATIONS

- Infections
- Bleeding
- Need for transfusions
- Sterility from treatment
- Severe drug side effects
- Relapse of leukemia

WHAT TO EXPECT

- Of patients younger than 60 years of age, 80% to 90% will have complete remission, and 35% to 60% will remain free of disease at 5 years.
- Some patients may receive bone marrow transplantation.

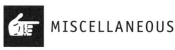 ## MISCELLANEOUS

PEDIATRIC

Bone growth and mental development can be affected by treatment.

PREGNANCY

Many chemotherapy drugs cause birth defects.

Leukemia, Acute Lymphoblastic in Adults (ALL)

Doctor
Office
Phone
Pager

Special notes to patient:

Light Sensitivity

 ## BASICS

DESCRIPTION
Light sensitivity, also called "sun poisoning," is a skin rash induced by exposure to sunlight. It is often a side effect of medication.

SIGNS AND SYMPTOMS
- Reddening
- Rash
- Blisters
- Usually develops shortly after sun exposure.
- Pain
- Itching

CAUSES
- Sunlight
- Phenothiazine
- Diuretics
- Tetracycline
- Sulfonamides
- Oral contraceptives
- Topicals: psoralens, coal tars, photoactive dyes (eosin, acridine orange)

SCOPE
Unknown

MOST OFTEN AFFECTED
All ages; males and females are affected equally

RISK FACTORS
Propensity to light sensitivity can be inherited in some inbred populations (e.g., Pima Indians).

 ## DIAGNOSIS

WHAT THE DOCTOR LOOKS FOR
The doctor will perform a physical examination to identify light sensitivity.

TESTS AND PROCEDURES
- Blood tests
- A sample of skin can be obtained by biopsy for laboratory analysis.
- Allergy testing can be done.

 ## TREATMENT

GENERAL MEASURES
- Avoid or limit exposure to sunlight.
- Use protective clothing and sunscreens.
- Use cold packs or cold water compresses.

ACTIVITY
Avoid sunlight.

DIET
No special diet

 ## MEDICATIONS

COMMONLY PRESCRIBED DRUGS (IF NEEDED)
- Topical corticosteroids
- Nonsteroidal antiinflammatory drugs (NSAIDs)
- Prednisone
- Antihistamines
- Sunscreens

CONTRAINDICATIONS
Read drug product information.

PRECAUTIONS
Read drug product information.

DRUG INTERACTIONS
Read drug product information.

 ## FOLLOW-UP

PATIENT MONITORING
See the doctor as often as necessary for persistent light allergy or recurrence of the condition.

PREVENTION
- Sunlight avoidance
- Wear protective clothing.
- Identify and avoid drugs that cause light sensitivity
- Sunscreens: apply before exposure to sunlight

WHAT TO EXPECT
Good outcome with avoidance and proper protection measures.

 ## MISCELLANEOUS

GERIATRIC
More likely to experience light sensitivity caused by drugs

Light Sensitivity

	Doctor
	Office
	Phone
	Pager

Special notes to patient:

Low Back Pain

 ## BASICS

DESCRIPTION
Low back pain, generally, is a self-limited condition of the aging spine that responds to conservative measures, including rest and pain management. Pain is typically at the belt-line, occasionally involving the buttocks, posterior thighs, or both areas. Low back pain is often the result of the stresses and demands placed on the low back area by everyday activities. In most cases, the condition does not last long and recovery is complete.

SIGNS AND SYMPTOMS
- Onset of low back pain begins suddenly after an injury or gradually over the next 24 hours.
- Variable pain at posterior belt-line, typically on both sides
- Pain may radiate to buttocks and posterior thighs
- Pain is aggravated by back motion, sitting, standing, lifting, bending, and twisting.
- Pain is relieved by rest

CAUSES
- Normal aging process of musculoskeletal system
- Acute event (injury)

SCOPE
At some point in their life, 80% of the population in the United States experience mechanical low back pain.

MOST OFTEN AFFECTED
Individuals 25 to 45 years of age; men and women affected equally

RISK FACTORS
- Age
- Activity
- Smoking
- Obesity
- Vibration (e.g., driving motor vehicles)
- Sedentary lifestyle
- Psychosocial factors

 ## DIAGNOSIS

WHAT THE DOCTOR LOOKS FOR
- The doctor will perform a thorough physical examination, with special emphasis on evaluating back function.
- Numerous other medical conditions that may be responsible for the symptoms should be investigated and ruled out.

TESTS AND PROCEDURES
- Blood tests
- X-ray study and bone scans can be done to assist in diagnosis.
- Magnetic resonance imaging (MRI) or computed tomography (CT) scan can be done.

 ## TREATMENT

GENERAL MEASURES
- Low back pain is managed in the outpatient setting.
- Initial short-term bedrest (2–3 days)
- Short-term pain relievers
- Nonsteroidal antiinflammatory drugs (NSAIDs)
- Muscle relaxants
- Physical therapy
- Manipulation

ACTIVITY
- Restricted activities for 3 to 6 weeks
- Resume activities of daily living as tolerated.

DIET
Weight reduction, if needed

 ## MEDICATIONS

COMMONLY PRESCRIBED DRUGS (IF NEEDED)
NSAIDs: ibuprofen, naproxen, salsalate

CONTRAINDICATIONS
Read drug product information.

PRECAUTIONS
- History of ulcer disease
- Elderly patients
- Kidney disease
- Heart disease

DRUG INTERACTIONS
Read drug product information.

 ## FOLLOW-UP

PATIENT MONITORING
- See the doctor as often as necessary.
- Care usually is for 1 to 6 weeks.

PREVENTION
- Smoking cessation
- Weight reduction
- General physical condition
- Avoid aggravating tasks (e.g., heavy lifting, bending, twisting, sudden unexpected movements)

COMPLICATIONS
- Incorrect diagnosis: missed disease
- Chronic low back pain
- Narcotic addiction
- Persistent psychosocial impairment

WHAT TO EXPECT
Normal activity without lasting symptoms, in most cases

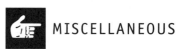 ## MISCELLANEOUS

PREGNANCY
Pregnancy is commonly associated with low back pain and sciatica. Treatment is conservative.

Low Back Pain

Doctor
Office
Phone
Pager

Special notes to patient:

Lumbar Disk Disorders

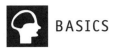 ## BASICS

DESCRIPTION
Many patients with low back pain have lumbar disk disease with involvement of surrounding spinal ligaments, muscles, and bones. Over time, disk degeneration, herniation, and arthritic changes can develop.

SIGNS AND SYMPTOMS
- Variable pain: usually dull, originating in the back, extending below knee
- Back pain decreases at night. Bedrest usually improves symptoms at least temporarily.
- Pain increases with sitting or standing.
- Sciatica can occur without back pain.
- Tingling, numbness, loss of sensation in legs and feet
- Muscle weakness
- Muscle spasm

CAUSES
- Injury
- Frequent lifting of heavy objects, especially if improper technique is used
- Vibration (e.g., driving motor vehicles)

SCOPE
In the United States, 60% to 90% of the population experience lumbar back disorder in their lifetime. It is one of the most common reasons for seeking medical attention.

MOST OFTEN AFFECTED
Individuals 25 to 45 years of age, with the first episode in 20s and 30s; infrequent before 20 or after 65 years of age. Men and women are affected with equal frequency.

RISK FACTORS
- Normal aging process after 20 years of age
- Cigarette smoking
- Spine disorders
- Stress, muscle tension
- Obesity

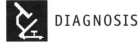 ## DIAGNOSIS

WHAT THE DOCTOR LOOKS FOR
- The doctor will perform a complete physical examination to evaluate back function.
- Numerous other disorders can cause similar symptoms, including strains, arthritis, fracture, poor posture, bursitis, cancers, infection, and other conditions.

TESTS AND PROCEDURES
- Blood tests
- X-ray study of affected area of the back
- Other special radiology procedures that can be done include myelography, computed tomography (CT) scan, magnetic resonance imaging (MRI), and bone scan.

 ## TREATMENT

GENERAL MEASURES
- Most cases of lumbar disk disorders are managed in the outpatient setting.
- Severe disability or surgery may require hospitalization.
- Initial: minimal bedrest, ordinary activities as tolerated, local heat, pelvic traction, sedation, physical therapy
- Chronic pain: Improve physical fitness with low impact aerobic exercise. Manipulation and physical therapy have shown to be beneficial.
- Transcutaneous electrical nerve stimulation (TENS): very short-term benefit
- Surgery may be required.

ACTIVITY
- After pain is controlled (2–4 days), begin a progressive walking program. Initially, take short walks four times a day and increase distance as tolerated.
- Return to work as soon as possible but avoid high-risk activities (e.g., heavy lifting, vibration, smoking).

DIET
Weight reduction, if appropriate

 ## MEDICATIONS

COMMONLY PRESCRIBED DRUGS (IF NEEDED)
- Pain relievers
- Nonsteroidal antiinflammatory medication (NSAIDs)
- Mild sedatives

CONTRAINDICATIONS
Read drug product information.

PRECAUTIONS
Elderly, hypertension, peptic ulcer disease or bleeding, kidney disease, liver disease, cardiac dysfunction may all impact the medications used to treat this condition.

DRUG INTERACTIONS
Read drug product information.

 ## FOLLOW-UP

PATIENT MONITORING
See the doctor about 10 days after the initial visit. Thereafter, the doctor should be seen every 2 weeks until full function returns.

PREVENTION
- Modification of jobs to reduce exposure to known risk factors.
- Selection of workers by strength testing for certain jobs
- Avoid smoking
- Use proper lifting technique.
- Use good posture.
- Control weight

COMPLICATIONS
- Foot drop, weakness of leg muscles
- Bladder and rectum weakness with retention or incontinence
- Limitation of movement and restricted activity
- Narcotic addiction

WHAT TO EXPECT
- Spontaneous recovery with conservative therapy.
- Chronic pain: Most patients respond to conservative management (e.g., manipulation, fitness, weight reduction, and good back care habits).
- Surgery produces good results in selected cases.

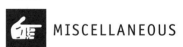 ## MISCELLANEOUS

PREGNANCY
Low back pain and sciatica are commonly associated with pregnancy. Treatment is conservative.

Lumbar Disk Disorders

	Doctor
	Office
	Phone
	Pager

Special notes to patient:

Lyme Disease

 ## BASICS

DESCRIPTION

- Lyme disease is a multisystem infection caused by a microbe transmitted by deer ticks. **Stage 1** includes a characteristic expanding, ringlike skin rash and flulike symptoms. **Stage 2** may involve one or more organ systems; neurologic and cardiac disease are most common. **Stage 3**, chronic Lyme disease, involves arthritis and chronic neurologic symptoms.

SIGNS AND SYMPTOMS

- Stage 1:
  - Expanding bull's-eye rash
  - Fever
  - Headache
  - Muscle and joint pain
  - May be no symptoms
- Stage 2:
  - Multiple ringlike rashes
  - Inflammation of facial nerves
  - Meningitis
  - Heart disorders
  - Inflammation of the testicles or liver
  - Arthritis
- Stage 3:
  - Recurring joint and muscle inflammation
  - Brain disorders (psychosis, dementia, memory loss, depression, strokelike symptoms)
  - Nerve disorders
  - Eye disorders

CAUSES

Infection with *Borrelia burgdorferi*, transmitted by the bite of a deer tick

SCOPE

Lyme disease affects 5.2 of 100,000 persons in the United States. It is most prevalent in Connecticut, Rhode Island, New York, New Jersey, Pennsylvania, Wisconsin, and Maryland.

MOST OFTEN AFFECTED

Lyme disease can occur in all ages, but it is most common in children under 15 years of age and in persons 25 to 44 years of age. Males and females are affected equally.

RISK FACTORS

Exposure to tick-infested area; most common from May to September

 ## DIAGNOSIS

WHAT THE DOCTOR LOOKS FOR

- The doctor will perform a physical examination to identify the presence of Lyme disease.
- Similar signs and symptoms can be caused by juvenile rheumatoid arthritis, viral infection, or many other diseases.

TESTS AND PROCEDURES

- Blood tests
- A sample of spinal fluids can be obtained by lumbar puncture (spinal tap).

 ## TREATMENT

GENERAL MEASURES

- Early stages of Lyme disease can be treated in the outpatient setting.
- Management of stages 2 and 3 may require more intensive treatment, based on symptoms.

ACTIVITY

No restriction

DIET

No special diet

 ## MEDICATIONS

COMMONLY PRESCRIBED DRUGS (IF NEEDED)

- Doxycycline (Vibramycin)
- Amoxicillin
- Ceftriaxone (Rocephin), cefotaxime (Claforan), penicillin G
- Steroids

CONTRAINDICATIONS

- Allergy to drug
- Doxycycline is contraindicated in children and in women who are pregnant or breast-feeding.

PRECAUTIONS

Read drug product information.

DRUG INTERACTIONS

- Can cause sensitivity to sunlight; use sunscreen
- Dosage of oral blood thinners (anticoagulants) may need to be reduced.
- Oral contraceptives can be less effective.

OTHER DRUGS

Cefuroxime (Ceftin)

 ## FOLLOW-UP

PATIENT MONITORING

Individuals with stages 2 and 3 disease should see the doctor often over a period of months to years, based on the severity of symptoms.

PREVENTION

- Prevention of infection is possible by careful examination of skin for ticks after outdoor activities. Be aware that deer ticks are extremely small.
- Remove ticks promptly.
- Wear clothing that covers the ankles in endemic areas.
- Use insect repellant.

COMPLICATIONS

- Recurrent inflammation
- Chronic neurologic symptoms
- See signs and symptoms of stage 3 disease

WHAT TO EXPECT

- Early treatment with antibiotics can shorten the duration of symptoms and prevent later disease.
- Response is variable for late-stage disease.

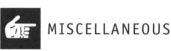 ## MISCELLANEOUS

OTHERS

Ticks are commonly found on deer. Hunters can be at increased risk.

PREGNANCY

Pregnant patients with active disease should receive intravenous (IV) antibiotics. Doxycycline should not be used in pregnant women.

FURTHER INFORMATION

Lyme Borreliosis Foundation, P.O. Box 462, Tolland, CT, 06084, (203) 871-2900

Lyme Disease

Doctor
Office
Phone
Pager

Special notes to patient:

Lymphoma, Burkitt's

 ## BASICS

DESCRIPTION
Burkitt's lymphoma is a cancer of the lymphatic system that can involve sites other than lymph nodes, particularly bone marrow and the central nervous system.

SIGNS AND SYMPTOMS
- Mouth pain
- Loose teeth
- Jaw mass
- Anemia
- Abdominal mass
- Abdominal pain

CAUSES
Unknown; is associated with Epstein-Barr virus

SCOPE
Burkitt's lymphoma is rare in the United States.

MOST OFTEN AFFECTED
Individuals 3 months to 16 years of age; more often in males than females

RISK FACTORS
Living in area where Burkitt's lymphoma occurs

 ## DIAGNOSIS

TESTS AND PROCEDURES
- Blood tests
- Specialized laboratory testing can be done.
- Tissue from a lymph node can be obtained by biopsy for laboratory analysis.
- Spinal fluids can be obtained by lumbar puncture (spinal tap).
- A sample of bone marrow can be obtained to assist in diagnosis.
- Computed tomography (CT) scan can be done to assess internal structures.

 ## TREATMENT

GENERAL MEASURES
- Staging surgery and chemotherapy requires hospitalization.
- After treatment, Burkitt's lymphoma is managed in the outpatient setting.
- Surgery is usually necessary.

ACTIVITY
As tolerated

DIET
- Patients may have difficulty swallowing or chewing; small meals of soft foods (protein milk shakes) help prevent malnutrition.
- Adequate fluid intake

 ## MEDICATIONS

COMMONLY PRESCRIBED DRUGS
Combination chemotherapy, according to most recent protocols

CONTRAINDICATIONS
Read drug product information.

PRECAUTIONS
Read drug product information.

DRUG INTERACTIONS
Read drug product information.

OTHER DRUGS
Intensive chemotherapy with or without bone marrow transplantation

FOLLOW-UP

PATIENT MONITORING
See the doctor as often as needed to monitor chemotherapy and detect recurrence of disease.

PREVENTION
Avoid areas where Burkitt's lymphoma is endemic.

COMPLICATIONS
Kidney failure

WHAT TO EXPECT
- Of patients, 70% to 90% experience long-term remission and possible cure.
- With newer treatments, some patients with more advanced disease have been cured also.
- Without treatment, prognosis is grave.

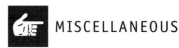 ## MISCELLANEOUS

PEDIATRIC
The pediatric population is a common age group for Burkitt's lymphoma.

GERIATRIC
Burkitt's lymphoma is unusual in the elderly.

FURTHER INFORMATION
Leukemia Society of America, 733 3rd Ave., New York, NY 10017, (212) 573-8424

Lymphoma, Burkitt's

	Doctor
	Office
	Phone
	Pager

Special notes to patient:

Lymphoma, Non-Hodgkin's

 BASICS

DESCRIPTION
Non-Hodgkin's lymphoma is a varied group of lymphatic cancers, distinct from Hodgkin's disease. Characteristics include widespread disease, painless enlargement of one or more lymph nodes. Usual course is progressive.

CAUSES
Malignant tumors of lymph tissues

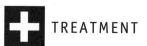 **TREATMENT**

GENERAL MEASURES
- Radiotherapy
- Chemotherapy

Lymphoma, Non-Hodgkin's

Doctor

Office

Phone

Pager

Special notes to patient:

Macular Degeneration, Age-Related (ARMD)

 ## BASICS

DESCRIPTION
Age-related macular degeneration (ARMD)–deterioration of a portion of the retina (the "screen" at the back of the eye that is responsible for vision)–leads to progressive vision loss. ARMD is the leading cause of irreversible, severe visual loss in persons above 65 years of age. The stages of ARMD are dry (nonexudative) and wet (exudative).

SIGNS AND SYMPTOMS
- Formation of small, yellowish-white spots on the retina (drusen)
- Atrophy of retinal pigment
- Distortion of central vision; straight lines (e.g., telephone poles) appear crooked

SCOPE
- Of individuals 52 years of age or older, 25% have signs of ARMD.
- Of patients above 65 years of age, 2.2% are blind in one or both eyes because of ARMD.

MOST OFTEN AFFECTED
- The prevalence of severe visual loss from ARMD increases with age.
- Primarily affects those 50 or more years of age
- Women affected more frequently than men

CAUSES
Exposure to light

RISK FACTORS
- Excess sunlight exposure
- Blue or light eye color
- Far-sightedness
- History of cardiovascular disease
- Short height
- History of lung infection
- Cigarette smoking

 ## DIAGNOSIS

WHAT THE DOCTOR LOOKS FOR
The doctor will perform a physical examination to identify the presence of macular degeneration.

TESTS AND PROCEDURES
Blood vessels of the eye can be assessed with a special radiology procedure called "angiography."

 ## TREATMENT

GENERAL MEASURES
- Macular degeneration is managed in the outpatient setting, including laser surgery.
- Hospitalization may be required for some surgical procedures.
- No specific treatment alters the course of deterioration.
- Vitamins A, E, C, and beta-carotene may be useful in preventing cellular damage.
- Oral zinc may retard visual loss.
- Laser treatment or other surgery may be an option.
- Low-vision aids may be helpful.

DIET
- A diet high in vitamins A, E, C, and beta-carotene along with zinc may be helpful.
- Eating dark green, leafy vegetables (spinach or collard greens), which are rich in carotenoids, may decrease the risk of developing the wet stage of ARMD.

 ## MEDICATIONS

COMMONLY PRESCRIBED DRUGS
- Zinc and antioxidants may be beneficial.
- Interferon (experimental)

PRECAUTIONS
Excess zinc ingestion can be associated with anemia and worsening of cardiovascular disease.

 ## FOLLOW-UP

PATIENT MONITORING
- After laser treatment, contact the doctor promptly if any new visual symptoms appear.
- The Amsler grid can aid in discovering visual disturbances.
- It is important to monitor vision, such as with the Amsler grid.
- If no new symptoms appear, see the doctor every 6 to 12 months.

PREVENTION
- Protect eyes from ultraviolet (UV) light.
- Eat a well-balanced diet that includes zinc and vitamins A, E, C, and beta-carotene.
- Routine visits to an ophthalmologist
- Use an Amster grid daily.
- Have an eye examination every 2 to 4 years when between 40 and 64 years of age and every 1 to 2 years after age 65 years.

COMPLICATIONS
Blindness

WHAT TO EXPECT
Increased risk of visual loss; individual outcomes vary

 ## MISCELLANEOUS

GERIATRIC
Prevalence increases with age.

FURTHER INFORMATION
American Academy of Ophthalmology, 655 Beach St., San Francisco, CA 94109-1336

Macular Degeneration, Age-Related (ARMD)

Doctor
Office
Phone
Pager

Special notes to patient:

Meniere's Disease

 ## BASICS

DESCRIPTION

- Meniere's disease is an inner ear disorder that results in recurrent attacks of hearing loss, tinnitus (ringing in the ears), and vertigo (dizziness).
- Usually occurs in one ear, but 10% to 50% of cases can involve the second ear later on
- Severity and frequency of symptoms may diminish over the years but with increasing loss of hearing.

SIGNS AND SYMPTOMS

- Ringing in the ears (tinnitus)
- Hearing loss
- Vertigo: spontaneous attacks, lasting 20 minutes to several hours
- Sensation of fullness in the ear
- Occurs as attacks, with intervening remission
- During severe attacks:
  - Pallor
  - Sweating
  - Nausea and vomiting
  - Falling
  - Prostration
  - Symptoms are aggravated by motion.

CAUSES

Unknown

SCOPE

Approximately 1,150 cases of Meniere's disease per 100,000 persons in the United States

MOST OFTEN AFFECTED

Usual onset occurs between 20 and 60 years of age; men and women are affected equally.

RISK FACTORS

- Caucasian race
- Stress
- Allergy
- Increased salt intake
- Noise

 ## DIAGNOSIS

WHAT THE DOCTOR LOOKS FOR

- The doctor will perform a physical examination to assess the presence of Meniere's disease.
- Conditions that can cause similar signs and symptoms should be investigated (e.g., acoustic tumor, multiple sclerosis, and other ear disorders).

TESTS AND PROCEDURES

- The ear can be examined by otoscopy.
- Hearing testing can be done.
- Magnetic resonance imaging (MRI) can be done to assist with diagnosis.

 ## TREATMENT

GENERAL MEASURES

- Meniere's disease is usually managed in the outpatient setting
- Surgery may involve hospitalization
- Medications are given primarily for symptomatic relief of vertigo and nausea. No medication is currently available that influences the disease process.
- For attacks, bedrest with eyes closed and protection from falling; attacks rarely last longer than 4 hours.
- Surgery may be required.

ACTIVITY

- Limit activity during attacks
- Between attacks, patient may be fully active.

DIET

Limit total food intake during attacks because of nausea. Otherwise, diet is usually not a factor, unless attacks are brought on by certain foods. A restricted salt diet may be useful in some cases.

MEDICATIONS

COMMONLY PRESCRIBED DRUGS

- Atropine
- Diazepam (Valium)
- Transdermal (skin patch) scopolamine
- Meclizine (Antivert, Bonine)
- Ergotamine-belladonna-phenobarbital (Bellergal-S)

CONTRAINDICATIONS

- Atropine: cardiac disease, especially supraventricular tachycardia and other arrhythmias
- Scopolamine: use with caution in children and the elderly

PRECAUTIONS

- Sedating drugs should be used with caution, particularly in the elderly. Do not operate motor vehicles while taking sedating drugs.
- Read drug product information.

DRUG INTERACTIONS

- Bellergal: oral anticoagulants, tricyclic antidepressants, phenothiazine, narcotics, beta-blockers, estrogens, and others
- Transdermal scopolamine: anticholinergics, belladonna products, antihistamines, tricyclic antidepressants

OTHER DRUGS

- Droperidol
- Promethazine (Phenergan)
- Diphenhydramine (Benadryl)
- Diphenidol (Vontrol)
- Chlorothiazide (Diuril)

Meniere's Disease

	Doctor
	Office
	Phone
	Pager

Special notes to patient:

Meniere's Disease

 ## FOLLOW-UP

PATIENT MONITORING

See the doctor as often as necessary. Hearing status should be monitored frequently.

PREVENTION

- Reduce stress.
- Reduce salt intake.
- Do not smoke.
- Avoid significant noise exposure, or use ear protectors.

COMPLICATIONS

- Failure to diagnose acoustic tumor
- Loss of hearing
- Injury during attack
- Inability to work

WHAT TO EXPECT

- Alternating attacks and remission
- Over time, balance improves but hearing worsens.
- Most cases can be managed successfully with medication.
- Of patients, about 5% to 10% require surgery for incapacitating vertigo.

 ## MISCELLANEOUS

PEDIATRIC

Unusual, but occasionally occurs in a child

GERIATRIC

Meniere's disease is less likely to occur in the elderly. Patients exposed to loud noise levels over many years are more susceptible.

OTHERS

Usual onset between 20 and 60 years of age

PREGNANCY

Not a common problem, but medications used to treat Meniere's disease pose risk of birth defects

Meniere's Disease

Doctor
Office
Phone
Pager

Special notes to patient:

Meningitis, Bacterial

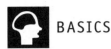 ## BASICS

DESCRIPTION
Bacterial meningitis is an inflammation of the lining of the brain and spinal cord caused by a bacterial infection. This condition must be identified and treated promptly. It constitutes a **medical emergency**.

SIGNS AND SYMPTOMS
- Fever
- Headache
- Vomiting
- Sensitivity to light
- Seizures
- Nausea
- Profuse sweating, "Shaking Chill"
- Weakness
- Altered mental function
- Confusion
- Rash

CAUSES
Bacterial infection

SCOPE
About 3 to 10 cases of bacterial meningitis occur annually per 100,000 persons in the United States.

MOST OFTEN AFFECTED
Newborns, infants, and the elderly; males and females affected equally

RISK FACTORS
- Immune system disorder
- Alcoholism
- Neurosurgical procedure or head injury
- Abdominal surgery

 ## DIAGNOSIS

WHAT THE DOCTOR LOOKS FOR
The doctor will perform a physical examination to identify the signs and symptoms of bacterial meningitis.

TESTS AND PROCEDURES
- A sample of spinal fluids can be obtained by lumbar puncture (spinal tap).
- Blood can be cultured for microbiological analysis.
- X-ray study of the head
- Computed tomography (CT) scan can be done to assist with the diagnosis.

 ## TREATMENT

GENERAL MEASURES
- Management of bacterial meningitis usually requires hospitalization, often in the intensive care unit.
- Antibiotic therapy

ACTIVITY
As tolerated in hospital and on discharge

DIET
Regular as tolerated

MEDICATIONS

COMMONLY PRESCRIBED DRUGS
- Ampicillin
- Cefotaxime, ceftriaxone
- Aminoglycoside (Tobramycin)
- Chloramphenicol
- Steroids: dexamethasone

CONTRAINDICATIONS
Allergies to antibiotics

PRECAUTIONS
- Ear damage
- Hearing loss
- Developmental abnormalities related to meningitis

DRUG INTERACTIONS
Read drug product information.

OTHER DRUGS
- Vancomycin
- Penicillin
- Aztreonam
- Quinolones (e.g., ciprofloxacin)

 ## FOLLOW-UP

PATIENT MONITORING
See the doctor as often as necessary.

PREVENTION
Prompt medical treatment for infections

COMPLICATIONS
- Seizures
- Brain damage
- Nerve disorders

WHAT TO EXPECT
- Patients often make a complete recovery with prompt diagnosis and treatment.
- Overall death rate is 14%.

 ## MISCELLANEOUS

GERIATRIC
May be less evident in elderly patients

FURTHER INFORMATION
American Academy of Pediatrics, 141 Northwest Point Blvd., P.O. Box 927, Elk Grove Village, IL 60009-0927, (800) 433-9016

Meningitis, Bacterial

Doctor
Office
Phone
Pager

Special notes to patient:

Meningitis, Viral

 ## BASICS

DESCRIPTION

Viral meningitis is a viral infection of the membrane covering the brain and spinal cord. It is usually acute (of short duration) but can be relapsing. Incidence peaks in the summer.

SIGNS AND SYMPTOMS

- Fever
- Headache, often severe
- Stiff neck
- Nausea and vomiting
- Sensitivity to light
- Generalized aches and pains
- Rash

CAUSES

Viral infection

SCOPE

An average of 10,000 cases of viral meningitis are reported annually in the United States.

MOST OFTEN AFFECTED

Can affect all ages, but most common in young adults; males and females affected equally

RISK FACTORS

- No specific risk factors are known.
- Immune system disorders

 ## DIAGNOSIS

WHAT THE DOCTOR LOOKS FOR

- The doctor will perform a physical examination to identify the presence of viral meningitis.
- Other conditions that cause similar signs and symptoms will be investigated (e.g., bacterial meningitis and other central nervous system disorders).

TESTS AND PROCEDURES

- A sample of spinal fluid can be obtained by lumbar puncture (spinal tap).
- An electroencephalograph (EEG) can be done to evaluate brain function.
- Computed tomography (CT) scan or magnetic resonance imaging (MRI) can be done to assist in diagnosis.

 ## TREATMENT

GENERAL MEASURES

- Viral meningitis is usually managed with hospitalization.
- Fever control
- Intravenous (IV) fluids, if oral intake is poor or vomiting occurs.

ACTIVITY

Bedrest initially, then activity as tolerated

DIET

Determined by symptoms; may be nothing by mouth because of nausea or vomiting, advancing to clear fluids and regular diet, as tolerated.

 ## MEDICATIONS

COMMONLY PRESCRIBED DRUGS

- Meperidine (Demerol), nalbuphine (Nubain), morphine
- Promethazine (Phenergan), prochlorperazine (Compazine)
- Acetaminophen-codeine, oxycodone-acetaminophen (Percocet)
- Antifever drugs: acetaminophen (Tylenol)
- Antibiotics

CONTRAINDICATIONS

Read drug product information.

PRECAUTIONS

- Aspirin should be avoided in children and adolescents because of its possible association with Reye's syndrome.
- Phenothiazines can produce a reaction, especially in adolescents.

DRUG INTERACTIONS

Read drug product information.

OTHER DRUGS

Symptomatic relief may be provided by a variety of antiemetics and analgesics (e.g., nonsteroidal antiinflammatory drugs).

 ## FOLLOW-UP

PATIENT MONITORING

See the doctor as often as necessary once the acute illness begins to resolve.

COMPLICATIONS

- Deafness
- Fatigue
- Irritability
- Muscle weakness
- Seizures (rare)

WHAT TO EXPECT

Complete recovery in 2 to 7 days; headaches and other uncomfortable symptoms may persist for 1 to 2 weeks.

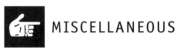 ## MISCELLANEOUS

GERIATRIC

Viral meningitis is rarely seen in the elderly.

FURTHER INFORMATION

American Academy of Pediatrics, 141 Northwest Point Blvd., P.O. Box 927, Elk Grove Village, IL 60009-0927, (800) 433-9016

Meningitis, Viral

Doctor
Office
Phone
Pager

Special notes to patient:

Menopause

 ## BASICS

DESCRIPTION

Menopause is the cessation of spontaneous menstrual cycles. Climacteric or the perimenopausal period is the time during which ovarian function declines. Although a woman can continue to have periodic uterine bleeding, such cycles may be without ovulation. During this time, hormone production diminishes and a woman may experience early signs of estrogen deficiency (e.g., "hot flashes"). Postmenopause is the period after menopause, usually accounting for more than a third of a woman's total lifespan.

SIGNS AND SYMPTOMS

- Cessation of menstruation: either abruptly or preceded by a period of irregular cycles, diminished bleeding, or both
- Vasomotor symptoms: hot flashes, sweating
- Psychological symptoms: depression, nervousness, insomnia
- Painful intercourse
- Urinary incontinence
- Skin atrophy: wrinkles
- Osteoporosis: fractures
- Arteriosclerosis: coronary artery disease

CAUSES

- Physiologic: normal depletion of ovary function
- Surgical: removal of ovaries, hysterectomy
- Medical: can result from treatment of endometriosis or breast cancer. Can occur after chemotherapy and be permanent or reversible.

SCOPE

Menopause is becoming more common as lifespan increases; symptoms currently affect more than 30 million American women.

MOST OFTEN AFFECTED

- Average age is 51 years; virtually all women will be postmenopausal by 58 years of age.
- Premature menopause occurs before 30 years of age and may be associated with abnormalities of the sex chromosomes.

RISK FACTORS

- Increasing age
- Pelvic surgery
- Sex chromosome abnormalities

 ## DIAGNOSIS

WHAT THE DOCTOR LOOKS FOR

- The doctor will take a history and perform a physical examination to identify the presence of menopause.
- Other conditions that can appear similar include pregnancy, ovarian disease, hormone disorders, and urinary tract disorders.
- The doctor will check for conditions known to be associated with menopause (e.g., osteoporosis and atherosclerosis).

TESTS AND PROCEDURES

- Blood tests
- A sample of tissue from the uterus can be obtained by biopsy for laboratory analysis.
- The reproductive tract can be examined by endoscopy.
- Computed tomography (CT) scan can be done to assist in diagnosis.
- Special test can be done to measure bone density.
- Pap smear

 ## TREATMENT

GENERAL MEASURES

- Menopause is managed by periodic office visits with primary care provider.
- To retard development of osteoporosis: adequate calcium intake; exercise; avoid smoking, excessive alcohol, and caffeine intake
- Estrogen replacement therapy

ACTIVITY

Actively exercise as much as possible. Some type of weightbearing exercise is recommended.

DIET

Increased calcium intake, adequate vitamin D (e.g. multivitamin and/or daily sunlight exposure)

 ## MEDICATIONS

COMMONLY PRESCRIBED DRUGS

- Estrogens: conjugated estrogen (Premarin)
- Progestogen: medroxyprogesterone acetate (Provera)
- Combinations: Prempro, Premphase

CONTRAINDICATIONS

- Estrogen-sensitive cancer
- Unexplained uterine bleeding
- History of clotting disorders
- Active liver disease

PRECAUTIONS

Read drug product information.

DRUG INTERACTIONS

Read drug product information.

OTHER DRUGS

- Oral: estropipate (Ogen), estradiol (Estrace)
- Transdermal (patch): estradiol (Estraderm, Vivelle, Climara)
- Vaginal: conjugated estrogens (Premarin cream)
- Progestogens (Depo-Provera)
- Clonidine (Catapres)
- Osteoporosis: alendronate (Fosamax)

 ## FOLLOW-UP

PATIENT MONITORING

- See the doctor as often as necessary.
- Annual Pap smear, pelvic and breast examinations
- Annual mammography

Menopause

Doctor
Office
Phone
Pager

Special notes to patient:

Menopause

PREVENTION

Menopause is a physiologic process that cannot be avoided, but the negative effects can be moderated or eliminated by estrogen replacement therapy.

COMPLICATIONS

- Vasomotor symptoms (flushing, sweating)
- Psychological symptoms
- Vaginal atrophy
- Skin wrinkles
- Osteoporosis
- Arteriosclerosis

WHAT TO EXPECT

- If untreated:
  - Flushing and sweating resolve over several years
  - Atrophy of reproductive and urinary systems
  - Osteoporosis: possible fractures especially of the hip, vertebrae, and wrists
  - Mortality rate associated with hip fractures is 15%.
  - Coronary artery disease
- If treated:
  - Minimal effects of menopause
  - Slower development of bone loss, reduced risk of coronary artery disease
  - Therapy can be continued indefinitely.

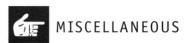

MISCELLANEOUS

FURTHER INFORMATION

- American College of Obstetricians and Gynecologists (ACOG), 409 12th St. S.W., Washington, D.C. 20024, (800) 673-8444
- American Academy of Family Physicians Foundation, P.O. Box 8418, Kansas City, MO 64114, (800) 274-2237, ext. 4400

Menopause

Doctor
Office
Phone
Pager

Special notes to patient:

_____
_____
_____
_____
_____
_____
_____
_____
_____
_____
_____
_____
_____
_____
_____
_____

Menorrhagia

 ## BASICS

DESCRIPTION
Menorrhagia is an excessive amount or duration of menstrual flow, occurring primarily at regular intervals of menstruation.

SIGNS AND SYMPTOMS
- "Excessive" menstrual flow varies greatly from woman to woman.
- Bleeding substantially heavier than the patient's usual flow
- Bleeding lasting more than 7 days
- Passage of significant clots
- Anemia

CAUSES
- Hypothyroidism
- Uterine disorders
- Blood-clotting disorders

SCOPE
Abnormal bleeding is common in the United States.

MOST OFTEN AFFECTED
- Women between menarche and menopause; about 50% of cases occur after 40 years of age.
- Abnormal bleeding is common in adolescence and near menopause.

RISK FACTORS
- Obesity
- Lack of ovulation
- Estrogen therapy

 ## DIAGNOSIS

WHAT THE DOCTOR LOOKS FOR
- The doctor will perform a complete physical examination seeking the cause of heavy menstrual flow.
- Other conditions (e.g., pregnancy and bleeding disorders) should be investigated and ruled out.

TESTS AND PROCEDURES
- Pregnancy test
- Blood tests
- A sample of uterine tissue can be obtained by biopsy for laboratory analysis.
- Ultrasound and computed tomography (CT) scan can be done to assist with the diagnosis.
- Pap smear
- The uterus can be examined by hysteroscopy.

 ## TREATMENT

GENERAL MEASURES
- Most women with menorrhagia can be managed as outpatients in the doctor's office or emergency department.
- Severe bleeding may require hospitalization.
- Pregnancy complications and nonuterine bleeding must be ruled out.

ACTIVITY
As tolerated. Resting with feet elevated may be helpful.

DIET
Iron supplementation may be needed to offset increased blood loss.

 ## MEDICATIONS

COMMONLY PRESCRIBED DRUGS
- Estrogen, conjugated (Premarin)
- Medroxyprogesterone acetate (Provera)

CONTRAINDICATIONS
- Pregnancy
- Breast or endometrial cancer
- Clotting disorder
- Liver failure

PRECAUTIONS
Nausea and vomiting are common.

DRUG INTERACTIONS
Read drug product information.

OTHER DRUGS
- Norethindrone acetate (Norlutin, Norlutate)
- Megestrol acetate (Megace)
- Naproxen sodium, mefenamic acid, ibuprofen
- Danazol (Cyclomen)

 ## FOLLOW-UP

PATIENT MONITORING
See the doctor as often as necessary.

PREVENTION
Annual Pap smear and pelvic examination

COMPLICATIONS
Anemia

WHAT TO EXPECT
- The outcome varies with the cause of bleeding.
- Most patients with hormonal causes will respond to hormone therapy.

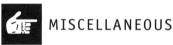

PEDIATRIC
Genital bleeding before puberty can result from trauma, foreign bodies, vaginal infection, or hormonal disorders.

GERIATRIC
Genital atrophy can predispose to bleeding with minimal trauma.

OTHERS
- In adolescence, irregular bleeding is common.
- After 35 to 40 years of age, endometrial dysplasia and cancer are significant causes of bleeding.

Menorrhagia

Doctor
Office
Phone
Pager

Special notes to patient:

Middle Ear Infection

 BASICS

DESCRIPTION

Otitis media is an inflammation of the middle ear. Acute otitis media (AOM) is usually a bacterial infection that is accompanied by an upper respiratory viral infection.

SIGNS AND SYMPTOMS

- Earache
- Fever
- Nasal discharge
- Cough common
- Decreased hearing
- Ear bleeding or discharge
- Irritability

SCOPE

By 7 years of age, 93% of American children have had one or more episodes of AOM; 39% have six or more episodes of AOM.

MOST OFTEN AFFECTED

Peak incidence is 6 to 12 months. Incidence declines after 7 years of age. AOM is rare in adults; males and females are affected equally.

CAUSES

- Bacterial, viral infection
- Allergy

RISK FACTORS

- Daycare
- Formula feeding
- Smoking in household
- Male gender
- Family history of middle ear disease

 DIAGNOSIS

WHAT THE DOCTOR LOOKS FOR

The doctor will perform a physical examination to identify the presence of otitis media.

TESTS AND PROCEDURES

Hearing tests can be performed.

 TREATMENT

GENERAL MEASURES

- Acute otitis media is managed in the outpatient setting, except for infants with fever and patients who require surgery.
- Antibiotics
- Surgery (tubes in eardrum, removal of adenoids) may be recommended.

ACTIVITY

No restrictions

DIET

No special diet

 MEDICATIONS

COMMONLY PRESCRIBED DRUGS

Amoxicillin

CONTRAINDICATIONS

Allergy to penicillins

PRECAUTIONS

Read drug product information.

DRUG INTERACTIONS

Read drug product information.

OTHER DRUGS

- Amoxicillin-clavulanate (Augmentin)
- Cefaclor (Ceclor)
- Cefixime (Suprax)
- Cefpodoxime (Vantin)
- Ceftriaxone (Rocephin)
- Clarithromycin (Biaxin)
- Trimethoprim-sulfamethoxazole (Septra, Bactrim)
- Erythromycin-sulfisoxazole (Pediazole)
- Sulfisoxazole

FOLLOW-UP

PATIENT MONITORING

See the doctor 2 to 4 weeks after diagnosis; for persistent otitis media, see the doctor monthly.

PREVENTION

- Breast-feeding decreases the incidence of AOM.
- Eliminate cigarette smoking in the household.

COMPLICATIONS

- Perforation of eardrum
- Bleeding from ear
- Nerve, bone, brain involvement
- Hearing loss

WHAT TO EXPECT

- The symptoms of acute otitis media usually improve in 48 to 72 hours; residual symptoms resolve within 3 months in 90% of cases.
- Recurring infections usually resolve by school age; only a small number of children have complications.

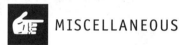 MISCELLANEOUS

PEDIATRIC

Otitis media is primarily a disease of childhood.

GERIATRIC

Otitis media is rare in adults: consider full evaluation to exclude tumors impinging on the eustachian tube.

Middle Ear Infection

Doctor
Office
Phone
Pager

Special notes to patient:

Migraine

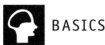
BASICS

DESCRIPTION

Migraine is an attack of headache lasting 4 to 72 hours. Frequency of episodes varies from more than once a week to fewer than one per year, with symptoms abating completely between attacks. Nonspecific symptoms, called "prodromal symptoms," can be felt hours to days before headache.

SIGNS AND SYMPTOMS

Symptoms of migraine vary from person to person and from attack to attack within the same individual.

- Five phases of a migraine:
  - Prodrome: warning signs preceding migraine (e.g., mood disruptions such as euphoria, irritability, depression), fatigue, muscle tension, food craving, bloating, yawning)
  - Aura: visual disruptions (e.g., spots, geometric patterns, and occasionally hallucinations). Headache typically begins within 1 hour after aura.
  - Headache: one-sided, throbbing pain lasting 4 to 72 hours, intensified by movement; accompanied by nausea, vomiting, diarrhea, light sensitivity, sound sensitivity, muscle tenderness, lightheadedness, dizziness
  - Headache termination: untreated, usually occurs with sleep
  - Postdrome: Headache pain has resolved but other symptoms linger (e.g., food intolerance, impaired concentration, fatigue, muscle soreness).

CAUSES

Exact cause is unknown.

SCOPE

- In the United States, 17.6% of women and 5.6% of men suffer from migraine.
- Childhood prevalence is unknown but may be significant.

MOST OFTEN AFFECTED

- Often begins in childhood and increases in early adolescence, through 30s and 40s; decreases with age, but attacks can persist into mature adulthood.
- May be more common among males in childhood, more common among females adolescents and adults.
- May be inherited; more than 80% of patients have a family history of migraines.

RISK FACTORS

- Specific foods, alcohol, missing meals, menstrual cycle, excessive sleep, fatigue, emotional stress
- Medications (estrogen replacement, vasodilators)
- Family history of migraine
- Female gender
- Young age
- History of childhood vomiting, abdominal pain, motion sickness

DIAGNOSIS

WHAT THE DOCTOR LOOKS FOR

- The doctor will take a history and do a physical examination to identify the presence of migraine.
- Other causes of similar symptoms include other types of headache, tumor, infection, epilepsy, and other conditions.

TESTS AND PROCEDURES

Blood tests

TREATMENT

GENERAL MEASURES

- Migraine is usually managed in the outpatient setting.
- Severe cases and individuals with complications may require hospitalization
- Compression to temple artery or tender areas of scalp or neck on affected side
- Cold compresses to area of pain
- Rest with pillows comfortably supporting head or neck in quiet, darkened area.
- Withdrawal from stressful surroundings
- Sleep
- Biofeedback and early psychologic intervention in appropriate cases or when pain behaviors are first identified
- Most attacks of migraine are managed with self-care.

ACTIVITY

Bedrest in a dark, quiet environment

DIET

Maintain fluid intake. Avoid dietary triggers of migraine.

MEDICATIONS

COMMONLY PRESCRIBED DRUGS

- Sumatriptan (Imitrex)
- Zulmitriptan (Zomig)
- Naratriptan (Amerge)
- Rizatriptan (Maxalt)
- Dihydroergotamine (DHE), metoclopramide, prochlorperazine
- Aspirin
- Acetaminophen
- Ibuprofen (Nuprin, Motrin)
- Naproxen (Naprosyn)
- Ketoprofen (Orudis)
- Ketorolac (Toradol)
- Isometheptene-dichloralphenazone-acetaminophen (Midrin)
- Acetaminophen-butalbital (Phrenilin)
- Acetaminophen-butalbital (Fioricet), acetaminophen-butalbital-codeine (Fiorinal)

CONTRAINDICATIONS

Drugs have many contraindications; read drug product information.

PRECAUTIONS

Read drug product information.

SIGNIFICANT POSSIBLE INTERACTIONS

- Other sedatives
- Analgesics
- Alcohol
- Decongestants

OTHER DRUGS

- Butorphanol (Stadol)

FOLLOW-UP

PATIENT MONITORING

See the doctor as often as necessary to monitor symptoms and drug therapy.

Migraine

Doctor
Office
Phone
Pager

Special notes to patient:

Migraine

PREVENTION

- Avoid triggers of attacks.
- Biofeedback and psychologic intervention may be helpful.
- Preventive therapy: If attacks significantly interfere with lifestyle or are not adequately controlled, daily preventive therapy with one of the following drugs may be appropriate:
  - Propranolol (Inderal)
  - Atenolol (Tenormin)
  - Nadolol (Corgard)
  - Timolol (Blocadren)
  - Metoprolol (Lopressor)
  - Amitriptyline (Elavil)
  - Nortriptyline (Pamelor)
  - Verapamil (Calan, Isoptin)
  - Isradipine (DynaCirc)
  - Methysergide (Sansert)
  - Cyproheptadine (Periactin)
  - Valproic acid (Depakene) or divalproex (Depakote)

- A referral to a specialist may be of benefit for patients who do not respond to standard treatment.

COMPLICATIONS

- Severe, persistent migraine (rare)
- Ministrokes (rare)
- Side effects of treatment

WHAT TO EXPECT

- With age: reduction in severity, frequency, and disability of attacks
- Most attacks subside within 72 hours.

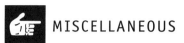 MISCELLANEOUS

PEDIATRIC

Recurrent abdominal pain and vomiting may be main symptoms; attacks may be of shorter duration; headache is not typical.

OTHERS

Migraine affects all races, social classes, and intelligence levels.

PREGNANCY

Attacks often diminish during pregnancy. No treatment drug has U.S. Food and Drug Administration approval for use in pregnancy; ergotamines are contraindicated.

Migraine

Doctor
Office
Phone
Pager

Special notes to patient:

Miscarriage

 ## BASICS

DESCRIPTION

Miscarriage, or spontaneous abortion, is the loss of a fetus before it can survive outside the womb. Miscarriage is "threatened" when vaginal bleeding occurs early in pregnancy, with or without uterine contractions.

SIGNS AND SYMPTOMS

- In a previously diagnosed pregnancy:
  - Vaginal bleeding (pink or brownish discharge)
  - Cramping
  - Cervical dilation
  - Ruptured membranes
  - Passage of nonviable products of conception
  - Fever
  - Shock

CAUSES

The cause of most spontaneous abortions is unknown.

SCOPE

- Of all fertilized ova, over 50% spontaneously miscarry.
- Of all recognized pregnancies, 10% to 15% end in miscarriage.

MOST OFTEN AFFECTED

- Women, under 15 years of age
- Advancing age: Women above 35 years of age have a threefold risk of miscarriage compared with women who are under 30 years of age.

RISK FACTORS

- Fetal chromosomal abnormalities
- Uterine abnormalities
- Maternal alcohol or drug ingestion
- Increasing maternal age
- Deteriorating health status (e.g., diabetes, thyroid disease)
- Infections
- Previous abortions

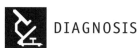 ## DIAGNOSIS

WHAT THE DOCTOR LOOKS FOR

- The doctor will perform a thorough physical examination to assess reproductive status, including a pelvic examination.
- Cervical polyps, cancer, or inflammatory conditions can cause vaginal bleeding.

TESTS AND PROCEDURES

- Cultures: for group B streptococcus, gonorrhea, and chlamydia
- Blood tests
- The products of conception can be retained for analysis.
- Ultrasound can be used to assist in the diagnosis.
- Fluid or tissue from the reproductive tract can be sampled for laboratory analysis.

 ## TREATMENT

GENERAL MEASURES

- Miscarriage can be managed in the outpatient setting or require hospitalization, depending on the nature of the condition.
- Threatened miscarriage: bedrest (usually at home) and insert nothing in the vagina. If bleeding is severe (i.e., more than a heavy period), hospitalization and close observation may be required.
- Surgical procedures (dilatation and curettage [D&C]) may be required.

ACTIVITY

If appropriate, bedrest until resolution

DIET

No special diet

 ## MEDICATIONS

COMMONLY PRESCRIBED DRUGS

- Oxytocin (Pitocin)
- Methylergonovine (Methergine)
- Analgesics, if needed
- Rho(D) immune globulin if mother is Rh negative
- Beta-agonists (e.g. isoxsuprine)
- Progesterone

CONTRAINDICATIONS

None

PRECAUTIONS

Read drug product information.

SIGNIFICANT POSSIBLE INTERACTIONS

Read drug product information.

 ## FOLLOW-UP

PATIENT MONITORING

- See the doctor as often as necessary.
- Subsequent pregnancy will require special care and attention.
- Counseling may be helpful for coping with emotional issues.

PREVENTION

- Any vaginal bleeding during pregnancy is abnormal and should be considered a "threatened" miscarriage until proved otherwise. In reality, vaginal bleeding in early pregnancy is common and often the bleeding source eludes diagnosis.
- Surgery for habitual miscarriage

COMPLICATIONS

- Complications of surgery include uterine perforation, infection, and bleeding.
- Recurrent miscarriage
- Depression and feelings of guilt

WHAT TO EXPECT

- In cases of threatened miscarriage where bleeding stops and pregnancy continues to progress normally, maternal prognosis is excellent.
- First-trimester bleeding is associated with preterm delivery, delivery of low-birthweight infants, and neonatal death.
- After surgery for incomplete or inevitable miscarriage and after complete miscarriage, the outcome is excellent.

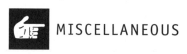 ## MISCELLANEOUS

PREGNANCY

A complication of pregnancy

FURTHER INFORMATION

American College of Obstetricians & Gynecologists, 409 12th St., SW, Washington, DC 20024-2188, (800) 762-ACOG

Miscarriage

Doctor
Office
Phone
Pager

Special notes to patient:

Mitral Valve Prolapse

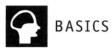 ## BASICS

DESCRIPTION

Mitral valve prolapse is a bulging that occurs to the mitral valve as the heart pumps, producing a distinctive sound that can be heard with a stethoscope. Mitral valve prolapse is usually harmless, causes no symptoms, and is not progressive. A few people with mitral valve prolapse develop related conditions (e.g., irregular heart rhythms, other cardiac disorders, or sudden death). Some have chest pain, palpitations, fatigue, shortness of breath, dizziness, anxiety, and panic attacks.

SIGNS AND SYMPTOMS

- May have no symptoms
- Chest pain: recurrent, located on left side or beneath the breastbone, duration varies from moments to hours
- Fatigue
- Fainting
- Shortness of breath
- Psychiatric symptoms, including anxiety and panic attacks

CAUSES

- Inherited
- Caused by any number of medical conditions

SCOPE

Mitral valve prolapse affects about 5% of the population in the United States.

MOST OFTEN AFFECTED

- Mitral valve prolapse is uncommon before adolescence and is usually detected in young adulthood. It is more common in females under 20 years of age and more common in men after 50 years of age.

RISK FACTORS

- Family history
- Connective tissue disorder

 ## DIAGNOSIS

WHAT THE DOCTOR LOOKS FOR

The doctor will perform a physical examination, with particular attention to assessing heart sounds with a stethoscope.

TESTS AND PROCEDURES

- Chest x-ray study
- An electrocardiogram (ECG) and echocardiogram can be done to assist in diagnosis.
- Other specialized tests can be done (e.g., the tilt-table studies, ECG stress test, and 24-hour monitoring of cardiac activity).

 ## TREATMENT

GENERAL MEASURES

- Mitral valve prolapse is usually managed in the outpatient setting.
- Of cases, 75% are not associated with any increase in illness or death, and no treatment is required.
- Complications tend to occur after age 50 years (more in men than in women) and include irregular heart rhythms and other conditions requiring surgery.
- People with mitral valve prolapse have an increased risk of developing infection of the mitral valve. Because dental procedures can release bacteria from dental plaque into the bloodstream, patients with mitral valve prolapse should take preventive antibiotics before and after dental procedures.
- Surgical repair or replacement of the valve may be necessary.

ACTIVITY

- Generally unrestricted
- Vigorous sports and dehydration can cause fainting.
- Competitive sports should be avoided in patients with severe symptoms.

DIET

- Adequate salt intake
- Caffeine, alcohol, and cigarettes should be avoided by individuals with palpitations.

 ## MEDICATIONS

COMMONLY PRESCRIBED DRUGS (IF NEEDED)

- Beta-blockers
- Aspirin
- Antibiotics
- Warfarin (coumadin)

CONTRAINDICATIONS

Read drug product information.

PRECAUTIONS

Beta-blockers will increase fatigue and dizziness.

DRUG INTERACTIONS

Read drug product information.

 ## FOLLOW-UP

PATIENT MONITORING

See the doctor as often as necessary.

PREVENTION

Preventive antibiotics before dental procedures

POSSIBLE COMPLICATIONS

Although uncommon, complications can include the following:

- Heart inflammation
- Stroke, ministroke
- Heart failure
- Irregular heart rhythms
- Sudden death
- Fainting

WHAT TO EXPECT

- Of people with mitral valve prolapse, 75% have an excellent outcome.
- The 25% of patients who become progressively worse, experience a long (25-year) period without symptoms followed by rapid deterioration requiring surgery.

 ## MISCELLANEOUS

PEDIATRIC

Mitral valve prolapse is rarely seen in young children.

GERIATRIC

Complications occur mostly in men above 50 years of age.

PREGNANCY

- Mitral valve prolapse itself is not a contraindication to pregnancy.
- Connective tissue diseases may be a contraindication to pregnancy.
- Symptoms of mitral valve prolapse may improve during pregnancy.

FURTHER INFORMATION

American Heart Association, 7320 Greenville Ave., Dallas, TX 75231, (214) 373-6300

Mitral Valve Prolapse

	Doctor
	Office
	Phone
	Pager

Special notes to patient:

Molluscum Contagiosum

 ## BASICS

DESCRIPTION

Molluscum contagiosum is a common, harmless viral skin disorder consisting of small skin elevations that tend to occur on the face, trunk, and extremities in children, and on the groin and genitalia in adults. The lesions can be extensive in a person with an immune system disorder.

SCOPE

Molluscum contagiosum is common in the United States.

MOST OFTEN AFFECTED

Children and young adults; males and females are equally affected

SIGNS AND SYMPTOMS

- Pearly to flesh-colored, firm elevations of skin
- Diameter 2 to 6 ml
- Usually grouped in one or two areas
- Lesions can be itchy or tender.
- Distribution: anywhere on the body; predilection for face, trunk, and extremities in children, and groin and genitalia in adults.

CAUSES

Viral infection

RISK FACTORS

- Close contact with infected persons
- In children, transmission can occur in swimming pools.
- In adults, sexual transmission is common.
- Immune system disorders

 ## DIAGNOSIS

WHAT THE DOCTOR LOOKS FOR

- The doctor will perform a physical examination to identify the presence of molluscum contagiosum.
- Similar signs can be caused by skin cancer, warts, and numerous other skin conditions.

TESTS AND PROCEDURES

A lesion can be sampled by biopsy for laboratory analysis.

 ## TREATMENT

GENERAL MEASURES

- Molluscum contagiosum is managed in the outpatient setting.
- Spontaneous resolution commonly occurs in 6 to 12 months. Individual lesions resolve in 2 months.
- Lesions may be surgically removed.
- Cryotherapy is also effective.

ACTIVITY

No restrictions

DIET

No special diet

 ## FOLLOW-UP

PATIENT MONITORING

- See the doctor 2 to 4 weeks after treatment.
- A complete course of treatment often requires two to four visits.

PREVENTION

In adults, avoid sexual contact with infected individuals.

COMPLICATIONS

- Disease can persist or spread.
- Can be transmitted to others
- People with immune system disorders can have extensive infections.

WHAT TO EXPECT

- Untreated, the condition is usually self-limited.
- Individual lesions spontaneously heal in 2 months; total resolution usually takes 6 to 12 months.
- Recurrences are uncommon.

 ## MISCELLANEOUS

PEDIATRIC

Commonly seen on face, trunk, and extremities; can be spread or acquired in swimming pools

OTHERS

Often, a sexually transmitted disease in adults

Molluscum Contagiosum

	Doctor
	Office
	Phone
	Pager

Special notes to patient:

Mononucleosis

 ## BASICS

DESCRIPTION
Mononucleosis, or "mono," is a viral illness caused by the Epstein-Barr virus (EBV). The illness is characterized by fatigue, fever, enlarged spleen, enlarged lymph nodes, and sore throat.

SIGNS AND SYMPTOMS
- Malaise
- Fatigue
- Headache
- Fever
- Enlarged lymph nodes
- Tonsillitis
- Swelling around eyes
- Rash
- Jaundice

CAUSES
Epstein-Barr virus

SCOPE
Of the population, 14% to 90% has been exposed to EBV.

MOST OFTEN AFFECTED
High school and college students; males and females in equal proportions

RISK FACTORS
- College and high school students
- Kissing
- Of people with mononucleosis, 70% to 90% continue to shed virus 2 to 6 months after the initial infection.

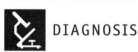 ## DIAGNOSIS

WHAT THE DOCTOR LOOKS FOR
The doctor will perform a physical examination to identify the presence of mononucleosis.

TESTS AND PROCEDURES
Blood tests

 ## TREATMENT

GENERAL MEASURES
- Mononucleosis is managed in the outpatient setting.
- No specific treatment
- Quarantine not indicated
- Gargling
- Surgery may be required.

ACTIVITY
- Rest
- Avoid contact sports, heavy lifting, strenuous athletics.

DIET
- Healthy diet is important.
- Drink milk shakes, fruit juices, and consume soft foods to ease sore throat.

 ## MEDICATIONS

COMMONLY PRESCRIBED DRUGS
- Antibiotics
- Pain relievers: acetaminophen (Tylenol), codeine
- Prednisone

CONTRAINDICATIONS
Aspirin should not be taken by young children because of the risk of Reye's syndrome.

PRECAUTIONS
Read drug product information.

DRUG INTERACTIONS
Read drug product information.

 ## FOLLOW-UP

PATIENT MONITORING
- See the doctor as often as necessary.
- See the doctor before resuming contact sports.

PREVENTION
Most likely spread by saliva

COMPLICATIONS
- Chronic infections (chronic fatigue syndrome; very controversial)
- Rupture of the spleen (rare)
- Anemia
- Blood-clotting disorders
- Seizures
- Brain damage
- Nerve disorders
- Coma
- Psychosis
- Heart disorders
- Airway obstruction
- Lung disorders
- Liver failure
- Digestive disorders
- Dermatitis
- Rash
- Kidney disorders
- Infection
- Jaundice

WHAT TO EXPECT
- Fever subsides in about 10 days.
- Enlarged lymph nodes and enlarged spleen subside in about 4 weeks.
- Children should be able to return to school when signs of infection have decreased; appetite returns; and alertness, strength, and sense of well-being allow.

 ## MISCELLANEOUS

PEDIATRIC
Children have mild infections.

Mononucleosis

Doctor
Office
Phone
Pager

Special notes to patient:

Motion Sickness

 ## BASICS

DESCRIPTION
Motion sickness is not a true illness, but a normal response to an abnormal situation in which a sensory conflict occurs about body motion and position. A mismatch between the visual, balance, and body-position senses results in motion sickness.

SIGNS AND SYMPTOMS
- Nausea
- Vomiting
- Profuse sweating
- Pallor
- Excessive production of saliva
- Yawning
- Rapid breathing
- Anxiety, panic
- Malaise
- Fatigue
- Weakness
- Confusion

CAUSES
Motion (e.g., auto, plane, boat, amusement rides)

RISK FACTORS
- Travel
- Visual stimuli (e.g., moving horizon)
- Poor ventilation (e.g., fumes, smoke, carbon monoxide)
- Emotions (e.g., fear, anxiety)
- Low or zero gravity (e.g., amusement park ride)
- Other illness or poor health

 ## DIAGNOSIS

WHAT THE DOCTOR LOOKS FOR
The doctor checks for conditions with similar signs and symptoms of motion sickness (e.g., mountain sickness, vestibular disease, gastroenteritis, metabolic disorders, and toxic exposure).

 ## TREATMENT

GENERAL MEASURES
- Remove triggers or stimuli of motion sickness.
- Minimize exposure (sit in middle of plane or boat)
- Improve ventilation

ACTIVITY
- Semireclining position
- Fix vision at 45° angle above horizon.
- Avoid fixation of vision on moving objects (e.g., waves).
- Avoid reading while in motion.

DIET
- Decrease oral intake or take frequent small feedings.
- Avoid alcohol.

 ## MEDICATIONS

COMMONLY PRESCRIBED DRUGS
Scopolamine

CONTRAINDICATIONS
Glaucoma

PRECAUTIONS
- Use scopolamine cautiously in:
  - Young children
  - Elderly
  - Pregnancy
  - Urinary obstruction
  - Pyloric obstruction

DRUG INTERACTIONS
- Sedatives (e.g., antihistamines, alcohol, antidepressants)
- Belladonna alkaloids

OTHER DRUGS
- Dimenhydrinate (Dramamine)
- Meclizine (Antivert)

 ## FOLLOW-UP

PREVENTION
- Minimize exposure (sit in middle of plane or boat).
- Improve ventilation.
- Semireclining position
- Fix vision at 45° angle above the horizon.
- Avoid fixation of vision on moving objects (e.g., waves).
- Avoid reading while in motion.
- Minimize food intake before travel.

COMPLICATIONS
- Low blood pressure
- Dehydration
- Depression
- Panic

WHAT TO EXPECT
- Symptoms should resolve when motion exposure ends.
- Resistance to motion sickness seems to increase with age.

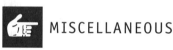 MISCELLANEOUS

PEDIATRIC
Children are particularly susceptible to motion sickness.

GERIATRIC
Age confers some resistance to motion sickness.

Motion Sickness

	Doctor
	Office
	Phone
	Pager

Special notes to patient:

Multiple Sclerosis

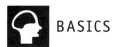 BASICS

DESCRIPTION

Multiple sclerosis (MS) is a progressive inflammatory disease of the brain and spinal cord that causes multiple and varied neurologic symptoms and signs. It is usually intermittent, progressive, and relapsing. It can be acute (brief duration) or slowly progressive. MS is a major cause of disability in young adults.

SIGNS AND SYMPTOMS

- Incoordination
- Neurologic disturbances
- Blurred, double or loss of vision in a single eye
- Muscle spasm
- Clumsiness
- Difficulty moving
- Mood swings
- Fatigue
- In women, loss of sensation in genital area
- Paralysis of the hands
- Paralysis of the right or left half of the body
- Loss of position sense
- Monoparesis
- Eye paralysis
- Loss of sensation, tingling
- Erectile dysfunction in men
- Urinary frequency, hesitancy, incontinence

CAUSES

Unknown; may be result of autoimmune disorder or viral infection

SCOPE

Annually, 25,000 new cases of MS are reported in the United States.

MOST OFTEN AFFECTED

Young adult (16 to 40 years of age); more frequent in females than males; may have a genetic component

RISK FACTORS

- Living in temperate climate
- Northern European descent
- Family history of MS

 DIAGNOSIS

WHAT THE DOCTOR LOOKS FOR

- The doctor will perform a physical examination to identify the signs and symptoms of MS.
- Conditions that may appear similar to MS include tumors, infections, and other nervous system disorders.

TESTS AND PROCEDURES

- A sample of spinal fluids can be obtained by lumbar puncture (spinal tap).
- Blood tests
- Special diagnostic procedures can be done to assess the nervous system, including visual-evoked response (VER), somatosensory-evoked potentials, and brain stem auditory-evoked responses.
- Magnetic resonance imaging (MRI) and computed tomography (CT) scan can be done to assist in diagnosis.

 TREATMENT

GENERAL MEASURES

- Should be managed in the outpatient setting for as long as possible.
- A long-term care facility may be required for physical therapy or complications.
- No specific treatment is available for multiple sclerosis. Remissions occur spontaneously.
- Emotional support, encouragement, and reassurances are necessary to help avoid a hopeless outlook.
- Occupational therapy
- Urologic evaluation including any sexual dysfunction problems (erectile dysfunction common in male patients)
- Self-catheterizations for inadequate bladder emptying
- Custodial care, in cases of cognitive impairment
- Physical therapy to maintain range of movement and strength and to avoid complications

ACTIVITY

- Maintain activity; avoid overwork and fatigue.
- Rest during periods of acute relapse.

DIET

If constipation is a problem, high-fluid intake plus a high-fiber diet

 MEDICATIONS

COMMONLY PRESCRIBED DRUGS

- Drug therapy is used to relieve symptoms:
- Methylprednisolone
- Baclofen, diazepam
- Stool softeners, bulk-producing agents, laxative suppositories
- Propantheline, oxybutynin chloride
- Antibiotics
- Primidone, clonazepam
- Haloperidol, lithium, amitriptyline
- Nonsteroidal antiinflammatory drugs (NSAIDs)
- Carbamazepine
- Azathioprine, ACTH (adrenocorticotropic hormone), methylprednisolone, cyclophosphamide, interferons, cyclosporine are all experimental

CONTRAINDICATIONS

Read drug product information.

PRECAUTIONS

Read drug product information.

SIGNIFICANT POSSIBLE INTERACTIONS

Read drug product information.

OTHER DRUGS

- Amantadine (no specific evidence that this drug is effective)
- Interferon (approved for limited cases)
- Copolymer-1, cladribine (experimental)

Multiple Sclerosis

Doctor
Office
Phone
Pager

Special notes to patient:

Multiple Sclerosis

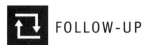 **FOLLOW-UP**

PATIENT MONITORING
See the doctor and other healthcare providers as often as necessary to maintain optimal health status.

PREVENTION
No known preventive measures. Avoid factors that can precipitate an attack, particularly stress from hot weather.

COMPLICATIONS
- Coma
- Delirium
- Mood swings
- Vision disturbances
- Paraplegia
- Sexual impotence (men)
- Urinary tract infections

WHAT TO EXPECT
- The outcome of MS is highly variable and unpredictable.
- About 70% of people with MS lead active, productive lives, with prolonged period of good health.
- MS can be disabling by early adulthood or cause death within months of onset.
- Average duration of the illness exceeds 25 years.
- Of individuals with MS, 30% have a relapse in 1 year, 20% in 5 to 9 years, 10% in 10 to 30 years.

 MISCELLANEOUS

PEDIATRIC
Multiple sclerosis is unlikely before puberty.

GERIATRIC
Remissions occur less frequent among the elderly.

PREGNANCY
Is a triggering factor for MS, in some cases

FURTHER INFORMATION
National Multiple Sclerosis Society, 205E 42nd St., New York, NY 10017, (800) 624-8236

Multiple Sclerosis

Doctor
Office
Phone
Pager

Special notes to patient:

Mumps

 ## BASICS

DESCRIPTION

Mumps is an acute infection usually presenting with inflammation of one or both parotid glands, which are located just behind the corner of the jaw. The swollen parotid glands can get very large, obscuring the normal contour of the cheek. Epidemics of mumps occur in late winter and spring. The virus that causes mumps is transmitted in the air. The incubation period is approximately 14 to 24 days.

SIGNS AND SYMPTOMS

- Pain and swelling in one or both parotid glands at the corner of the jaw
- Pre-illness syndrome of fever, neck muscle ache, malaise
- Swelling peaks in 1 to 3 days; lasts 3 to 7 days.
- Sour foods cause pain.
- Moderate fever, usually not above 104°F (40.0°C)
- Can affect joints, testicles (orchitis), thyroid, breasts, pancreas
- Rash
- Up to 50% of cases have no symptoms.

CAUSES

Viral infection

SCOPE

Mumps is common in the United States.

MOST OFTEN AFFECTED

Most mumps cases (80%) occur in people under 15 years of age. The illness is more severe in adults. Males and females are affected with equal frequency

RISK FACTORS

- Urban epidemics, nonvaccinated population
- Usual contagious period is 2 days before, to 6 to 10 days after onset.

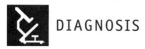 ## DIAGNOSIS

WHAT THE DOCTOR LOOKS FOR

- The doctor will perform a physical examination to determine the presence of mumps.
- Numerous other medical conditions can cause signs and symptoms similar to mumps.

TESTS AND PROCEDURES

- Blood tests
- Body fluids can be cultured for laboratory analysis.
- A sample of spinal fluids can be obtained by lumbar puncture (spinal tap).

 ## TREATMENT

GENERAL MEASURES

- Without complications, mumps is managed in the outpatient setting.
- General care is supportive and symptomatic.
- For orchitis (inflammation of the testis), cold packs to scrotum can help relieve pain.
- Scrotal support with adhesive bridge while lying down and athletic supporter while walking

ACTIVITY

Mumps orchitis: bedrest and local supportive clothing (e.g., such as wearing two pairs of briefs or an adhesive-tape bridge)

DIET

Liquids, if the patient cannot chew

 ## MEDICATIONS

COMMONLY PRESCRIBED DRUGS

- Corticosteroids
- Nonsteroidal antiinflammatory drugs (NSAIDs)
- Acetaminophen

CONTRAINDICATIONS

Read drug product information.

PRECAUTIONS

Avoid aspirin for pain in children because of the risk of Reye's syndrome.

DRUG INTERACTIONS

Read drug product information.

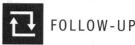 ## FOLLOW-UP

PATIENT MONITORING

Most cases of mumps are mild. Monitor fluid intake to prevent dehydration.

PREVENTION

Mumps vaccine is recommended for active immunization at 15 months of age and at entry to middle school.

COMPLICATIONS

Can affect the brain, heart, pancreas, kidneys, ears, eyes, testicles, ovaries, and other body systems.

WHAT TO EXPECT

- Usually, complete recovery; immunity is permanent.
- Temporary hearing loss occurs in 4% of adults.
- Rarely recurs

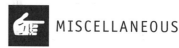 ## MISCELLANEOUS

PEDIATRIC

- In adolescents, orchitis is more common.
- Most cases of acute epidemic mumps occur in children 5 to 15 years of age. It is unusual in children under 2 years of age. Most infants under 1 year of age are immune.
- Not likely to develop complications

GERIATRIC

Most elderly persons are immune to mumps.

OTHERS

Most complications occur in the postpubertal group.

PREGNANCY

- Although no complications of vaccine administration to pregnant women have been noted, theoretically it should not be given in pregnancy because it is a "live" vaccine.
- Disease can increase rate of miscarriage in first trimester.

Mumps

Doctor
Office
Phone
Pager

Special notes to patient:

Nail Fungus

 ## BASICS

DESCRIPTION
A fungus can cause infectious inflammation of the skin folds surrounding the fingernail or toenail. This condition is also called "paronychia." It can be acute (brief) or chronic (long-lasting).

SIGNS AND SYMPTOMS
- Separation of nail fold from nail plate
- Red, painful swelling of skin around nail plate
- Pus, drainage
- Changes of nail plate
- Greenish tint to nail

CAUSES
Infection by bacteria, *Candida albicans*, other fungi, or molds

SCOPE
Common

MOST OFTEN AFFECTED
All ages; three times more frequent in females than males

RISK FACTORS
- Trauma to skin surrounding the nail
- Ingrown nails
- Frequent immersion of hands in water
- Diabetes mellitus

 ## DIAGNOSIS

WHAT THE DOCTOR LOOKS FOR
The doctor will identify the presence of nail fungus.

TESTS AND PROCEDURES
Nail tissue can be sampled for laboratory analysis.

 ## TREATMENT

GENERAL MEASURES
- Acute: warm compresses or soaks, elevation
- Chronic: keep fingers dry
- Surgical incision and drainage of any abscess present.
- Partial or complete removal of nail may be necessary.

ACTIVITY
Full activity

DIET
No special diet

 ## MEDICATIONS

COMMONLY PRESCRIBED DRUGS
- Dicloxacillin
- Cloxacillin
- Erythromycin
- Cephalexin (Keflex)
- Mupirocin
- Econazole
- Ketoconazole
- Itraconazole
- Fluconazole

CONTRAINDICATIONS
Allergy to antibiotic

PRECAUTIONS
Erythromycin can cause significant gastrointestinal upset.

DRUG INTERACTIONS
Numerous interactions; read drug product information.

 ## FOLLOW-UP

PATIENT MONITORING
See the doctor routinely until the condition has healed.

PREVENTION
- Avoid frequent wetting of hands, wear rubber gloves with cloth liner.
- Good diabetic control

COMPLICATIONS
- Acute: abscess under nail
- Chronic: ridging, thickening, and discoloration of nail; nail loss

WHAT TO EXPECT
With adequate treatment and prevention, healing can be expected.

 ## MISCELLANEOUS

PEDIATRIC
Can be related to thumb or finger sucking

Nail Fungus

Doctor
Office
Phone
Pager

Special notes to patient:

Nosebleed

 ## BASICS

DESCRIPTION
Nosebleed, or epistaxis, is a hemorrhage from the nostril, nasal cavity, or nasal portion of the throat.

SIGNS AND SYMPTOMS
Usually bleeding from the nostril. However, nose can bleed to the back of the throat and not be apparent, resulting in nausea, the spitting or vomiting of blood, or the appearance of dark, tarry stool.

CAUSES
- Unknown (most common)
- Injury: nose picking, low humidity, foreign body
- Infection
- Vascular abnormalities
- Cancer
- High blood pressure
- Blood clotting disorders
- Deviation or perforation of the nasal septum

SCOPE
Unknown

MOST OFTEN AFFECTED
Children younger than 10 years of age or adults above 50 years of age; males and females are affected equally.

RISK FACTORS
Hay fever

 ## DIAGNOSIS

WHAT THE DOCTOR LOOKS FOR
Epistaxis is a symptom or a sign, not a disease; the underlying cause of nosebleed should be identified and treated.

TESTS AND PROCEDURES
- Blood tests
- X-ray study of the sinuses
- Special imaging of blood vessels (angiography) can be done (rare).

 ## TREATMENT

GENERAL MEASURES
- Nosebleed is usually managed in the outpatient setting.
- Nasal packing may be required.
- Management of severe bleeding may require hospitalization.
- Elderly patient may require hospitalization.
- Provide first aid as needed
- Pinch nostrils together to help reduce bleeding.
- If nosebleeds persist, the doctor may stop prescribing sedation, pain relievers, or high blood pressure medication.

ACTIVITY
Bedrest with head at 45° to 90° angle

DIET
No alcohol or hot liquids

MEDICATIONS

COMMONLY PRESCRIBED DRUGS
- Antibiotics
- Decongestants
- Iron supplement

CONTRAINDICATIONS
Drug allergies

PRECAUTIONS
Read drug product information.

DRUG INTERACTIONS
Read drug product information.

 ## FOLLOW-UP

PATIENT MONITORING
See the doctor as often as needed.

PREVENTION
- Apply petroleum jelly (Vaseline) to nostril to prevent drying and picking.
- Humidification at night
- Cut fingernails.

COMPLICATIONS
- Sinusitis
- Airway obstruction
- Injury to nasal structures by treatment
- Drug side effects

WHAT TO EXPECT
The outcome is good with proper treatment.

Nosebleed

Doctor
Office
Phone
Pager

Special notes to patient:

Obesity

 ## BASICS

DESCRIPTION

Obesity is a condition of increased body weight (consisting of both lean and fat tissue) that leads to increased illness and death. Obesity is also defined as weight 20% greater than an individual's desirable weight or BMI > 28.

Obesity threshold (BMI = 28)

Height	Weight (lb)
5'0"	143
5'4"	163
5'8"	184
6'0"	206
6'4"	230

SIGNS AND SYMPTOMS

Increased body weight and adipose tissue

CAUSES

- Multiple factors
- May have genetic cause
- Imbalance between food intake and energy expenditure
- Medical conditions (pancreatic disease, thalamus disorder, Cushing's syndrome)
- Drug side effects

SCOPE

In the United States, 20% to 30% of men and 30% to 40% of women are overweight.

MOST OFTEN AFFECTED

Obesity affects all ages; females affected more frequently than males; 20% to 25% of tendency to obesity is inherited.

RISK FACTORS

- Parental obesity
- Pregnancy
- Sedentary lifestyle
- High-fat diet
- Low socioeconomic status

 ## DIAGNOSIS

TESTS AND PROCEDURES

- Blood tests
- Body mass index (BMI) can be calculated.

 ## TREATMENT

GENERAL MEASURES

- Healthcare providers should assess the degree of health risk from obesity; help set goals for therapy; counsel or refer to a registered dietitian or weight loss program for in-depth work on diet, exercise, and behavior modification.
- Behavior modification, which can improve dietary adherence and long-term results of weight loss, should be included in any weight-loss program.
- Many reputable commercial and community programs offer weight reduction treatment. Look for programs with diets that meet the recommended daily allowance (RDA) for nutrients, include exercise counseling, behavior modification, and provisions for long-term maintenance.
- Occasionally, patients with severe obesity are treated with a gastric bypass or stapling procedure. This complex procedure should only be done in a center skilled in this treatment. Surgical treatment is the most effective long-term weight-loss treatment available for morbid obesity.

ACTIVITY

Exercise alone rarely causes significant weight loss. It can improve long-term results of weight-loss treatment and should be an integral part of any weight-loss program.

DIET

- Diet restriction is the cornerstone of obesity management: maintain a low-fat, high-complex carbohydrate, and high-fiber diet.
- A 500 kilocalorie (kcal) reduction in calorie intake per day will result in approximately 1 pound of weight loss per week.
- Very low-calorie diets (400–800 kcal/day) are usually based on liquid formulas and cause more rapid weight loss. However, they can cause serious medical complications, and medical supervision is important.
- Avoid fad diets and miracle cures.

 ## MEDICATIONS

COMMONLY PRESCRIBED DRUGS

- Drug treatment is not usually recommended.
- Appetite suppressants may be indicated for short-term use (few weeks) along with a weight-toss regimen:
  - Diethylpropion
  - Phentermine
  - Fenfluramine
  - Mazindol
  - Dexfenfluramine (Redux)
  - Phendimetrazine
  - Benzphetamine

CONTRAINDICATIONS

Advanced atherosclerosis, cardiovascular disease, hypertension, hyperthyroidism, glaucoma, history of drug abuse, agitated states, use of monoamine oxidase (MAO) inhibitors

PRECAUTIONS

- Abuse potential
- Weight gain after discontinuation of drug

OTHER DRUGS

- Phenylpropanolamine (PPA) is used in over-the-counter weight-loss preparations.
- Orlistat (Xenical)

Obesity

Doctor
Office
Phone
Pager

Special notes to patient:

Obesity

 ## FOLLOW-UP

PATIENT MONITORING

Long-term follow-up and management is crucial to prevent further weight gain or regain after weight loss.

PREVENTION

Regular exercise and prudent diet with regular follow-up, especially in children and young adults and individuals with a family history of obesity or diabetes mellitus

COMPLICATIONS

- Increased risk of death caused mainly by cardiovascular disease
- Diabetes mellitus
- High blood pressure
- High levels of lipids in the bloodstream
- Gallbladder disease with stone formation
- Osteoarthritis
- Gout
- Blood clot formation
- Breathing problems and sleep apnea
- Poor self-esteem
- Discrimination

WHAT TO EXPECT

- Long-term maintenance of weight loss is extremely difficult.
- If a person is not motivated, successful weight loss is unlikely.

 ## MISCELLANEOUS

PEDIATRIC

Prevalence of obesity is increasing in children, in part, because of decreased physical activity and increased television viewing.

GERIATRIC

Acceptable weight ranges increase with age.

OTHERS

Prepuberty and young adulthood appear to be sensitive periods for the development of obesity.

PREGNANCY

Pregnancy is a common time for onset of or increase in obesity.

Obesity

Doctor
Office
Phone
Pager

Special notes to patient:

Obsessive-Compulsive Disorder

 ## BASICS

DESCRIPTION

- Obsessive-compulsive disorder (OCD) is a psychiatric condition characterized by intrusive thoughts (obsessions) and compulsions. **Compulsions** are ritualistic behaviors that relieve the anxiety of obsessions.
- Common obsessive themes:
  - Violence (e.g., harming a child)
  - Doubt (e.g., whether doors or windows are locked or iron turned off)
  - Blasphemous thoughts (e.g., in a devoutly religious person)
  - Contamination, dirt, or disease
  - Symmetry or orderliness
- Common rituals or compulsions:
  - Handwashing
  - Checking
  - Counting
  - Hoarding
  - Repeating (e.g., dressing rituals)

SIGNS AND SYMPTOMS

- Obsessions, compulsions, or both that consume more than 1 hour a day and cause significant distress or impairment
- Neither obsessions nor compulsions are related to another mental disorder.
- Compulsions (actions) are repetitive, purposeful behaviors that are performed in an attempt to neutralize intrusive thoughts (e.g., checking in response to doubt, such as locks, doors, windows, or driving back over route to check for any possible damage inadvertently done while driving one's car)
- Repeated handwashing or ritualistic handwashing in response to fear of contamination
- Of patients, 80% to 90% have obsessions and compulsions.
- Of patients with OCD, 10% to 19% are purely obsessional.
- Only 5% of patients perform rituals until they "feel right" and may not have an identifiable obsession.

CAUSES

Disorder of neurotransmitter serotonin

SCOPE

About 2.5% of the population in the United States will experience obsessive-compulsive behavior in their lifetime.

MOST OFTEN AFFECTED

- Average age of 20 years
- One third of cases present by age 15 years.
- New cases after 50 years of age are rare
- Family history in 20% of cases
- Males and females are affected equally.

RISK FACTORS

Family history of OCD

 ## DIAGNOSIS

WHAT THE DOCTOR LOOKS FOR

The doctor will evaluate for the presence of obsessive-compulsive behavior or other mental health disorders.

TESTS AND PROCEDURES

- Psychological testing can be done.
- Positron emission tomography (PET) can be done to assist in the diagnosis.

 ## TREATMENT

GENERAL MEASURES

- Counseling by psychiatrist or other mental health professional
- Drug therapy
- Psychosurgery (last resort)

ACTIVITY

No restriction

 ## MEDICATIONS

COMMONLY PRESCRIBED DRUGS

- Fluoxetine (Prozac)
- Sertraline (Zoloft)
- Paroxetine (Paxil)
- Fluvoxamine (Luvox)

CONTRAINDICATIONS

Read drug product information.

PRECAUTIONS

Many precautions; read drug product information.

DRUG INTERACTIONS

Drugs have many possible interactions; read drug product information.

OTHER DRUGS

Clomipramine

 ## FOLLOW-UP

PATIENT MONITORING

See the doctor as often as necessary to monitor the disorder and drug therapy.

COMPLICATIONS

- Depression
- Phobias
- Anxiety and paniclike episodes

WHAT TO EXPECT

Chronic waxing and waning course for most people

 ## MISCELLANEOUS

PEDIATRIC

Adolescent onset in 15%; at this age, males outnumber females 3:1.

GERIATRIC

OCD is not usually diagnosed after age 50 years.

PREGNANCY

- Onset OCD has been noted after delivery.
- Safety of fluoxetine and clomipramine has not been established in pregnancy or lactation.

FURTHER INFORMATION

- OCD Foundation, P.O. Box 9573, New Haven, CT 06535, (203) 772-0565
- Obsessive-Compulsive Anonymous, P.O. Box 215, New Hyde Park, NY 11040, (516) 741-4901

Obsessive-Compulsive Disorder

	Doctor
	Office
	Phone
	Pager

Special notes to patient:

Osteoporosis

 ## BASICS

DESCRIPTION

Osteoporosis is a skeletal disease characterized by severe bone loss sufficient to predispose to fractures of the vertebral column, leg, arm, pelvis, and ribs.

SIGNS AND SYMPTOMS

- Backache, pain
- Curvature of the spine
- Fractures in the absence of trauma
- Loss of height
- Depression
- Gastrointestinal symptoms

CAUSES

Multiple factors; in many cases, the exact cause is unknown

SCOPE

About 30% to 40% of women and 5% to 15% of men will develop osteoporosis.

MOST OFTEN AFFECTED

Osteoporosis can be diagnosed in individuals from 8 years of age to old age. It is more common in females than males and in whites and Asians than in African-Americans or Latinos.

RISK FACTORS

- Dietary: inadequate calcium, excessive phosphate or protein; inadequate vitamin D
- Physical: immobilization, sedentary lifestyle
- Alcohol, smoking, caffeine
- Medical: chronic diseases, malabsorption, hormone disorders
- Drug therapy: corticosteroids, thyroid hormone replacement, heparin, chemotherapy, diuretics, anticonvulsants, radiation therapy
- Heredity

 ## DIAGNOSIS

WHAT THE DOCTOR LOOKS FOR

- The doctor will assess the presence and degree of osteoporosis.
- Numerous diseases can cause similar signs and symptoms, including cancers and other bone disorders.

TESTS AND PROCEDURES

- Blood tests
- Urinalysis
- X-ray study
- Specialized radiology procedures can be done, including bone mineral density (BMD) measurement.
- A sample of bone tissue can be obtained for laboratory analysis (rare).

 ## TREATMENT

GENERAL MEASURES

- Osteoporosis is usually managed in the outpatient setting.
- Acute back pain may require hospitalization, especially for vertebral fractures and upper leg and pelvic fractures.
- Nursing home or home care may be needed following fractures.
- Treatment is directed at relief of pain and disability (e.g., heat, pain relievers, physical therapy).

ACTIVITY

- Walk 1 mile twice a day. If possible, try swimming and bicycling.
- Avoid exercises and maneuvers that increase compressive forces and mechanical stress on bone.
- Rehabilitation may be prescribed for back muscle spasm and walking.

DIET

- Reducing diet if overweight.
- Calcium intake 1,500 mg/day from all sources, if not contraindicated.
- Avoid excess phosphate or protein intake (i.e., avoid phosphoric acid-containing beverages and excess meat intake).
- Consume 600 to 800 international units (IU) of vitamin D daily from all sources.

MEDICATIONS

COMMONLY PRESCRIBED DRUGS

- Hormone replacement therapy (HRT: estrogen/progesterone)
- Synthetic salmon calcitonin nasal spray (Miacalcin)
- Oral synthetic salmon calcitonin (Osteocalcin, Calcimar, Miacalcin)
- Alendronate (Fosamax)

CONTRAINDICATIONS

Numerous contraindications; read product information.

PRECAUTIONS

Numerous precautions; read drug product information.

DRUG INTERACTIONS

None

OTHER DRUGS

- Etidronate disodium
- Sodium fluoride
- Tamoxifen
- Raloxifene
- Hormones

Osteoporosis

Doctor
Office
Phone
Pager

Special notes to patient:

Osteoporosis

FOLLOW-UP

PATIENT MONITORING

- See the doctor monthly during start of therapy, then every 2 to 4 months thereafter.
- Annual gynecologic examination, breast examination, and mammography
- Repeat x-ray study every 3 years; more often when indicated
- Annual or every-other-year bone mineral density test

PREVENTION

- Diet, exercise, and HRT at menopause
- Increased calcium intake and adequate vitamin D intake
- Correction of treatable medical conditions and other risk factors

COMPLICATIONS

- Severe disabling pain
- Nerve disorder caused by vertebral fracture (rare)
- Disability or death from complications of upper leg fractures

WHAT TO EXPECT

- In 70% patients, treatment will lead to stabilization.
- Small increases in bone mass occur in many cases.
- Reduced pain, increased mobility

MISCELLANEOUS

PEDIATRIC

A juvenile form of osteoporosis exists.

PREGNANCY

Osteoporosis of pregnancy exists, but rarely.

FURTHER INFORMATION

National Osteoporosis Foundation, 2100 M St., Suite 602, Washington, DC 20037

Osteoporosis

	Doctor
	Office
	Phone
	Pager

Special notes to patient:

Ovarian Cancer

 ## BASICS

DESCRIPTION
Ovarian cancer is composed of a variety of malignancies that arise from the ovary.

SIGNS AND SYMPTOMS
- Vague gastrointestinal symptoms
- Bloating, heartburn
- Abdominal swelling, pain, and distention
- Occasional vaginal discharge
- Irregular vaginal bleeding
- Pelvic mass
- Painful intercourse
- Weight loss

CAUSES
Unknown

SCOPE
Ovarian cancer is responsible for 12,000 deaths each year in the United States. It is the fifth leading cause of cancer death in women.

MOST OFTEN AFFECTED
- The most common form of ovarian cancer affects women 40 to 75 years of age.
- Other types of ovarian cancer affect women 12 to 40 years of age.
- May have a genetic component

RISK FACTORS
- Risk decreases as the number of childbirths increases.
- Late pregnancies (>30 years of age)
- Family history

 ## DIAGNOSIS

WHAT THE DOCTOR LOOKS FOR
The doctor will perform a physical examination to identify the presence of ovarian cancer and associated conditions.

TESTS AND PROCEDURES
- Blood tests
- Other radiologic procedures can be used, including mammogram, barium enema, computed tomography (CT) scan, and upper gastrointestinal (GI) series.
- Pelvic ultrasound can be used to assist in diagnosis.
- A sample of ovarian tissue can be obtained for laboratory analysis.
- Surgery may be necessary for diagnosis and staging.

 ## TREATMENT

GENERAL MEASURES
- Ovarian cancer is usually managed by hospitalization.
- Surgical staging and debulking are critical.
- Chemotherapy and radiotherapy may be recommended by the oncologist.
- Other surgical procedures (e.g. hysterectomy) may be necessary.

ACTIVITY
As tolerated

DIET
High-protein diet

 ## MEDICATIONS

COMMONLY PRESCRIBED DRUGS
- Platinum-based regimen (cisplatin or carboplatin)
- Cyclophosphamide (Cytoxan)
- Paclitaxel (Taxol)
- Other drugs based on current protocol

CONTRAINDICATIONS
Cisplatin: impaired kidney function, hearing loss, nerve disease

PRECAUTIONS
All drugs cause bone marrow suppression. Cisplatin is toxic to the eyes, kidney, and peripheral nerves.

DRUG INTERACTIONS
Read drug product information.

OTHER DRUGS
- Etoposide
- 5-Fluorouracil
- Doxorubicin (Adriamycin)
- Melphalan, hexamethylmelamine, ifosfamide, thiotepa
- Ondansetron (Zofran), dronabinol (Marinol), metoclopramide (Reglan), and others for nausea

 ## FOLLOW-UP

PATIENT MONITORING
See the doctor as often as needed to assess health and monitor drug therapy.

PREVENTION
Oral contraceptive agents may provide some protection.

COMPLICATIONS
- Lung disorders
- Thyroid disorder
- Accumulation of fluid in the abdomen
- Radiotherapy and chemotherapy adverse reactions
- Bowel obstruction

WHAT TO EXPECT
- Five-year survival rate depends on cancer cell type, stage, and residual disease:
  - Stage I, 80%
  - Stage II, 60%
  - Stage III, 15% to 30%
  - Stage IV, 10%

Ovarian Cancer

Doctor
Office
Phone
Pager

Special notes to patient:

Painful Intercourse

 ## BASICS

DESCRIPTION
Painful intercourse (dyspareunia) is recurring and persistent genital pain associated with intercourse, in either the man or woman.

SIGNS AND SYMPTOMS
Pelvic or genital pressure, aching, tearing, or burning

CAUSES
- Vaginal or pelvic disorders (e.g., decreased lubrication, infection)
- Gastrointestinal disorders (e.g., inflammatory bowel disease, constipation)
- Urinary tract disorders (e.g., cystitis)
- Male reproductive disorder (e.g., muscle spasm, infection, prostate condition)
- Psychological disorders (e.g., fear, anxiety, phobias)

SCOPE
- Most women who are sexually active will experience dyspareunia at some time in their lives. Approximately 15% of adult women will have dyspareunia on a few occasions during a year. About 1% to 2% of women will have painful intercourse more than occasionally.
- Prevalence among men is unknown.

MOST OFTEN AFFECTED
All ages, women more frequently than men

RISK FACTORS
- Diabetes
- Estrogen deficiency
- Alcohol or marijuana use
- Menopause
- Medroxyprogesterone use

 ## DIAGNOSIS

WHAT THE DOCTOR LOOKS FOR
- The doctor will take a history and perform a physical examination.
- Causes of dysfunction should be identified and treated (e.g., such as vaginismus—spasm of muscles of the vaginal opening).

TESTS AND PROCEDURES
- Urinalysis
- Fluid from the urinary or reproductive tract can be sampled for laboratory analysis.
- For female patient, a Pap smear can be done.
- The urinary system can be assessed with a test called "voiding cystourethrogram."
- X-ray study of the digestive system can be done to assist in diagnosis.
- The reproductive, urinary, or intestinal systems can be visually examined by endoscopy.

 ## TREATMENT

GENERAL MEASURES
- Dyspareunia is managed in the outpatient setting.
- The first step in treatment is to educate the patient and partner about the nature of the problem and reassure them that the problem can be solved.
- Referral for long-term therapy may be necessary (e.g., behavioral therapy, individual therapy, couple therapy).

ACTIVITY
Routine

DIET
- Regular

 ## MEDICATIONS

COMMONLY PRESCRIBED DRUGS
Depends on the cause. Can include antibiotics, estrogen, pain relievers, and lubricants

CONTRAINDICATIONS
Read drug product information.

PRECAUTIONS
Read drug product information.

DRUG INTERACTIONS
Read drug product information.

FOLLOW-UP

PATIENT MONITORING
See the doctor as frequently as needed for therapy, every 6 to 12 months once the problem has been resolved.

PREVENTION
Avoid alcohol and tobacco products.

WHAT TO EXPECT
Most cases respond to treatment.

 ## MISCELLANEOUS

GERIATRIC
The incidence of dyspareunia increases dramatically in the postmenopausal woman who is not receiving hormone replacement therapy (HRT). More than half of women who are sexually active report dyspareunia.

PREGNANCY
Episiotomy can result in dyspareunia.

Painful Intercourse

	Doctor
	Office
	Phone
	Pager

Special notes to patient:

Pancreatitis

 ## BASICS

DESCRIPTION

Pancreatitis is an inflammation of the pancreas, which can be acute (brief) or chronic (long-lasting).

SIGNS AND SYMPTOMS

- Abdominal pain: upper abdominal pain may radiate to back
- Nausea and vomiting
- Mild abdominal distention
- Fever (100°F to 101°F [37.7°C to 38.3°C])
- Shock
- Jaundice
- Discoloration of the flank or navel
- Discoloration around the navel

CAUSES

- Gallstones
- Alcoholism and acute intoxication
- Medications
- Metabolic disorders
- Peptic ulcer (rare)
- Trauma or surgery
- Infection
- Tumor
- Systemic lupus erythematosus
- Mumps
- Cystic fibrosis
- Acquired immunodeficiency syndrome (AIDS)
- Insect or animal sting

SCOPE

About 10 to 22 cases of pancreatitis per 100,000 persons are reported in the United States annually.

MOST OFTEN AFFECTED

Acute pancreatitis can affect all ages; chronic pancreatitis primarily affects individuals 35 to 45 years of age (usually related to alcohol). Males and females are affected equally.

RISK FACTORS

Listed under *Causes*

 ## DIAGNOSIS

WHAT THE DOCTOR LOOKS FOR

The doctor will assess for the presence of pancreatitis and other conditions that can cause similar signs and symptoms.

TESTS AND PROCEDURES

- Blood tests
- X-ray study of the abdomen
- Ultrasound
- Computed tomography (CT) scan
- The pancreas can be examined by endoscopy.

 ## TREATMENT

- Acute pancreatitis: hospitalization, unless very mild and the patient can maintain oral intake
- Chronic pancreatitis: outpatient treatment except for complications

GENERAL MEASURES

- Acute pancreatitis usually requires hospitalization but mild cases can be managed on an outpatient basis.
- Chronic pancreatitis is managed on an outpatient basis, except for complications.
- Surgery may be required.

ACTIVITY

- Acute pancreatitis: usually bedrest, although sitting in a chair may be more comfortable.
- Chronic pancreatitis: not restricted

DIET

- Acute pancreatitis: small amounts of high-carbohydrate, low-fat, and low-protein foods
- Chronic pancreatitis: small meals high in protein

 ## MEDICATIONS

COMMONLY PRESCRIBED DRUGS

- Meperidine (Demerol)
- Analgesics: acetaminophen (Tylenol), oxycodone-acetaminophen (Tylox), hydrocodone-acetaminophen (Vicodin), propoxyphene napsylate
- Pancreatic enzyme (Pancrease MT, Creon)
- Antacids (e.g. ramitidine)

CONTRAINDICATIONS

Read drug product information.

PRECAUTIONS

Narcotic addiction

DRUG INTERACTIONS

Read drug product information.

 ## FOLLOW-UP

PATIENT MONITORING

- See the doctor as often as needed.
- The cause of pancreatitis should be identified and treated.

PREVENTION

Avoid alcohol.

COMPLICATIONS

Pancreas damage with subsequent diabetes mellitus

WHAT TO EXPECT

- Acute pancreatitis:
  - Of patients, the condition resolves spontaneously in 85% to 90%; mortality rate is 3% to 5%.
- Chronic pancreatitis:
  - Patients may have recurrent acute episodes.

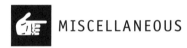 ## MISCELLANEOUS

PEDIATRIC

Pancreatitis can sometimes accompany mumps.

FURTHER INFORMATION

National Digestive Diseases Information Clearinghouse, Box NDDIC, Bethesda, MD 20892, (301) 468-6344

Pancreatitis

Doctor
Office
Phone
Pager

Special notes to patient:

Parkinson's Disease

 ## BASICS

DESCRIPTION

Parkinson's disease is a degenerative disorder of the central nervous system that affects adults. The condition is marked by tremors at rest, rigidity, and slow movement.

SIGNS AND SYMPTOMS

- Tremor
- Slow movement
- Rigidity
- Speech is poorly enunciated, low volume, clipped
- Eye abnormalities: decreased blinking, spasm of eyelid
- Seborrhea
- Constipation, incontinence, sexual dysfunction
- Depression
- Dementia
- Walking disturbances: no arm swing, problems standing up from chair
- Neglect of swallowing, with drooling

CAUSES

Unknown

SCOPE

Parkinson's disease affects 50,000 persons annually in the United States.

MOST OFTEN AFFECTED

Individuals 60 years of age and older; slightly more common in men; may be inherited

RISK FACTORS

Unknown

 ## DIAGNOSIS

WHAT THE DOCTOR LOOKS FOR

- The doctor will perform a physical examination to identify the signs and symptoms of Parkinson's disease.
- Numerous other conditions that can appear similar to Parkinson's disease should be ruled out (including Alzheimer's, drug side effects, atherosclerosis, certain toxins, etc.).

TESTS AND PROCEDURES

Computed tomography (CT) scan, magnetic resonance imaging (MRI), or positron emission tomography (PET) can be done to assist in diagnosis.

 ## TREATMENT

GENERAL MEASURES

- Parkinson's disease is managed in the outpatient setting, except for complications or elective surgery.
- Drugs can have both therapeutic and toxic effects.
- Worsening symptoms may indicate noncompliance with drug therapy, depression, or another illness.
- Course is progressive, with or without drugs. Life-long therapy is directed toward control of symptoms and treatment of disability.
- Physical, occupational, and speech therapy may be useful.
- Patient's physical limitations may require many adjustments in the home (e.g., special chairs, elevated toilet seat, eating utensils, assistance with dressing).
- Surgery may be recommended.

ACTIVITY

Maintain activity to whatever degree possible; use cane for walking.

DIET

- Small, frequent meals, if eating is difficult
- High-liquid intake is important; high-bulk foods
- Reduced protein diet is unnecessary.

 ## MEDICATIONS

COMMONLY PRESCRIBED DRUGS

- Levodopa-carbidopa (Sinemet, Sinemet SR)
- Bromocriptine
- Pergolide
- Trihexyphenidyl (Artane)
- Benztropine (Cogentin)
- Amantadine
- Tolcapone
- Entacapone

CONTRAINDICATIONS

Read drug product information.

PRECAUTIONS

Numerous precautions; read drug product information.

DRUG INTERACTIONS

Most of the drugs have additive therapeutic and side effects.

OTHER DRUGS

- Tricyclic antidepressants
- Apomorphine
- Clozapine

 ## FOLLOW-UP

PATIENT MONITORING

The doctor should see the patient frequently to monitor health status, drug therapy, and physical therapy.

PREVENTION

Avoid drugs known to cause tardive dyskinesia (e.g., such as fluphenazine, perphenazine, prochlorperazine, thiopropazate, trifluoperazine, promazine, thioridazine, haloperidol, droperidol, benperidol, fluspirilene, pimozide, trifluperidol, chlorprothixene, clopenthixol, and thiothixene).

WHAT TO EXPECT

Parkinson's disease is slowly progressive.

COMPLICATIONS

Dementia, depression, pneumonia, falls, freezing, movement difficulty; also associated with a twofold increase in risk of death

 ## MISCELLANEOUS

GERIATRIC

Common among elderly

FURTHER INFORMATION

- United Parkinson Foundation, 360 W. Superior St., Chicago, IL 60610, (312) 664-2344
- Parkinson's Education Program-USA, 3900 Birch St., 105, Newport Beach, CA 92660, (800) 344-7872

Parkinson's Disease

Doctor
Office
Phone
Pager

Special notes to patient:

Parvovirus B19 Infection

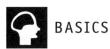 ## BASICS

DESCRIPTION
Human parvovirus B19 is the primary cause of erythema infectiosum (EI; also called "fifth disease"). It can cause arthritis and joint pain and, in some persons, aplastic anemia. In a pregnant woman, the virus can cross the placenta and infect the fetus.

SIGNS AND SYMPTOMS
- Rash on the face ("slapped cheek appearance") followed 1 to 4 days later by a second-stage rash on the trunk and limbs
- Itching and mild joint pain
- Headache, sore throat, runny nose, joint and muscle aches, and gastrointestinal disturbances are more frequent and severe in adults.
- Of adults, 80% may experience arthritis or joint pain.
- In children, joint symptoms are less common.

CAUSES
Viral infection; virus can be transmitted to the fetus during pregnancy

SCOPE
- Parvovirus is extremely common: 50% of adults have evidence of prior infection.
- Parvovirus infection is most common as a community epidemic in winter and spring in nontropical regions.

MOST OFTEN AFFECTED
- Infection is common in childhood.
- Peak age for illness is 4 to 12 years of age. Males and females are affected equally.

RISK FACTORS
- Anemia
- Immune system disorders
- Intrauterine infection

 ## DIAGNOSIS

WHAT THE DOCTOR LOOKS FOR
- The doctor will perform a physical examination to identify the presence of parvovirus infection.
- Numerous other conditions that can cause similar signs and symptoms should be ruled out, including rubella (german measles), other viral infections, systemic lupus erythematosus, drug reaction, Lyme disease, and rheumatoid arthritis.

TESTS AND PROCEDURES
- Blood tests
- If the patient is pregnant, fetal ultrasound, amniocentesis, or chorionic villus sampling (CVS) can be done.

 ## TREATMENT

GENERAL MEASURES
- Parvovirus infection is usually managed in the outpatient setting.
- Individuals with severe symptoms may require hospitalization

ACTIVITY
- Unrestricted
- Individuals with arthritis may require physical therapy or an exercise program.

DIET
No special diet

 ## MEDICATIONS

Usually, no treatment is needed.

COMMONLY PRESCRIBED DRUGS (IF NEEDED)
- Intravenous immune globulin (IVIG)
- Blood transfusions
- Antiinflammatory agents may alleviate arthritic symptoms.

CONTRAINDICATIONS
Read drug product information.

PRECAUTIONS
Read drug product information.

DRUG INTERACTIONS
Read drug product information.

 ## FOLLOW-UP

PATIENT MONITORING
See the doctor often for repeat blood tests.

PREVENTION
- Standard hygienic practices can minimize spread.
- Because the illness is so common, it is not possible to avoid exposure completely.
- Pregnant healthcare workers should avoid caring for patients with bone marrow disorders.
- Pregnant child care workers are at some increased risk; however, exclusion from the workplace will not eliminate this risk, and exclusion is not recommended.

COMPLICATIONS
- Complications are rare, but they are seen more commonly in adults than in children.
- Arthritis
- Persistent anemia
- Blood disorders
- Lung inflammation
- Brain disease
- Reports of birth defects, but no clear-cut association

WHAT TO EXPECT
- Usually self-limited
- Joint symptoms subside in weeks
- Full recovery in 2 to 3 weeks

 ## MISCELLANEOUS

GERIATRIC
None known

PREGNANCY
See above

Parvovirus B19 Infection

Doctor
Office
Phone
Pager

Special notes to patient:

Pelvic Inflammatory Disease (PID)

 BASICS

DESCRIPTION

Pelvic inflammatory disease (PID) is caused by bacterial infection of the female reproductive tract. PID is a broad term that includes a variety of upper genital tract infections unrelated to pregnancy or surgical procedures.

SIGNS AND SYMPTOMS

- May cause no symptoms
- Lower abdominal pain
- Fever and malaise
- Vaginal discharge
- Irregular bleeding
- Urinary discomfort
- Bowel inflammation
- Nausea and vomiting
- Abdominal tenderness
- Tender cervix

CAUSES

Bacterial infection

SCOPE

An estimated 1 million women are treated for PID annually in the United States.

MOST OFTEN AFFECTED

Females 16 to 40 years of age

RISK FACTORS

- Sexually active, reproductive age
- Most common in adolescents
- Multiple sexual partners
- Use of an intrauterine device (IUD)
- Previous history of PID
- Cervicitis
- Gonorrhea
- Condoms and vaginal spermicides lessen the risks of PID.
- Oral contraceptives may reduce the risk of PID.

 DIAGNOSIS

WHAT THE DOCTOR LOOKS FOR

- The doctor will perform a physical examination to identify PID.
- Other possible causes of similar signs and symptoms should be ruled out (e.g., ectopic pregnancy, appendicitis, or other medical disorders).

TESTS AND PROCEDURES

- Pregnancy test
- Blood tests
- Urinalysis
- The uterus can be sampled for culture.
- Pelvic ultrasound can be done.
- The reproductive tract can be examined by laparoscopy.

 TREATMENT

GENERAL MEASURES

- PID is usually managed in the outpatient setting.
- Hospitalization may be required for severe cases or other special factors.
- Avoid sexual intercourse until treatment is completed.
- Sex partners should be evaluated and treated.
- Surgery may be required.

ACTIVITY

According to severity of illness

DIET

According to severity of illness

 MEDICATIONS

COMMONLY PRESCRIBED DRUGS

Antibiotics

CONTRAINDICATIONS

Read drug product information.

PRECAUTIONS

Read drug product information.

DRUG INTERACTIONS

Read drug product information.

 FOLLOW-UP

PATIENT MONITORING

- Individuals with fever or other severe symptoms should be followed closely.
- See the doctor as often as necessary.
- Ultrasonography should be repeated.

PREVENTION

- Use safe sex practices.
- Use barrier contraceptives, especially condoms, and spermicidal creams or sponges.
- Evaluation and treatment of sex partners
- Comply with management instructions.
- Seek medical care early when genital lesions or discharge appear.
- Seek routine check-ups for sexually transmitted diseases (STDs) if not in a mutually monogamous relationship

COMPLICATIONS

- Abscess
- Recurrent infection
- Increased risk of ectopic pregnancy
- Tubal infertility
- Chronic pelvic pain

WHAT TO EXPECT

- PID has a wide variation in outcome, with good prognosis if early, effective therapy is instituted and further infection is avoided.
- Poor prognosis is related to late therapy and continued unsafe lifestyle.

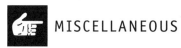 MISCELLANEOUS

PEDIATRIC

- PID is rare before puberty.
- Adolescents are highly vulnerable to STDs, including PID.

GERIATRIC

PID is rare after menopause.

PREGNANCY

PID is rare during pregnancy but occurs occasionally.

FURTHER INFORMATION

Information Services, Centers for Disease Control, E06, Atlanta, GA 30333, (404) 639-1819

Pelvic Inflammatory Disease (PID)

Doctor

Office

Phone

Pager

Special notes to patient:

Peptic Ulcer Disease

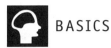 BASICS

DESCRIPTION

A peptic ulcer is an ulcer in the lining of the gastrointestinal tract.

SIGNS AND SYMPTOMS

- Gnawing or burning upper abdominal pain 1 to 3 hours after meals, relieved by food or antacids
- Nocturnal pain causing early morning awakening
- Dyspepsia: belching, bloating, abdominal distention, food intolerance
- Heartburn
- Dizziness, fainting, blood in vomit, tarry stool
- Feeling full early in meal
- Weight loss

CAUSES

The cause of ulcers involves multiple factors. The bacteria, *Helicobacter pylori*, is found in 75% to 90% or more of patients with an ulcer. Other physiologic factors are involved.

SCOPE

Between 200,000 and 500,000 new cases of peptic ulcer disease are reported annually in the United States.

MOST OFTEN AFFECTED

Individuals 25 to 75 years of age; slightly more common in males than females

RISK FACTORS

- Cigarette smoking
- Drugs (e.g., nonsteroidal antiinflammatory drugs [NSAIDs])
- Family history of ulcer
- Stress
- Lower socioeconomic status
- Manual labor
- Poorly or not associated: dietary spices, alcohol, caffeine, acetaminophen

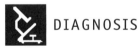 DIAGNOSIS

WHAT THE DOCTOR LOOKS FOR

- The doctor will take a history and perform a physical examination to identify the presence of a peptic ulcer.
- Numerous other conditions that can cause similar signs and symptoms should be investigated.

TESTS AND PROCEDURES

- Blood tests
- Special tests can be done to assess gastric function.
- The stomach can be examined by endoscopy.
- A sample of the digestive tract lining can be obtained by biopsy for laboratory analysis.
- Exploratory surgery may be recommended.

 TREATMENT

GENERAL MEASURES

- Hospitalization and surgery may be required for ulcer perforation or bleeding.
- Avoid cigarette smoking.
- Reduce use of NSAIDs.
- Reduce stress.

ACTIVITY

Fully active for uncomplicated disease; exercise to tolerance after hemorrhage

DIET

Three regular meals daily, with avoidance of dietary irritants

 MEDICATIONS

COMMONLY PRESCRIBED DRUGS

- H_2 blockers: ranitidine, nizatidine, cimetidine, famotidine
- Omeprazole, lansoprazole
- Antibiotics to treat *H. pylori*

CONTRAINDICATIONS

Allergies to antibiotics

PRECAUTIONS

Antibiotic-related side effects include diarrhea, nausea and vomiting, unpleasant taste in mouth, rash, colitis, and severe allergic reaction.

DRUG INTERACTIONS

Many drug interactions; read drug product information.

OTHER DRUGS

- Sucralfate
- Antacids: magnesium hydroxide, aluminum hydroxide

 FOLLOW-UP

PATIENT MONITORING

See the doctor as often as needed to assess health status and monitor treatment.

PREVENTION

- Eradication of *H. pylori*
- Maintenance therapy
- Bleeding ulcers may require continued maintenance therapy even if *H. pylori* organisms are eradicated.

COMPLICATIONS

- Hemorrhage
- Perforation
- Intestinal obstruction

WHAT TO EXPECT

- Relapse rates are low after antibiotic treatment.
- Reinfection rate is less than 1% per year.

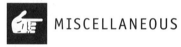 MISCELLANEOUS

PEDIATRIC

Peptic ulcers are uncommon before puberty.

PREGNANCY

Medications should be used with caution in pregnancy.

FURTHER INFORMATION

National Digestive Diseases Information Clearinghouse, Box NDDIC, Bethesda, MD 20892, (301) 468-6344

Peptic Ulcer Disease

Doctor
Office
Phone
Pager

Special notes to patient:

Pink Eye

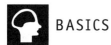 ## BASICS

DESCRIPTION

Conjunctivitis, also called "pink eye," is inflammation of the inner surface of the eyelid or the "white" of the eye.

SIGNS AND SYMPTOMS

- Red eyes
- Burning sensation
- Foreign body sensation
- Itching
- Excessive tearing
- Matting of eyelashes
- Swelling
- Drooping of the eyelid
- Sensitivity to light
- Visual impairment does **not** occur

CAUSES

- Bacteria, including *Chlamydia* organisms
- Viral
- Allergic reaction
- Irritation (home or industrial chemicals, wind, smoke, ultraviolet light)
- Other infections

SCOPE

Conjunctivitis is common in the United States.

MOST OFTEN AFFECTED

Affects all ages, males and females equally

RISK FACTORS

Numerous, including trauma from wind, cold, and heat; chemicals; and foreign body

 ## DIAGNOSIS

WHAT THE DOCTOR LOOKS FOR

The doctor will examine the eye for signs of conjunctivitis, as well as for a foreign body or other conditions.

TESTS AND PROCEDURES

Fluid from the eye can be obtained for laboratory analysis.

 ## TREATMENT

GENERAL MEASURES

- Conjunctivitis is managed in the outpatient setting.
- See *Medications*
- Ophthalmologic referral may be needed if an ulcer or herpes is present or if the condition worsens after 24 hours of treatment.
- Compresses: warm if infective, cold if allergic or irritative
- Remove material and debris (may require frequent irrigation).
- Discontinue use of contact lenses.

ACTIVITY

No restrictions

DIET

No restrictions

 ## MEDICATIONS

COMMONLY PRESCRIBED DRUGS

- Antibiotics: tobramycin, gentamicin, sodium sulfacetamide, erythromycin ophthalmic ointment
- Antivirals: trifluridine, acyclovir
- Chlamydial: doxycycline
- Allergic: naphazoline, antazoline (Albalon-A, Vasocon-A), oral antihistamines

CONTRAINDICATIONS

Read drug product information.

PRECAUTIONS

- Read drug product information.
- It is important to avoid contamination of medication eyedropper. Do not touch the eye with the eyedropper.

DRUG INTERACTIONS

Read drug product information.

OTHER DRUGS

Other antibiotics

 ## FOLLOW-UP

PATIENT MONITORING

See the doctor if the eye condition worsens after 24 hours of treatment.

PREVENTION

- Avoid listed causes when possible.
- Wash hands often.

COMPLICATIONS

- Scarring and other eye conditions
- Bacterial superinfection

WHAT TO EXPECT

- Bacterial: resolves within 10 to 14 days without treatment, 2 to 4 days with treatment
- Some forms of conjunctivitis can take 3 to 9 months to resolve without treatment, 3 to 5 weeks with treatment.

 ## MISCELLANEOUS

GERIATRIC

Elderly individuals are more likely to have the diseases or problems listed in *Causes*.

Pink Eye

Doctor
Office
Phone
Pager

Special notes to patient:

Pinworms

 ## BASICS

DESCRIPTION

Pinworms are parasites that infect the gastrointestinal tract and cause anal itching. Itching is usually worse at night.

SIGNS AND SYMPTOMS

- Perianal itching
- Perineal itching
- Vulvovaginitis
- Bed-wetting
- Abdominal pain
- Insomnia

CAUSES

The intestinal parasite *Enterobius* (Oxyuris) *vermicularis*

SCOPE

Pinworms affect about 20% of children 5 to 10 years of age.

MOST OFTEN AFFECTED

Children 5 to 14 years of age; girls affected more often than boys

RISK FACTORS

- Institutionalization (50% to 90% of institutionalized children have pinworms.)
- Crowded living conditions
- Poor hygiene
- Warm climate

 ## DIAGNOSIS

WHAT THE DOCTOR LOOKS FOR

- The doctor may perform a physical examination to identify pinworms.

TESTS AND PROCEDURES

Pinworms can be directly observed; tape test can be done to identify the parasite.

 ## TREATMENT

GENERAL MEASURES

- All symptomatic family members should be treated simultaneously.
- Bedclothes and underwear of infected individuals should be washed in hot water at the time of treatment (eggs can remain viable for 2 to 3 weeks in a moist environment).
- Strict handwashing can help prevent transmission.
- Practice good hygiene (showers, nail cleaning)
- Topical use of antiitch creams or ointments may help relieve itch.

ACTIVITY

No restrictions

DIET

No restrictions

 ## MEDICATIONS

COMMONLY PRESCRIBED DRUGS

- Mebendazole (Vermox)
- Pyrantel pamoate (Antiminth)
- Thiabendazole (Mintezol)
- Albendazole (Albenza)

CONTRAINDICATIONS

Read drug product information.

PRECAUTIONS

- All family members should be treated.
- Take medicine on empty stomach.
- Medication can cause diarrhea and nausea.

DRUG INTERACTIONS

Read drug product information.

 ## FOLLOW-UP

PATIENT MONITORING

Unnecessary, unless symptoms persist after drug therapy

PREVENTION

- Careful handwashing; keep nails short and clean.
- Wash anus and genitals at least once a day, preferably in a shower.
- Do not scratch anus or put fingers near nose or mouth.

COMPLICATIONS

- Perianal scratching can cause infection.
- Young girls: infection of reproductive tract
- Urinary tract infections

WHAT TO EXPECT

- Carriers of pinworms often have no symptoms.
- Infections are cured more than 90% of the time with drug therapy.
- Reinfection is common.

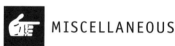 MISCELLANEOUS

PEDIATRIC

Pinworms are commonly found in children.

PREGNANCY

Drug therapy is contraindicated in pregnancy.

FURTHER INFORMATION

Centers for Disease Control, Department of Health and Human Services, Office of Public Affairs, Atlanta, GA 30333, (404) 329-3534

Pinworms

Doctor
Office
Phone
Pager

Special notes to patient:

Pneumonia, Bacterial

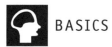 ## BASICS

DESCRIPTION
Bacterial pneumonia is an acute (brief) bacterial infection of the lung.

SCOPE
About 1,200 cases of bacterial pneumonia per 100,000 persons occur annually in the United States. Among hospitalized individuals, 800/100,000 cases of acquired bacterial pneumonia occur annually.

MOST OFTEN AFFECTED
Extremes of age: the very young and the very old; more frequent in males

SIGNS AND SYMPTOMS
- Cough and fever
- Chest pain (pleuritic)
- Chill, with sudden onset
- Dark, thick or rusty (bloody) sputum
- Rapid (or slow) heart rate
- Rapid breathing rate
- Bluish discoloration around eyes, lips, and nail beds
- Changes in the level of consciousness
- Anxiety, confusion, restlessness, and meningeal signs
- Abdominal pain
- Loss of appetite
- Profuse sweating
- Muscle aches
- Pinpoint bruises

CAUSES
Bacterial infection, spread by air or blood

RISK FACTORS
- Recent viral infections
- Extremes of age
- Alcoholism
- Acquired immune deficiency syndrome (AIDS) or other immune system disorders
- Smoking
- Kidney failure
- Cardiovascular disease
- Lung disease
- Diabetes mellitus
- Malnutrition
- Cancer
- Occupational exposure

 ## DIAGNOSIS

WHAT THE DOCTOR LOOKS FOR
- The doctor will perform a physical examination to identify pneumonia.
- Bacterial pneumonia can be caused by a number of different organisms; many other respiratory diseases appear similar to pneumonia.

TESTS AND PROCEDURES
- Blood tests
- Blood culture
- Chest x-ray study
- Fluid from the airway can be sampled for culture.
- The lower airway can be examined by bronchoscopy.
- The fluids from the chest cavity can be obtained by thoracentesis for laboratory analysis.

 ## TREATMENT

GENERAL MEASURES
- Mild cases of bacterial pneumonia are managed in the outpatient setting.
- Severe cases require hospitalization.
- Antibiotic therapy
- Respiratory support, as needed
- Maintain fluid and salt balance.
- Pain relievers
- Respiratory isolation if tuberculosis suspected

ACTIVITY
Bedrest, reduced activity, or both during acute phase

DIET
- Nothing by mouth if a risk of respiratory failure exists.
- Consider soft, easy-to-eat foods

 ## MEDICATIONS

COMMONLY PRESCRIBED DRUGS
Antibiotics

CONTRAINDICATIONS
Allergy to prescribed drugs

PRECAUTIONS
Read drug product information.

DRUG INTERACTIONS
Read drug product information.

OTHER DRUGS
Other antibiotics

 ## FOLLOW-UP

PATIENT MONITORING
- See the doctor every day during the acute phase. Contact primary care provider if no improvement or IF condition worsens in 48 to 72 hours.
- Repeat chest x-ray study

PREVENTION
- Reduce risk factors, where possible.
- Avoid use of antibiotics during minor viral infections.
- Annual flu vaccine for individuals at high risk
- Pneumococcal vaccine

COMPLICATIONS
- Severe infection
- Multiple organ failure
- Adult respiratory distress syndrome (ARDS)

WHAT TO EXPECT
- Usual course in otherwise healthy individual is improvement and fever resolution in 1 to 3 days.
- Overall death rate is about 5%.
- Poorest prognosis: extremes of age, spread of infection to blood, presence of other medical disease, immune system disorders

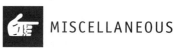 ## MISCELLANEOUS

PEDIATRIC
The risk of illness and death is high in children under 1 year of age.

GERIATRIC
The risk of illness and death is high among those above 70 years of age, especially when other disease or risk factors are present.

FURTHER INFORMATION
American Lung Association, 1740 Broadway, New York, NY 10019 (212) 315-8700

Pneumonia, Bacterial

Doctor
Office
Phone
Pager

Special notes to patient:

Pneumonia, Viral

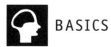 **BASICS**

DESCRIPTION

Viral pneumonia is an inflammatory disease of the lungs caused by viral infection.

SIGNS AND SYMPTOMS

- Fever
- Chills
- Cough (with or without sputum production)
- Difficulty breathing
- Noisy breathing
- Altered breath sounds
- Chest pain
- Headache
- Muscle ache
- Malaise
- Gastrointestinal symptoms

CAUSES

Viral infection

SCOPE

- About 90% of childhood pneumonia is from a viral infection.
- In adults, 4% to 39% of pneumonia cases are caused by a virus.
- Prevalence is unknown and variable because of seasonal variation, although it is more common in winter months.
- Mixed infections with bacteria is common.

MOST OFTEN AFFECTED

More common in children than in adults; males and females are affected equally.

RISK FACTORS

- Immune system disorders
- Living in close quarters
- Seasonal: epidemic upper respiratory illness
- Elderly
- Heart disease
- Chronic lung disease
- Recent upper respiratory infection

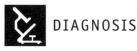 **DIAGNOSIS**

WHAT THE DOCTOR LOOKS FOR

- The doctor will perform a physical examination to assess the presence of viral pneumonia.
- Similar signs and symptoms can be caused by other forms of pneumonia, cancer, and other lung diseases.

TESTS AND PROCEDURES

- Blood tests
- Sputum culture
- Chest x-ray study
- The throat can be swabbed for laboratory analysis.
- The lower airway can be examined by bronchoscopy.

 TREATMENT

GENERAL MEASURES

- Most cases of viral pneumonia are managed in the outpatient setting.
- Infants under 4 months of age, the elderly, and individuals with severe infection are managed by hospitalization.
- Encourage coughing and deep breathing exercises to clear secretions.
- Carefully dispose of secretions and body fluids.
- Maintain adequate fluid intake.
- Respiratory isolation for highly contagious viruses

ACTIVITY

Rest

DIET

Increase fluids; eat a high-calorie, high-protein, soft diet

 MEDICATIONS

COMMONLY PRESCRIBED DRUGS

- Amantadine (Symmetrel)
- Acyclovir (Zovirax)
- Ganciclovir (Cytovene)
- Ribavirin (Virazole)
- Zanamivir (Relenza)
- Oseltamivir (Tamiflu)

CONTRAINDICATIONS

Read drug product information.

PRECAUTIONS

- Amantadine should be used cautiously in patients with liver disease, epilepsy, kidney disease, or eczema and in individuals with a history of psychotic illness.
- Ribavirin causes birth defects and should not be taken by pregnant women.

DRUG INTERACTIONS

Read drug product information.

OTHER DRUGS

- Rimantadine (Flumadine)
- Antibiotics
- Foscarnet (Foscavir)
- Immune globulin, intravenous (IVIG)

 FOLLOW-UP

PATIENT MONITORING

See the doctor as often as necessary.

PREVENTION

- Influenza A and B vaccine
- For those patients unable to receive influenza vaccine (egg allergy or other) and are at high risk, amantadine or rimantadine can be given.
- Healthcare workers who are pregnant need to take proper precautions to avoid infectious patients.
- Measles vaccine
- Varicella zoster vaccine

COMPLICATIONS

- Bacterial infections
- Respiratory failure
- Adult respiratory distress syndrome (ARDS)

WHAT TO EXPECT

- Usually, favorable prognosis, with illness lasting several days to a week
- Postviral fatigue is common.
- Death can occur, especially in pediatric or bone-marrow transplant infections or among the elderly stricken with influenza.

 MISCELLANEOUS

PEDIATRIC

Some viral infections in children are serious.

GERIATRIC

The elderly have the greatest risk of illness and death.

PREGNANCY

Pregnant women should avoid contact with persons who may have viral infections.

FURTHER INFORMATION

American Lung Association, 1740 Broadway, New York, NY 10019, (212) 315-8700

Pneumonia, Viral

Doctor
Office
Phone
Pager

Special notes to patient:

Posttraumatic Stress Disorder (PTSD)

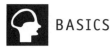

BASICS

DESCRIPTION

Posttraumatic stress disorder (PTSD) is a condition seen in people who have experienced an event that would be extremely distressing to most human beings. For example:

- Serious threat to one's life, physical, or psychological integrity
- Serious threat or harm to one's children, spouse, siblings, parents, or other close relatives or friends
- Sudden destruction of one's home or community
- Seeing another person who has recently been (or is being) injured or killed as a result of a man-made violent act or natural disaster.

SIGNS AND SYMPTOMS

- Recurrent and intrusive distressing recollections of the event
- Recurrent distressing dreams of the event
- Acting or feeling as if the traumatic event were recurring
- Reactions (e.g., increased heart rate, changes in blood pressure, discoloration of the skin, blurred vision, nausea, vomiting, diarrhea, urinary urgency).
- Efforts to avoid thoughts, feelings, or conversations associated with the trauma
- Efforts to avoid activities, places, or people that arouse recollections of the trauma
- Inability to recall an important aspect of the trauma (psychogenic amnesia)
- Diminished interest in significant activities
- Feelings of detachment or estrangement from others
- Sense of a foreshortened future (e.g., does not expect to have a career, marriage, or a normal lifespan)
- Difficulty falling or staying asleep (insomnia)
- Irritability or outbursts of anger
- Difficulty in concentrating
- Hypervigilance
- Exaggerated startle response
- Symptom(s) lasting longer than 1 month
- Causes significant impairment in social, occupational, or other areas of functioning

CAUSES

Events that threaten one's personal integrity, self-esteem, and security are psychologically traumatic and can lead to PTSD.

SCOPE

Up to 30% of victims of disasters develop PTSD. Up to 14% of the population of the United States experiences PTSD at some point.

MOST OFTEN AFFECTED

The elderly and the very young are more vulnerable to PTSD.

RISK FACTORS

Individuals with a history of childhood neglect, abuse, or dysfunctional families and children of alcoholic parents are predisposed and more susceptible to developing PTSD in response to trauma.

DIAGNOSIS

WHAT THE DOCTOR LOOKS FOR

The doctor will assess the person to determine whether PTSD exists, or whether symptoms are caused by some other emotional, mental, or behavioral disorder.

TESTS AND PROCEDURES

- Neuropsychological testing
- Electroencephalograph (EEG) to rule out brain damage
- Sleep studies
- Computed tomography (CT) scan and magnetic resonance imaging (MRI) can be done.

TREATMENT

GENERAL MEASURES

- As indicated by the individual's general condition, treatment includes individual psychotherapy, group therapy, hypnotherapy, narcoanalysis and narcosynthesis, and behavior therapy.
- Crisis intervention shortly after the traumatic event is valuable for the immediate distress and may prevent the development of a chronic or delayed form of PTSD.
- Relaxation exercises to help reduce anxiety and improve sleep have been found to be helpful.

ACTIVITY

- As indicated by patient's physical condition
- Restoration of regular sleep at night is essential in cases of insomnia.

DIET

A healthy diet consisting of complex carbohydrates, proteins, multivitamins, and minerals; avoid fatty foods.

MEDICATIONS

COMMONLY PRESCRIBED DRUGS

- Fluoxetine
- Sertraline
- Paroxetine
- Citalopram
- Venlafaxine
- Doxepin
- Nortriptyline
- Imipramine
- Desipramine
- Amitriptyline
- Trimipramine
- Protriptyline
- Amoxapine
- Maprotiline
- Phenelzine
- Trazodone
- Nefazodone
- Bupropion
- Neuroleptics
- Benzodiazepines

CONTRAINDICATIONS

- Allergic reactions to specific drugs
- Use with caution in alcoholic patients with poor liver function.

PRECAUTIONS

- Do not mix tricyclic antidepressants with monoamine oxidase (MAO) inhibitors.
- Long-term use of benzodiazepines can lead to increased tolerance and drug dependency.

DRUG INTERACTIONS

MAO inhibitors can interact with other antidepressants. Stimulants (e.g., pseudoephedrine) and many foods interact with tyramine.

OTHER DRUGS

- Clomipramine
- Fluvoxamine
- Fluoxetine
- Buspirone
- Propranolol
- Clonidine

Posttraumatic Stress Disorder (PTSD)

Doctor
Office
Phone
Pager

Special notes to patient:

Posttraumatic Stress Disorder (PTSD)

 FOLLOW-UP

PATIENT MONITORING

Psychotherapy for at least 1 hour per week is necessary in the first phase of treatment.

PREVENTION

Crisis intervention immediately after the traumatic event involving intensive support and treatment may prevent the development of chronic PTSD later.

COMPLICATIONS

Suicide, self-inflicted violence

WHAT TO EXPECT

- The lack of crisis intervention immediately following the trauma can lead to symptom persistence.
- If symptoms persist over 3 months, patients can develop chronic PTSD, which can lead to loss of job, marital conflicts, total disability, and repeated or lengthy hospitalizations.
- The onset of symptoms can be 6 months or more after the traumatic event.

 MISCELLANEOUS

PEDIATRIC

Young children are susceptible to abuse and neglect and can develop chronic PTSD, with subsequent failure to progress and grow in a healthy way.

GERIATRIC

The elderly have fewer social support resources and their adjustment to trauma is less flexible. Also, they are more sensitive to medication.

PREGNANCY

Avoid drugs in the first trimester. Try nondrug treatment techniques (e.g., psychotherapy, hypnotherapy, relaxation therapy).

Posttraumatic Stress Disorder (PTSD)

Doctor

Office

Phone

Pager

Special notes to patient:

Preeclampsia

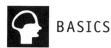
BASICS

DESCRIPTION
Preeclampsia is hypertension associated with edema and acute excessive weight gain, which develops during pregnancy after 20 weeks' gestation.

SIGNS AND SYMPTOMS
- Elevated blood pressure
- Swelling
- Rapid excessive weight gain (more than 5 lb/week)
- Epigastric pain
- Headache
- Visual disturbances
- Apprehension
- Amnesia
- Scant or absent urine

CAUSES
- Altered cardiovascular reaction
- Disorders of blood or blood vessels
- Hypertension

SCOPE
Preeclampsia affects 5% to 10% of all pregnant women.

MOST OFTEN AFFECTED
- Young women who are pregnant for the first time. Women above 35 years of age

RISK FACTORS
- Family history of preeclampsia
- Lower socioeconomic status
- Multiple fetuses
- Teenage mother
- Connective tissue disorders
- Above 35 years of age
- First pregnancy
- Diabetes mellitus of pregnancy
- Chronic hypertension
- History of kidney disease

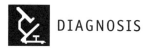
DIAGNOSIS

WHAT THE DOCTOR LOOKS FOR
- The doctor will assess for the presence of preeclampsia.
- Other factors will be considered (e.g., preexisting hypertension that may have been induced or worsened by pregnancy).

TESTS AND PROCEDURES
- Blood tests
- Urinalysis

TREATMENT

GENERAL MEASURES
- A mild case of preeclampsia can be managed in the outpatient setting.
- Moderate or changing case of preeclampsia requires hospitalization.
- If preeclampsia is severe, fetus should be delivered as soon as possible

ACTIVITY
- Bedrest on left side
- Walk only to bathroom

DIET
- No salt restriction
- Protein: 80 to 100 g/day

MEDICATIONS

COMMONLY PRESCRIBED DRUGS
Magnesium sulfate

CONTRAINDICATIONS
Read drug product information.

PRECAUTIONS
Read drug product information.

DRUG INTERACTIONS
Read drug product information.

OTHER DRUGS
- Hydralazine (Apresoline)
- Diazoxide
- Diazepam (Valium)

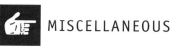
FOLLOW-UP

PATIENT MONITORING
See the doctor often for monitoring of health status.

PREVENTION
Weight control

COMPLICATIONS
- Eclampsia (seizures)
- Hypertensive crisis
- Acute kidney disease
- Acute liver disease
- Acute lung disease

WHAT TO EXPECT
Prevention of seizures and delivery of viable baby with prompt and appropriate treatment

MISCELLANEOUS

PEDIATRIC
An increased risk of preeclampsia is found among pregnant teenagers.

OTHERS
Older pregnant women (>35 years of age) have an increased risk of preeclampsia.

Preeclampsia

Doctor
Office
Phone
Pager

Special notes to patient:

Premature Labor

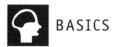 BASICS

DESCRIPTION
Premature labor occurs before the completion of 36 weeks' gestation.

SIGNS AND SYMPTOMS
- Regular uterine contractions, with or without pain, continuing for 1 hour
- Dull, low backache, pressure, or pain
- Intermittent lower abdominal or thigh pain
- Intestinal cramping, with or without diarrhea or indigestion
- Change in vaginal discharge
- Palpable contractions on examination
- Dilatation of the cervix
- Effacement (thinning) of the cervix
- Signs of ruptured membranes

CAUSES
- Infections
- Uterine abnormalities
- Uterine overdistention
- Premature membrane rupture
- Trauma
- Unknown

SCOPE
Premature labor affects 8% to 12% of all births in the United States.

MOST OFTEN AFFECTED
Women of childbearing age

RISK FACTORS
- Prior preterm delivery
- Multiple gestation
- Three or more first-trimester abortions
- Previous second-trimester abortion
- Abdominal surgery during pregnancy
- Uterine or cervical disorders
- Complications of pregnancy
- Fetal abnormalities
- Serious maternal infection
- Second-trimester bleeding
- Low prepregnancy weight: less than 45 kg (100 lb)
- Single parent
- No prenatal care
- Substance abuse
- Lower socioeconomic status

 DIAGNOSIS

WHAT THE DOCTOR LOOKS FOR
- The doctor will assess the degree of premature labor.
- The doctor will look for signs and symptoms of associated conditions (e.g., dehydration, infection, and muscular back pain).

TESTS AND PROCEDURES
- Urinalysis and urine culture
- Testing for infection
- Amniocentesis can be done.
- Ultrasound

 TREATMENT

GENERAL MEASURES
- Premature labor can be managed in the outpatient setting or by hospitalization, depending on circumstances.
- Underlying risk factors should be treated with appropriate measures (antibiotics, hydration).
- If delivery is inevitable, but not immediate, mother can be transported to a tertiary care center or hospital equipped with a neonatal intensive care unit.
- No sexual intercourse

ACTIVITY
- Bedrest. Discontinue work or other physical activities.
- Hospitalization may be necessary.

DIET
Liquids only, if delivery seems imminent

 MEDICATIONS

COMMONLY PRESCRIBED DRUGS
- Terbutaline
- Ritodrine
- Magnesium sulfate
- Glucocorticoids: betamethasone, dexamethasone, hydrocortisone
- Nifedipine
- Indomethacin

CONTRAINDICATIONS
Read drug product information.

PRECAUTIONS
Read drug product information.

DRUG INTERACTIONS
Read drug product information.

 FOLLOW-UP

PATIENT MONITORING
Women at high risk for preterm labor should see the doctor weekly.

PREVENTION
Close observation; call the doctor or go to the hospital if contractions last for more than an hour or if low back pain, change in vaginal discharge, "menstrual cramping," or intestinal cramping occur.

COMPLICATIONS
Premature birth

WHAT TO EXPECT
- If membranes are ruptured, delivery generally occurs within 3 to 7 days.
- If membranes are intact, the woman is treated until 37 weeks of gestation.

 MISCELLANEOUS

PREGNANCY
Premature labor is a problem of pregnancy.

Premature Labor

Doctor
Office
Phone
Pager

Special notes to patient:

Premenstrual Syndrome (PMS)

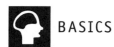 BASICS

DESCRIPTION
Premenstrual syndrome (PMS) is a constellation of symptoms that occurs before menstruation and is severe enough to interfere significantly with the patient's life.

SIGNS AND SYMPTOMS
- Depressed mood
- Mood swings
- Irritability
- Difficulty concentrating
- Fatigue
- Swelling
- Breast tenderness
- Headaches
- Sleep disturbances

CAUSES
Unknown, presumed hormonal

SCOPE
Almost all women have some symptoms before menses. A few have actual PMS.

MOST OFTEN AFFECTED
Women in the childbearing years, worse during the late 20s and 30s

RISK FACTORS
- Other diseases (e.g., depression)
- Caffeine and high-fluid intake
- Stress
- Increasing age

 DIAGNOSIS

WHAT THE DOCTOR LOOKS FOR
The doctor will take a thorough history and perform an examination to identify the presence of PMS.

TESTS AND PROCEDURES
The individual may be asked to track symptoms for several months.

 TREATMENT

GENERAL MEASURES
- Increase daily exercise.
- Eat regular, balanced meals.
- Stop smoking.
- Get regular sleep.
- Reduce stress.
- Individual or couples counseling
- Support groups
- Photo therapy

ACTIVITY
- No restrictions
- Exercise is recommended.

DIET
- Frequent, small meals
- Low-salt, high-carbohydrate diet
- Reduce caffeine intake.

 MEDICATIONS

No single drug works for all women.

COMMONLY PRESCRIBED DRUGS
- Diuretics
- Pain relievers
- Antidepressants: fluoxetine, sertraline, clomipramine, or nortriptyline
- Alprazolam
- Buspirone
- Magnesium
- Calcium
- Vitamin B_6
- Vitamin E
- Evening primrose oil
- Bromocriptine
- Danazol

CONTRAINDICATIONS
Read drug product information.

PRECAUTIONS
Read drug product information.

DRUG INTERACTIONS
Read drug product information.

OTHER DRUGS
Oral contraceptives may help.
Progesterone

 FOLLOW-UP

PATIENT MONITORING
See the doctor as often as necessary for general support and further patient education.

WHAT TO EXPECT
Many patients adequately control their symptoms.

Premenstrual Syndrome (PMS)

Doctor
Office
Phone
Pager

Special notes to patient:

Prostate Cancer

 ## BASICS

DESCRIPTION
Cancer occurring in the prostate, which is a walnut-sized gland located at the base of the urinary bladder of men

SIGNS AND SYMPTOMS
- May have no symptoms
- Difficulty with urination
- Blood in urine (rare)
- Urinary tract infection
- Bone pain
- Weight loss
- Anemia
- Shortness of breath
- Enlarged lymph nodes

CAUSES
Unknown

SCOPE
Prostate cancer affects 69 of 100,000 men in the United States.

PREDOMINANT AGE
Primarily affects men 50 to 60 years of age

RISK FACTORS
- Genetic predisposition
- Hormonal influences
- Exposure to chemical carcinogens
- Sexually transmitted diseases
- Man above 60 years of age
- Increased risk with vasectomy has been newly proposed, but is unsupported.

 ## DIAGNOSIS

WHAT THE DOCTOR LOOKS FOR
The doctor will perform a physical examination, including a rectal examination, to identify the presence of prostate cancer.

TESTS AND PROCEDURES
- Blood tests: prostate-specific antigen (PSA)
- Urinalysis
- Computerized tomography (CT) scan and magnetic resonance imaging (MRI) can be done.
- Ultrasound
- A sample of prostate, lymph node, or bone can be obtained for laboratory analysis.

 ## TREATMENT

GENERAL MEASURES
- Prostate cancer is managed in the outpatient setting, except for any surgery that requires hospitalization.
- Conservative or palliative treatment for men above 70 years of age
- Radiation therapy
- Hormone therapy
- Surgery may be required.

ACTIVITY
Full activity

DIET
No special diet

 ## MEDICATIONS

COMMONLY PRESCRIBED DRUGS
- Flutamide (Eulexin)
- Leuprolide (Lupron)
- Goserelin (Zoladex)

CONTRAINDICATIONS
None

PRECAUTIONS
- Disease flare
- Fluid retention
- Nausea
- Vomiting
- Hot flashes
- Liver changes

DRUG INTERACTIONS
Read drug product information.

OTHER DRUGS
None

FOLLOW-UP

PATIENT MONITORING
See the doctor every 3 months for 1 year (including blood tests), then every 6 months for a year, then annual examinations thereafter.

PREVENTION
None

COMPLICATIONS
- Cardiac failure
- Phlebitis
- Fractures

WHAT TO EXPECT
- With early diagnosis and treatment, prostate cancer should be curable.
- Advanced, unresponsive disease progresses in an average of 18 months.

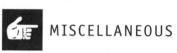 ## MISCELLANEOUS

PEDIATRIC
Does not occur in children

FURTHER INFORMATION
National Kidney & Urologic Diseases Information Clearinghouse, Box NKUDIC, Bethesda, MD 20893, (301) 468-6345

Prostate Cancer

	Doctor
	Office
	Phone
	Pager

Special notes to patient:

Prostatic Hyperplasia, Benign (BPH)

 ## BASICS

DESCRIPTION
Benign prostatic hypertrophy (BPH) is the overgrowth of the prostate, the walnut-sized gland at the base of the urinary bladder of men. BPH can obstruct the flow of urine from the bladder.

SIGNS AND SYMPTOMS
- Decrease force or caliber of urine stream
- Hesitancy
- Dribbling
- Sensation of incomplete bladder emptying
- Incontinence
- Inability to voluntarily stop stream
- Urinary retention
- Frequent urination
- Urination during sleep hours
- Urgency

CAUSES
Exact cause is unknown, but evidence suggests BPH occurs because of a hormonal imbalance.

SCOPE
BPH is a universal phenomenon seen in older men.

MOST OFTEN AFFECTED
BPH is rarely seen in men under 40 years of age; it affects 50% of men above 50 years of age and 80% of men above 70 years of age.

RISK FACTORS
- Aging (rare in men under 40 years of age)
- No dietary, environmental, or sexual practices currently implicated.

 ## DIAGNOSIS

WHAT THE DOCTOR LOOKS FOR
The doctor will perform a physical examination to identify the presence of BPH.

TESTS AND PROCEDURES
- Blood tests
- Urinalysis, culture
- Tissue from the prostate can be obtained by biopsy for laboratory analysis.
- The urinary system can be evaluated with a special diagnostic procedure, called an "intravenous pyelogram."
- Computed tomography (CT) scan or magnetic resonance imaging (MRI) can be done.
- Ultrasound
- Special tests can be done to measure the flow and pressure of urine to assist in diagnosis.
- The urinary tract can be examined by cystoscopy.

 ## TREATMENT

GENERAL MEASURES
- BPH is managed in the outpatient setting.
- Surgery may be required.

ACTIVITY
No restriction

DIET
Avoid caffeinated or alcoholic beverages and excessively spiced foods.

 ## MEDICATIONS

COMMONLY PRESCRIBED DRUGS
- Prazosin (Minipress), terazosin, doxazosin
- Flutamide, leuprolide, finasteride (Proscar)

CONTRAINDICATIONS
Read drug product information.

PRECAUTIONS
Read drug product information.

DRUG INTERACTIONS
Read drug product information.

 ## FOLLOW-UP

PATIENT MONITORING
- Symptoms should be monitored every 1 to 6 months.
- Urine testing every 3 to 12 months.
- Digital rectal examination annually
- PSA test annually

PREVENTION
Prostatic hypertrophy appears to be part of the aging process.

COMPLICATIONS
- Bladder stones
- Prostatitis
- Kidney failure

WHAT TO EXPECT
- Symptoms improve or stabilize in 70% to 80% of patients; 20% to 30% require treatment because of worsening symptoms.
- Of men with BPH, 11% to 33% have prostate cancer.

 ## MISCELLANEOUS

GERIATRIC
BPH is much more common in elderly men.

FURTHER INFORMATION
National Kidney & Urologic Diseases Information Clearinghouse, Box NKUDIC, Bethesda, MD 20893, (301) 468-6345

Prostatic Hyperplasia, Benign (BPH)

Doctor
Office
Phone
Pager

Special notes to patient:

Psoriasis

 ## BASICS

DESCRIPTION
Psoriasis is a common chronic disease characterized by reddened, dry, scaling patches of skin. The condition tends to recur and improve unpredictably over time, with flares possibly related to systemic or environmental factors.

SCOPE
About 1,000 to 2,000 cases of psoriasis per 100,000 people in the United States.

MOST OFTEN AFFECTED
- Individuals 16 to 22 and 57 to 60 years of age
- Can develop in infants; males and females affected equally
- May be inherited

SIGNS AND SYMPTOMS
- Arthritis
- Itching
- Silvery scales on red plaques
- Affects the knees, elbows, and scalp
- Finger and toe nails may appear stippled and pitted.

CAUSES
Possible genetic defect

RISK FACTORS
- Trauma or skin irritation
- Infection
- Hormone changes
- Stress (physical and emotional)
- Sudden withdrawal of psoriasis drugs
- Alcohol use
- Obesity

 ## DIAGNOSIS

WHAT THE DOCTOR LOOKS FOR
- The doctor will perform a physical examination to identify the signs and symptoms of psoriasis.
- Numerous other conditions can appear similar to psoriasis.

TESTS AND PROCEDURES
Blood tests

 ## TREATMENT

GENERAL MEASURES
- Psoriasis is usually managed in the outpatient setting.
- Hospitalization may be required for severe or resistant cases.
- Medication to soften scales, followed by soft brushing while bathing.
- Oatmeal baths for itching
- Tar shampoos
- Avoid excessive sun exposure.
- Desert climates provide a favorable effect for some patients.
- Wet dressings may help relieve itching.
- Ultraviolet light (including sunlight) is effective and may be the best treatment option during pregnancy or in young children. Lamps are available for home use.
- For severe psoriasis that resists treatment, a referral to a specialist in psoriatic therapy is suggested.

ACTIVITY
No restrictions

DIET
No special diet

 ## MEDICATIONS

COMMONLY PRESCRIBED DRUGS
- Emollients: soft yellow paraffin or aqueous cream; petrolatum or Aquaphor cream
- Corticosteroids
- Coal tar (Estar, PsoriGel)
- Salicylic acid
- Anthralin ointment
- Methotrexate
- PUVA (psoralen plus ultraviolet light)
- Etretinate
- Isotretinoin
- Triamcinolone
- Vitamin D analogs
- Cyclosporine, tacrolimus
- Betamethasone valerate mousse

CONTRAINDICATIONS
Read drug product information.

PRECAUTIONS
Read drug product information.

DRUG INTERACTIONS
Read drug product information.

OTHER DRUGS
Mycophenolate mofetil (CellCept) for resistant cases.

 ## FOLLOW-UP

PATIENT MONITORING
- See the doctor as often as necessary.
- Medications used in treatment require close follow-up.
- Blood tests may be repeated on a monthly basis.

PREVENTION
- Avoid alcoholic beverages.
- Avoid irritating drugs.
- Avoid stimulating drugs or antimalarial medications.

COMPLICATIONS
- Severe psoriasis or other skin disorders
- Topical corticosteroids can cause skin side effects.

WHAT TO EXPECT
- Psoriasis is usually benign.
- Life-threatening forms do occur.
- Can be resistant to treatment

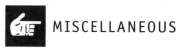 ## MISCELLANEOUS

PEDIATRIC
The onset of psoriasis is common before 10 years of age, but rare before 3 years of age.

GERIATRIC
- About 3% of patients with psoriasis acquire the disease after 65 years of age.
- Elderly patients may have difficulty applying topical preparations over all affected body parts.

PREGNANCY
Pregnancy has an unpredictable effect on psoriasis. Avoid tars, topical corticosteroids, calcipotriene, and systemic therapies. Etretinate is toxic to fetus.

FURTHER INFORMATION
- American Academy of Family Physicians Foundation, P.O. Box 8418, Kansas City, MO 64114, (800) 274-2237, ext. 4400
- National Psoriasis Foundation, Suite 300, 6600 S.W. 92nd Ave., Portland, OR 97223, (503) 244-7404; toll free (800) 723-9166; fax (503) 245-0626; E-mail 76135.2746@compuserve.com

Psoriasis

Doctor
Office
Phone
Pager

Special notes to patient:

Rabies

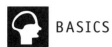 ## BASICS

DESCRIPTION
Rabies is a rapidly progressive infection of the central nervous system caused by a virus. The disease is essentially 100% fatal once symptoms develop. Infection can be prevented by prompt treatment.

SIGNS AND SYMPTOMS
- Usually proceed through five stages, although they can overlap:
- Incubation period: often, 1 to 3 months
- Prodrome (2–10 days):
  - Pain or tingling at bite site
  - Fever
  - Headache
- Acute neurologic period (2–10 days):
  - Episodes of hyperactivity
  - Paralysis
- Coma
- Death
- Usually occurs within 3 weeks of the onset of complications

CAUSES
Rabies virus present in saliva of infected animals.

SCOPE
About five cases of rabies occur per year in humans; about 30,000 people receive treatments after exposure.

MOST OFTEN AFFECTED
Rabies can affect all ages; males and females affected equally.

RISK FACTORS
- Professions or activities that may expose a person to wild or domestic animals (e.g., animal handlers, some laboratory workers, veterinarians, spelunkers [cave explorers])
- International travel to countries where canine rabies is endemic (most common risk factor)
- In the United States, most cases seem to be caused by exposure to bats.

 ## DIAGNOSIS

WHAT THE DOCTOR LOOKS FOR
- The diagnosis of rabies should be considered if an individual has been bitten by an animal capable of transmitting the disease; however, most patients in the United States do not recall exposure.
- Other conditions that can cause similar signs and symptoms should be identified and treated.

TESTS AND PROCEDURES
- Blood tests
- Spinal fluid can be obtained by lumbar puncture (spinal tap).
- The rabies virus can be isolated from saliva or spinal fluid.
- A sample of skin from the bite area can be obtained for laboratory analysis.
- X-ray study

 ## TREATMENT

GENERAL MEASURES
- The management of rabies requires hospitalization.
- Immediate and thorough washing of all bite wounds and scratches with soap and water
- Because no treatment is available for rabies, care is directed at preventing the disease following exposure to potentially rabid animals.

ACTIVITY
As tolerated

DIET
No restrictions

 ## MEDICATIONS

COMMONLY PRESCRIBED DRUGS
- Rabies immune globulin, human (HRIG)
- Rabies vaccine, human diploid cell (HDCV)
- Rabies vaccine adsorbed (RVA)

 ## FOLLOW-UP

PATIENT MONITORING
No follow-up is required in most cases; see the doctor as often as necessary for wound care.

PREVENTION
- Avoid travel to areas where rabies is endemic.
- Avoid wild or unfamiliar animals that act strange or unusual.
- If bitten or scratched by an animal suspected of having rabies, seek prompt medical attention.

COMPLICATIONS
None

WHAT TO EXPECT
No failures of after-exposure treatment have been reported in the United States since the 1970s.

Rabies

Doctor
Office
Phone
Pager

Special notes to patient:

Rape (Sexual Assault)

BASICS

DESCRIPTION

Sexual assault is defined as follows, although definitions can vary by state:

- Sexual contact: touching of a person's intimate parts (including thighs) or the clothing covering such areas for the purpose of sexual gratification
- Sexual conduct: vaginal intercourse between a male and female, or anal intercourse, fellatio, or cunnilingus between persons, regardless of gender
- Rape: any sexual penetration; however slight, using force or coercion against the person's will
- Corruption of a minor: sexual conduct by an individual 18 years of age or older with an individual aged less than 16 years

SIGNS AND SYMPTOMS

- In adults:
  - History of sexual penetration
  - Sexual contact or sexual conduct without consent or with the use of force
- In children:
  - Actual observation of, or suspicion of, sexual penetration, sexual contact, or sexual conduct
  - Signs include evidence of the use of force or evidence of sexual contact (e.g., presence of semen or sperm).

SCOPE

More than 100,000 cases of alleged rape are reported in the United States every year. It is estimated that only 10% to 20% of adult cases and only 5% to 7% of pediatric cases are reported.

MOST OFTEN AFFECTED

- Most adult victims are women in their teens and 20s.
- Child victims can be of either gender, with a predominance of females.
- Increasing numbers of adult male victims are presenting for treatment.
- Overall, females are victims more often than males.

RISK FACTORS

- Numerous risk factors
- About 50% of rapes occur in the home, with one third of these involving a male intruder.

DIAGNOSIS

WHAT THE DOCTOR LOOKS FOR

The doctor will perform a physical examination to assess the nature of sexual contact and look for signs of penetration, force, and other evidence of sexual assault.

TESTS AND PROCEDURES

- The vagina can be swabbed to test for the presence of semen.
- Pregnancy test

TREATMENT

GENERAL MEASURES

- Contact appropriate social services agency or rape crisis center.
- Most adult victims can be treated as outpatients unless associated trauma (physical or mental) requires hospital admission.
- Most pediatric sexual assault or abuse victims require admission or outside placement until the appropriate social agency can evaluate home environment.
- All sexual assault cases must be reported immediately to the appropriate law enforcement agency.
- Sedation and tetanus prevention may be given.
- Sexually transmitted disease prevention for gonorrhea and Chlamydia should be administered.
- Consider possible pregnancy; "morning-after" pills should be offered.
- Testing for exposure to the human immunodeficiency virus (HIV); possibly, testing for hepatitis B.

ACTIVITY

No restrictions

DIET

No restrictions

MEDICATIONS

COMMONLY PRESCRIBED DRUGS

- Ceftriaxone, cefixime
- Spectinomycin
- Ciprofloxacin, norfloxacin, ofloxacin
- Ampicillin/probenecid, amoxicillin/probenecid
- Azithromycin (Zithromax)
- Doxycycline, tetracycline, erythromycin

CONTRAINDICATIONS

Read drug product information.

PRECAUTIONS

Read drug product information.

DRUG INTERACTIONS

Read drug product information.

FOLLOW-UP

PATIENT MONITORING

- See the doctor in 7 to 10 days for follow-up care, including pregnancy testing and counseling by a gynecologist or appropriate gynecologic clinic.
- Follow-up tests for pregnancy and sexually transmitted diseases in 5 to 6 weeks and at 6 months after initial treatment
- Referral to agencies that can provide counseling and legal services should be provided.

Rape (Sexual Assault)

Doctor
Office
Phone
Pager

Special notes to patient:

Rape (Sexual Assault)

PREVENTION

Assertiveness and self-defense training

COMPLICATIONS

- Sexually transmitted disease
- Pregnancy (with the possibility of abortion)
- Trauma (physical and mental)

WHAT TO EXPECT

- Acute phase (usually 1–3 weeks following rape):
  - Shaking, pain, wound healing, mood swings, appetite loss, crying. Also, feelings of grief, shame, anger, fear, revenge, or guilt.
- Late or chronic phase:
  - Female victim may develop fear of intercourse, fear of men, nightmares, sleep disorders, daytime flashbacks, fear of being alone, loss of self-esteem, anxiety, depression, posttraumatic stress syndrome
- Recovery may be prolonged. Individuals who are able to talk about their feelings seem to recover faster.

MEDICATIONS

PEDIATRIC

Assure the child that he or she is a good person and was not the cause of the incident.

FURTHER INFORMATION

National Institute of Mental Health, Public Inquiries Branch, Office of Scientific Information, Department of Health and Human Services, Parklawn Bldg., Room 15C-05, 5600 Fishers Lane, Rockville, MD 20857, (301) 443-4513

Rape (Sexual Assault)

Doctor
Office
Phone
Pager

Special notes to patient:

Rash (Urticaria)

BASICS

DESCRIPTION

A rash consisting of a single or multiple itchy raised bumps on the skin, typically pale with a red halo. A rash can subside rapidly, resulting in no scars or change in pigmentation, and can recur.

- Acute urticaria:
  - Reaction to many stimuli
  - Can be an unusual response to drug exposure
  - Subsides over several hours
- Chronic urticaria:
  - Persists more than 6 weeks in 30% of cases
  - Cold urticaria: results from cooling and rewarming; can be fatal. Another form can affect several members of a family with fever, chills, joint and muscle pain, and headache.
  - Heat urticaria: small (5–10 ml) spots on upper trunk from overheating, hot shower
  - Exercise-induced urticaria: from extreme exercise; marked by swelling, wheezing, low blood pressure. Often is associated with eating food to which person is allergic.
  - Linear urticaria: results from scratching the skin
  - Solar urticaria: results from exposure to sunlight. Onset in minutes; subsides in 1 to 2 hours.
  - Delayed pressure urticaria: occurs 4 to 6 hours after pressure to skin (e.g., elastic, shoes)
  - Water urticaria: occurs after contact with water at any temperature (rare)

SIGNS AND SYMPTOMS

- Urticaria can appear alone or with swelling.
- Can occur with generalized allergic reaction, potentially fatal
- Single or multiple raised, pale spots surrounded by a red halo
- Intense itching
- Can occur anywhere on the body
- Spots are variably sized.
- Acute urticaria develops rapidly, resolves spontaneously in fewer than 48 hours

CAUSES

- Can be allergic or nonallergic
- Allergy-triggering substance may be inhaled, eaten, or contacted by the skin.
- Drug reaction
- Food or food additive allergy
- Insect bite, sting
- Infection
- Vascular disease
- Physical trauma (e.g., heat, cold, sunlight)
- Emotional stress (reported; little supporting evidence)

SCOPE

Urticaria affects about 1 in 1,000 persons (15% to 20% of the population in the United States) at some time during a lifetime.

MOST OFTEN AFFECTED

Urticaria can affect all ages. Acute urticaria is seen mainly in children and young adults. Males and females are affected with equal frequency, although chronic rash is more common in older women.

RISK FACTORS

See *Causes*

DIAGNOSIS

WHAT THE DOCTOR LOOKS FOR

- Conditions known to be associated with rash (e.g., angioedema and allergic reaction)
- Possible causes of urticaria (e.g., insect bites or skin diseases)
- A cause is identified in 10% to 25% of chronic cases.

TESTS AND PROCEDURES

- Urinalysis
- Blood tests can be done to identify signs of infection or inflammation.
- A sample of skin tissue obtained by biopsy can be examined microscopically.
- Tests can be done to evaluate allergies to foods or other substances.
- Special tests include:
  - Cold urticaria: ice cube test (ice cube placed on skin 5 minutes, observed 10–15 minutes)
  - Exercise-induced urticaria: exercise challenge; methacholine skin test
  - Solar urticaria: exposure to defined wavelengths of light.
  - Delayed pressure urticaria: apply a sandbag (5–10 lb) for 3 hours, then observe
  - Water urticaria: apply tap water at different temperatures
  - Vibratory urticaria: apply vibration 4 to 5 minutes with a laboratory mixing device, then observe

TREATMENT

GENERAL MEASURES

- Acute cases usually do not require a full workup.
- Cool, moist compresses help control itching.
- Avoid known substances that provoke allergies. Use antihistamines if accidentally reexposed.

ACTIVITY

As desired. Avoid overheating.

DIET

As desired. Avoid foods suspected as possible allergy triggers.

MEDICATIONS

COMMONLY PRESCRIBED DRUGS

- First-generation antihistamines
  - Older children and adults: hydroxyzine or diphenhydramine
  - Children under 6 years of age: diphenhydramine
- Second-generation drugs are equally effective as antihistamines and are less sedating but more expensive.
  - Fexofenadine (Allegra)
  - Astemizole (Hismanal)
  - Loratadine (Claritin)
  - Acrivastine (Semprex)
  - Cetirizine (Zyrtec)

PRECAUTIONS

- First-generation drugs can cause drowsiness.
- Second-generation H_1-blockers should be used with caution in pregnant women and the elderly.
- Antihistamines, in children, can cause unexpected agitation.

Rash (Urticaria)

	Doctor
	Office
	Phone
	Pager

Special notes to patient:

Rash (Urticaria)

DRUG INTERACTIONS
Read drug product information.

OTHER DRUGS
- Doxepin (Sinequan)
- H_2-blockers (e.g., cimetidine, ranitidine) may be helpful in treating chronic urticaria.
- Corticosteroids (prednisone) for unresponsive, nonacute cases

FOLLOW-UP

PATIENT MONITORING
- No follow-up is necessary after an initial episode of rash.
- See the doctor if symptoms persist or recur.

PREVENTION
If a cause is identified, avoidance is the best solution.

COMPLICATIONS
Severe systemic allergic reaction

WHAT TO EXPECT
About 70% of people with urticaria improve in fewer than 72 hours. About 30% develop chronic urticaria. Urticaria becomes chronic in 75% of persons with both rash and swelling. About 20% have attacks for more than 20 years.

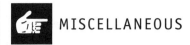

MISCELLANEOUS

PEDIATRIC
Isolated acute cases are frequent, but chronic urticaria is rare.

GERIATRIC
Less likely to occur in this age group

PREGNANCY
A chronic rash can develop during pregnancy.

Rash (Urticaria)

Doctor
Office
Phone
Pager

Special notes to patient:

Raynaud's Phenomenon

 ## BASICS

DESCRIPTION

Raynaud's phenomenon, or cold intolerance, is a disorder marked by attacks of extreme pallor, then a bluish discoloration of the fingers (rarely, of the toes) brought on by cold exposure. With warming, intense redness develops, followed by swelling, throbbing, and tingling. Sometimes accompanies emotional upset.

SIGNS AND SYMPTOMS

- Pallor or whiteness of fingertips with cold exposure, followed by a bluish discoloration, then redness and pain with warming
- Ulceration of fingertips, progressing to finger loss in severe, prolonged cases (10% to 13% of cases)

CAUSES

Unknown

SCOPE

Of the population, 4% to 10% experience cold intolerance.

MOST OFTEN AFFECTED

Individuals 40 years of age or older; women affected more frequently than men

RISK FACTORS

- Smoking
- Immune or connective tissue disorder
- Alcohol use (women only)

 ## DIAGNOSIS

WHAT THE DOCTOR LOOKS FOR

- The doctor will do a physical examination to discern the signs and symptoms of cold intolerance.

TESTS AND PROCEDURES

- Blood tests
- X-ray studies
- Special diagnostic tests can be done to assess response to cold.

 ## TREATMENT

GENERAL MEASURES

- Dress warmly, wear gloves, avoid cold
- No smoking
- Avoid beta-blockers, amphetamines, ergot alkaloids, and sumatriptan
- Biofeedback training can help increase hand temperature.
- Finger guards over ulcerated fingertips

ACTIVITY

Avoidance of situations in which exposure to cold is likely; avoid vibrating tools

DIET

No special diet

 ## MEDICATIONS

COMMONLY PRESCRIBED DRUGS

Nifedipine

CONTRAINDICATIONS

- Allergy to drug
- Pregnancy
- Congestive heart failure

PRECAUTIONS

Can cause headache, dizziness, lightheadedness

DRUG INTERACTIONS

Read drug product information.

OTHER DRUGS

- Diltiazem, verapamil, reserpine, methyldopa, prazosin
- Captopril (not approved by the US Food and Drug Administration)
- Prostacyclin
- Nitroglycerin patches may also be helpful, but they may cause severe headache.
- Amlodipine, isradipine, nicardipine, felodipine

 ## FOLLOW-UP

PATIENT MONITORING

The doctor should be seen as often as necessary.

PREVENTION

- Avoid trauma to fingertips
- Avoid exposure to cold
- Smoking cessation

COMPLICATIONS

Gangrene, amputation of fingertips

WHAT TO EXPECT

Cold intolerance usually follows a prolonged course with recurrent attacks and formation of fingertip ulcers.

 ## MISCELLANEOUS

GERIATRIC

Appearance of Raynaud's phenomenon after age 40 almost always indicates an underlying disease.

Raynaud's Phenomenon

	Doctor
	Office
	Phone
	Pager

Special notes to patient:

Renal Failure, Acute (ARF)

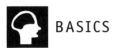 ## BASICS

DESCRIPTION

Acute renal failure (ARF) is a syndrome of rapidly deteriorating kidney function with the accumulation of wastes in the bloodstream.

SIGNS AND SYMPTOMS

- Loss of appetite
- Back pain
- Coma
- Delirium
- Diarrhea
- Difficulty breathing
- Bruising
- Swelling
- Brain damage
- Nosebleed
- Fatigue
- Gastrointestinal bleeding
- Headache
- Hiccups
- High blood pressure
- Lethargy
- Muscle cramps, spasm
- Nausea
- Scant urine production
- Rash
- Eye disease
- Seizure
- Sleepiness
- Rapid heart rate
- Rapid breathing rate
- Urine-like odor from body
- Vomiting
- Weakness
- Dry mouth

CAUSES

- Severe illness (e.g., heart failure, cirrhosis of liver)
- Kidney disease
- Vascular disease
- Urinary tract obstruction

SCOPE

Of individuals admitted to hospitals in the United States, 5% develop acute renal failure.

MOST OFTEN AFFECTED

All ages are affected by ARF, males and females equally

RISK FACTORS

- Surgery
- Volume depletion (especially in diabetes)
- Drug side effect
- Medical illness

 ## DIAGNOSIS

WHAT THE DOCTOR LOOKS FOR

See *Causes*

TESTS AND PROCEDURES

- Urinalysis
- Blood tests
- A sample of kidney tissue can be obtained by biopsy for laboratory analysis.
- Special radiology procedures that can be done include angiogram, renal scan, ultrasound, and computed tomography (CT) scan.
- The urinary tract can be examined by cystoscopy.

 ## TREATMENT

GENERAL MEASURES

Acute renal failure requires hospitalization.

ACTIVITY

As tolerated

DIET

- Restrict fluids.
- Eliminate potassium, if serum level is increased.
- Increase carbohydrates.

 ## MEDICATIONS

COMMONLY PRESCRIBED DRUGS

- Intravenous (IV) saline solution
- Mannitol
- Furosemide (Lasix)
- Calcium channel blockers

PRECAUTIONS

Read drug product information.

DRUG INTERACTIONS

Read drug product information.

 ## FOLLOW-UP

PATIENT MONITORING

See the doctor and other health professionals, as needed.

PREVENTION

See *Risk Factors*

COMPLICATIONS

- Severe, life-threatening infection (leading cause of death)
- Convulsions
- Swelling
- Fluid in lungs
- Congestive heart failure
- Paralysis
- Irregular heart rhythms
- Death
- Heart disorders
- Blood poisoning
- Bleeding

WHAT TO EXPECT

Recovery usually occurs in days to 6 weeks. Mortality rate is high (5% to 80%), depending on cause, severity, and age.

 ## MISCELLANEOUS

GERIATRIC

Greater occurrence of ARF among the elderly, especially after surgery

FURTHER INFORMATION

- National Kidney & Urologic Diseases Information Clearinghouse, Box NKUDIC, Bethesda, MD 20893, (301) 468-6345
- The National Kidney Foundation, Inc., 30 East 33rd St., New York, NY 10016

Renal Failure, Acute (ARF)

	Doctor
	Office
	Phone
	Pager

Special notes to patient:

Retinal Detachment

 ## BASICS

DESCRIPTION
Retinal detachment is the separation of the sensory retina (the "screen" at the back of the eye) from the underlying retinal tissue, with an accumulation of fluid between them.

SIGNS AND SYMPTOMS
- Flashes
- Floaters
- Visual field loss (typically, a "curtain" across a portion of the visual field)

CAUSES
- Normal aging
- Tumors
- Inflammatory diseases
- Trauma, foreign bodies
- Miscellaneous (e.g., uveal effusion, malignant hypertension)

SCOPE
- Annually, 10 per 100,000 persons experience retinal detachment without surgery or injury.
- Retinal detachment is rare before 30 years of age and is seen in 63% of patients above 70 years of age; males and females affected equally.

RISK FACTORS
- Nearsightedness
- Absence of lens
- Trauma
- Retinal detachment in other eye
- Retinal degeneration

 ## DIAGNOSIS

WHAT THE DOCTOR LOOKS FOR
The doctor will examine the eyes to evaluate the status of the retina.

 ## TREATMENT

GENERAL MEASURES
- Referral to a retina specialist for examination and repair
- Surgery is required.

ACTIVITY
In some cases, bedrest and patching of both eyes

DIET
No special diet

 ## MEDICATIONS

COMMONLY PRESCRIBED DRUGS
- Intraocular gases
- Perflurocarbon liquids
- Silicone oil

 ## FOLLOW-UP

PATIENT MONITORING
See the doctor as often as necessary.

PREVENTION
Regular eye examination by an ophthalmologist

COMPLICATIONS
Partial or total loss of vision

WHAT TO EXPECT
- Untreated, visual loss continues, and, ultimately, complete blindness results.
- With current techniques, 90% to 95% of retinal detachments can be repaired.
- Outcome depends on the severity of underlying disorder causing detachment.

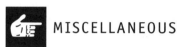

PREGNANCY
Preeclampsia and eclampsia may predispose to with retinal detachment.

FURTHER INFORMATION
American Academy of Ophthalmology (415) 561-8500

Retinal Detachment

	Doctor
	Office
	Phone
	Pager

Special notes to patient:

Rhinitis, Allergic

 ## BASICS

DESCRIPTION

Allergic rhinitis, or hay fever, is a reaction to airborne allergens. The condition can be seasonal or perennial, depending on climate and individual response. Seasonal responses are usually to grasses, trees, and weeds. Perennial responses are to house-dust mites, mold antigens, and animal body products.

SIGNS AND SYMPTOMS

- Nasal stuffiness and congestion
- Sneezing, often in spasms
- Watery eyes
- Dark circles under eyes, "allergic shiners"
- Long eyelashes
- Sensation of plugged ears
- Sleeping difficulties
- Fatigue
- Mouth breathing
- Scratchy throat
- Voice change
- Irritating cough
- Postnasal drip
- Loss or alteration of smell
- Itchy nose, eyes, ears, and palate

CAUSES

- Animal and plant proteins: pollens, molds, mite dust, animal danders, dried saliva, and urine
- Insect debris: cockroach, locusts, fish food

SCOPE

Allergic rhinitis affects 8% to 12% of the population in the United States.

MOST OFTEN AFFECTED

Onset usually occurs before 30 years of age; average age of onset is 10 years

PREDOMINANT SEX

Males and females are affected in equal proportion.

RISK FACTORS

- Family history
- Repeated exposure to offending antigen
- Exposure to multiple allergens
- Presence of other allergies (e.g., asthma, rash)
- Noncompliance with therapy

 ## DIAGNOSIS

WHAT THE DOCTOR LOOKS FOR

- The doctor will perform a physical examination to identify the presence of rhinitis.
- Numerous other conditions can produce signs and symptoms similar to rhinitis, including nasal polyps, foreign bodies, drug side effects, and infections.

TESTS AND PROCEDURES

- Blood tests
- Nasal secretions can be sampled for laboratory analysis.
- Allergy testing
- Hearing testing may be performed
- X-ray study of the head
- The interior of the nose can be examined by rhinoscopy.

 ## TREATMENT

GENERAL MEASURES

- Rhinitis is managed in the outpatient setting.
- Limit exposure to offending allergen.
- Specific causes should be identified.
- Intensity of treatment is determined by disease severity.
- Immunotherapy may be beneficial.
- Surgical repair of the nose may be required.

ACTIVITY

No specific restrictions. Avoid activity in areas of allergen exposure.

DIET

No special diet, unless food allergies are suspected.

 ## MEDICATIONS

COMMONLY PRESCRIBED DRUGS

- Antihistamines:
  - Diphenhydramine (Benadryl), clemastine (Taoist), chlorpheniramine, brompheniramine, tripelennamine (PBZ), hydroxyzine (Atarax), promethazine (Phenergan), methdilazine (Tacaryl), astemizole (Hismanal)
- Decongestants:
  - Pseudoephedrine, phenylephrine
- Nasal sprays:
  - Saline solution, cromolyn sodium (Nasalcrom), beclomethasone (Beconase AQ, Vancenase AQ), flunisolide (Nasalide, AeroBid), triamcinolone (Nasacort), budesonide (Rhinocort)
- Steroids

CONTRAINDICATIONS

Read drug product information.

PRECAUTIONS

The elderly often require less aggressive treatment.

DRUG INTERACTIONS

Numerous interactions; read drug product information.

Rhinitis, Allergic

Doctor
Office
Phone
Pager

Special notes to patient:

Rhinitis, Allergic

 ## FOLLOW-UP

PATIENT MONITORING

See the doctor as often as needed.

PREVENTION

- Avoidance: not sufficient to control symptoms for most people
- Air conditioning and limited outside exposure during season is helpful.
- House cleaning (particularly in the bedroom) tactics and control for dust mites for patients sensitive to this allergen
- Minimize exposure to animals. House pets are discouraged.
- Avoid environmental irritants (e.g., smoke and fumes).
- Use an air purifier.
- Use allergy control covers on mattresses and pillows.

COMPLICATIONS

- Infection
- Sinusitis
- Nosebleed
- Impaired lung function
- Appearance change

WHAT TO EXPECT

- For many people, symptoms can be well controlled.
- Treatment should be tailored to the specific individual.
- Symptoms often ease over time.

 ## MISCELLANEOUS

PEDIATRIC

Environmental control can include carpet and drape removal, removal of house plants, pet control, and so on.

GERIATRIC

- Increased medication side effects
- Symptoms may decrease among the elderly.

PREGNANCY

Pregnancy can aggravate rhinitis.

FURTHER INFORMATION

Asthma & Allergy Foundation of America. 1717 Massachusetts Ave., Suite 305, Washington, DC 20036, (800) 7-ASTHMA

Rhinitis, Allergic

Doctor
Office
Phone
Pager

Special notes to patient:

Rocky Mountain Spotted Fever

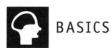# BASICS

DESCRIPTION

Rocky Mountain spotted fever (RMSF), an acute, potentially fatal illness transmitted by tick bite, is marked by headache, fever, and rash.

SIGNS AND SYMPTOMS

- Fever
- Rash
- Headache
- Nausea, vomiting
- Abdominal pain
- Muscle and joint pain
- Enlarged lymph nodes
- Cough
- Central nervous system dysfunction (e.g., stupor, confusion, coma)

CAUSES

RMSF is caused by *Rickettsia rickettsii*, which is transmitted by a tick bite.

SCOPE

About 600 new cases are reported each year in the United States. Peak incidence is in late spring and summer.

MOST OFTEN AFFECTED

Highest incidences occur among children and young adults, but all ages are susceptible. RMSF is more common in males than females, because they participate in more outdoor activities.

RISK FACTORS

- Outdoor activity during warm months
- Contact with dogs

DIAGNOSIS

WHAT THE DOCTOR LOOKS FOR

- The doctor will perform a physical examination to identify the presence of illness.
- Numerous other conditions that can cause similar signs and symptoms should be ruled out (e.g., viral infection, Lyme disease, and other disorders).

TESTS AND PROCEDURES

- Blood tests
- Chest x-ray study
- Tissue can be sampled by biopsy for laboratory analysis.

TREATMENT

GENERAL MEASURES

- Individuals who are moderately ill are usually hospitalized.
- Individuals with mild disease are treated as outpatients.
- Supportive care, as needed

ACTIVITY

Bedrest until symptoms subside.

DIET

Small, frequent meals may be necessary to maintain nutritional levels.

MEDICATIONS

COMMONLY PRESCRIBED DRUGS

- Doxycycline (Vibramycin)
- Tetracycline
- Chloramphenicol

CONTRAINDICATIONS

- Tetracycline should not be used in children under 9 years of age.
- Doxycycline and tetracycline are contraindicated in pregnancy.

PRECAUTIONS

Can cause sensitivity to light; use a sunscreen

DRUG INTERACTIONS

Tetracycline can interact with milk products, iron preparations, or antacids containing aluminum or magnesium.

FOLLOW-UP

PATIENT MONITORING

If not hospitalized, see the doctor every 2 to 3 days until symptoms have fully resolved.

PREVENTION

- Wear occlusive clothing.
- Use insect repellants.
- After possible exposure, all body areas should be carefully inspected for ticks, especially legs, groin, and belt lines. Risk of infection increases with the duration of tick attachment.
- Ticks should be removed from humans or animals with caution; gloves should be worn or instruments used to minimize direct contact. Place a drop of oil, alcohol, gasoline, or kerosine on the tick first. Hands should be washed thoroughly afterward.

COMPLICATIONS

- Brain disease, usually temporary
- Seizures
- Kidney failure
- Hepatitis
- Heart failure
- Respiratory failure

WHAT TO EXPECT

- When treated promptly, the usual outcome is excellent, with symptoms resolving over several days and no lasting effects.
- Death is rare when appropriate therapy is instituted promptly.
- If complications develop, the course may be more severe and long-term effects (e.g., neurologic disorders) can result.

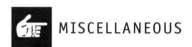# MISCELLANEOUS

GERIATRIC

Mortality risk is higher among the elderly.

Rocky Mountain Spotted Fever

Doctor
Office
Phone
Pager

Special notes to patient:

Rosacea

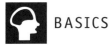 ## BASICS

DESCRIPTION
Rosacea is a chronic skin eruption with flushing and dilation of small blood vessels in the face, especially the nose and cheeks.

SIGNS AND SYMPTOMS
- Skin flushing
- Redness: lower half of nose; sometimes, entire nose, forehead, cheeks, and chin
- Reddened eyes (sometimes)
- Dusky, reddened skin
- Blood vessels in involved area collapse under pressure
- Acne
- "Spider veins"
- Bulging or overgrowth of nose

CAUSES
- No proven cause. Possibilities include:
- Hormone disturbance
  - Alcohol, coffee, tea, spiced food overindulgence (unproved)
  - Parasite (suspected)
  - Exposure to cold, heat, hot drinks
  - Emotional stress
  - Disorder of the gastrointestinal tract

SCOPE
Rosacea is common in the United States.

MOST OFTEN AFFECTED
Persons 30 to 50 years of age; women affected more frequently than men

 ## DIAGNOSIS

WHAT THE DOCTOR LOOKS FOR
- The doctor will perform a physical examination to assess the presence of rosacea.
- Numerous other conditions that can cause skin eruptions similar to rosacea should be investigated (including Seborrhea, bleparitis, drug-induced rash, acne, etc.).

 ## TREATMENT

GENERAL MEASURES
- Reassurance
- Psychological stress should be treated, if present.
- Avoid oil-based cosmetics.
- Treat permanently dilated blood vessels
- Surgical repair of nose may be necessary.

ACTIVITY
No restrictions. Physical fitness is encouraged.

DIET
Avoid any food or drink that causes facial flushing (e.g., hot drinks, spiced food, alcohol).

 ## MEDICATIONS

COMMONLY PRESCRIBED DRUGS
- Tetracycline
- Alcohol-sulfur (Liquimat), sulfur (Fostril), resorcinol-sulfur (Rezamid), sulfacetamide-sulfur (Sulfacet-R)
- Metronidazole (topical)
- Erythromycin (topical)
- Clindamycin (topical)

CONTRAINDICATIONS
- Tetracycline: not for use in pregnant women or in children under 9 years of age
- Isotretinoin: causes birth defects; not for use in pregnant women or in women of reproductive age who are not using a reliable birth control method

PRECAUTIONS
Tetracycline: can cause sensitivity to sunlight; use a sunscreen

DRUG INTERACTIONS
- Tetracycline: avoid antacids, dairy products, and iron
- Broad-spectrum antibiotics: can reduce the effectiveness of oral contraceptives

 ## FOLLOW-UP

PATIENT MONITORING
See the doctor as often as needed.

PREVENTION
No preventive measure is known.

COMPLICATIONS
- Thickened, bulbous skin on nose, especially in men
- Conjunctivitis (pink eye)
- Blepharitis
- Keratitis

WHAT TO EXPECT
- Is usually slowly progressive.
- Sometimes rosacea subsides spontaneously.

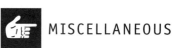 ## MISCELLANEOUS

PEDIATRIC
Uncommon among children

GERIATRIC
Uncommon after 60 years of age

PREGNANCY
Use of isotretinoin is contraindicated during pregnancy.

FURTHER INFORMATION
American Academy of Dermatology
(708) 330-0230

Rosacea

Doctor
Office
Phone
Pager

Special notes to patient:

Salmonella Infection

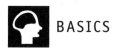 ## BASICS

DESCRIPTION
Salmonella infection, caused by *Salmonella* bacteria, produces severe gastrointestinal symptoms. In its most common form, the infection is transmitted by eating food contaminated with *Salmonella* organisms.

SCOPE
About 55 outbreaks of salmonella infections are reported annually in the United States. The peak frequency occurs in July through November.

MOST OFTEN AFFECTED
- Salmonella infection is most common in individuals younger than 20 or older than 70 years of age.
- Highest incidence occurs in infants younger than 1 year of age.
- Males and females are affected equally.

SIGNS AND SYMPTOMS
- Nausea, vomiting, diarrhea
- Abdominal cramps
- Headache, muscle pain
- Fever to 102°F (39°C); may be persistent
- Bone or joint inflammation
- Wound infection
- Inflammation of heart or blood vessels
- Pneumonia
- Shock
- Urinary tract infection

CAUSES
- Ingestion of contaminated food (e.g., poultry, meat, eggs, dairy products) or water
- Person-to-person spread
- Contact with infected animal (e.g., poultry, cows, pigs, birds, sheep, seals, donkeys, lizards, snakes) and pets (e.g., turtles, cats, dogs, mice, guinea pigs, hamsters)
- Contact with chronic carrier
- Ulcerative colitis
- Systemic lupus erythematosus
- Gallstones
- Kidney stones
- Drugs: antibiotics, purgatives, opiates

RISK FACTORS
- Anemia
- Cancer
- Immune system disorder
- Pets (snakes, iguanas)

 ## DIAGNOSIS

WHAT THE DOCTOR LOOKS FOR
The doctor will perform a physical examination to identify salmonella poisoning.

TESTS AND PROCEDURES
- Blood tests and culture
- A stool sample can be obtained for laboratory analysis.
- A radiology procedure, called an "angiography," can be performed on patients above 50 years of age.

 ## TREATMENT

GENERAL MEASURES
- Uncomplicated cases of salmonella infection are managed in the outpatient setting; severe cases may require hospitalization.
- Correct fluid and salt imbalances.
- Relief of symptoms (pain, nausea, vomiting)
- Surgery may be required.

ACTIVITY
As tolerated

DIET
Oral rehydration solution during diarrhea phase; advance to normal diet, as tolerated

 ## MEDICATIONS

COMMONLY PRESCRIBED DRUGS
- Ampicillin
- Trimethoprim-sulfamethoxazole (Bactrim, Septra)
- Cefotaxime (Claforan), ciprofloxacin (Cipro), norfloxacin
- Chloramphenicol
- Azithromycin (Zithromax)

CONTRAINDICATIONS
Known drug allergy; read drug product information.

PRECAUTIONS
Read drug product information.

DRUG INTERACTIONS
Read drug product information.

OTHER DRUGS
Ofloxacin (Floxin)

 ## FOLLOW-UP

PATIENT MONITORING
See the doctor as needed; stool culture should be repeated 5 months and 1 year after infection.

PREVENTION
- Maintain proper hygiene during preparation and storage of food. Wash hands, utensils, and surfaces (countertops, serving dishes) thoroughly with soap and hot water after contact with raw meat, especially poultry.
- Keep hot foods hot and cold foods cold during picnics, buffets, and so on.
- Do not eat raw eggs or foods prepared with raw or undercooked eggs (e.g., caesar salad, hollandaise sauce).
- Handle animals carefully and avoid contact with animal feces.
- Wash hands thoroughly.

Salmonella Infection

Doctor
Office
Phone
Pager

Special notes to patient:

Salmonella Infection

COMPLICATIONS
- Severe colon disorder
- Shock
- Severe infection
- Brain involvement

WHAT TO EXPECT
- Prognosis for gastrointestinal symptoms is excellent. Exceptions include the very young, the very old, and those who are debilitated or hospitalized.
- Prognosis for brain or heart involvement is poor, unless effective treatment is given early.

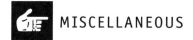 MISCELLANEOUS

PEDIATRIC
Children, especially newborns, are more likely to become chronic carriers.

GERIATRIC
Patients above 60 years of age also have high carrier rate.

OTHERS
Contaminated marijuana is an important source of infection, particularly in young adults.

FURTHER INFORMATION
Food Safety and Inspection Service, Office of Public Awareness, Department of Agriculture, Room 1165-S, Washington, DC 20205, (202) 447-9351

Salmonella Infection

Doctor
Office
Phone
Pager

Special notes to patient:

Scabies

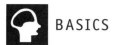 ## BASICS

DESCRIPTION
Scabies is a contagious disease caused by infestation of the skin by the mite *Sarcoptes scabiei*.

SIGNS AND SYMPTOMS
- Generalized itching
- Itching during sleep hours
- Mites burrow between the fingers, and into the skin of wrists, hands, feet, penis, scrotum, buttocks, and waistline.
- Blisters and welts
- Peeling skin
- Reddening

CAUSES
Skin infestation by *S. scabiei*

SCOPE
Common in the United States

MOST OFTEN AFFECTED
Children and young adults; males and females are affected equally

RISK FACTORS
- Personal skin-to-skin contact (e.g., sexual promiscuity, crowding, poverty, nosocomial infection)
- Immune system disorders
- Eczema

 ## DIAGNOSIS

WHAT THE DOCTOR LOOKS FOR
The doctor will examine for the presence of scabies; numerous other skin conditions that look similar must be ruled out.

TESTS AND PROCEDURES
A sample of skin can be obtained by biopsy for analysis (rare).

 ## TREATMENT

GENERAL MEASURES
- Treat all intimate contacts and close household and family members.
- Wash all clothing, bed linens, and towels in a normal wash cycle.

ACTIVITY
Full activity

DIET
No special diet

 ## MEDICATIONS

COMMONLY PRESCRIBED DRUGS
- Permethrin (Elimite)
- Lindane (Kwell, Scabene)
- Crotamiton (Eurax)

CONTRAINDICATIONS
Lindane should be avoided in premature, malnourished, or emaciated children, and in individuals with severe skin disease or a history of seizures.

PRECAUTIONS
- Do not overuse the medication when applying it to the skin.
- For medications other than permethrin, use a second application only when specifically advised to do so by the doctor.

OTHER DRUGS
- Sulfur ointment (5%)
- Ivermectin

FOLLOW-UP

PATIENT MONITORING
See the doctor weekly, if rash or itching persist.

COMPLICATIONS
- Eczema
- Other skin disorders
- Itching
- Scabies nodules

WHAT TO EXPECT
- Lesions begin to heal in 1 to 2 days, along with the worst itching.
- Some itching commonly persists for 10 to 14 days and can be treated with topical or oral medication.
- Nodules

 ## MISCELLANEOUS

PEDIATRIC
Infants often have more widespread involvement.

GERIATRIC
The elderly are at greater risk for extensive infestations; they often itch more severely.

PREGNANCY
Lindane should be used cautiously and no more than twice during pregnancy.

Scabies

Doctor
Office
Phone
Pager

Special notes to patient:

Schizophrenia

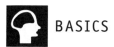 ## BASICS

DESCRIPTION

Schizophrenia is a major psychiatric disorder with symptoms of delusions, hallucinations, disturbed emotion, and impaired thought processes, lasting at least 6 months.

SIGNS AND SYMPTOMS

- Withdrawal from reality
- Delusions, paranoia
- Reference (people or things have unusual significance)
- Patient believes that he or she can hear person's thoughts or put thoughts into another person or control another person
- Grandiose or religious delusions
- Hallucinations, usually auditory
- Flat or inappropriate emotion
- Much speech but conveys little information

CAUSES

Unknown. Schizophrenia is not initiated or maintained by an organic factor. It is probably caused by a complex interaction between inherited and environmental factors.

SCOPE

About 1% of the population in the United States suffers schizophrenia at some point in their lifetime.

MOST OFTEN AFFECTED

Onset before 45 years of age; highest prevalence in lower socioeconomic classes; males and females affected equally

RISK FACTORS

Relative with schizophrenia

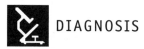 ## DIAGNOSIS

WHAT THE DOCTOR LOOKS FOR

The doctor will evaluate the patient to arrive at the diagnosis of schizophrenia; mental illnesses are subject to strict definitions.

TESTS AND PROCEDURES

- Blood tests, urinalysis
- Psychological testing can be done.
- Electroencephalogram (EEG) to rule out seizure disorder, brain damage, and so forth.
- Computed tomography (CT) scan and magnetic resonance imaging (MRI) can be done to assist in the diagnosis.
- A sample of spinal fluid can be obtained by lumbar puncture (spinal tap).

 ## TREATMENT

GENERAL MEASURES

- Management of schizophrenia often involves hospitalization for initial assessment and treatment.
- Can be managed in the outpatient setting if the person is not dangerous to self or others, is able to cooperate with treatment, and has a supportive family
- Ensure safety of patient and others; the patient may act on delusional thinking.

ACTIVITY

Establish safe environment.

DIET

No special diet

 ## MEDICATIONS

COMMONLY PRESCRIBED DRUGS

- Phenothiazine
- Haloperidol
- Thiothixene
- Risperidone
- Clozapine
- Olanzapine
- Quetiapine

CONTRAINDICATIONS

Read drug product information.

PRECAUTIONS

Numerous precautions; read drug product information.

DRUG INTERACTIONS

Read drug product information.

OTHER DRUGS

- Benzodiazepines
- Anticonvulsants

 ## FOLLOW-UP

PATIENT MONITORING

The doctor should see the patient as often as necessary.

COMPLICATIONS

- Drug side effects
- Self-inflicted trauma
- Combative behavior toward others

WHAT TO EXPECT

- Chronic course: good and bad periods
- Guarded prognosis, although 30% recover completely
- The negative symptoms (decreased ambition, energy, and emotional responsiveness) are often the most difficult to treat.

 ## MISCELLANEOUS

PEDIATRIC

Unusual before puberty

FURTHER INFORMATION

Education and support groups for patient and family available from National Alliance for the Mentally Ill (NAMI), 2101 Wilson Blvd., Suite 302, Arlington, VA 22201, (703) 524-7600

Schizophrenia

Doctor
Office
Phone
Pager

Special notes to patient:

Scoliosis

 ## BASICS

DESCRIPTION

Scoliosis is a curvature in the thoracic, lumbar, or thoracolumbar segment of the spine. It may be associated with kyphosis (humpback) or lordosis (swayback). Scoliosis usually causes no other symptoms.

SIGNS AND SYMPTOMS

CAUSES

- Unknown
- Congenital spine defects
- Musculoskeletal disorders
- Poor posture
- Uneven leg length

MOST OFTEN AFFECTED

The most common type of scoliosis usually begins at about 8 to 10 years of age; it is more common in girls than boys.

 ## DIAGNOSIS

WHAT THE DOCTOR LOOKS FOR

The doctor may take several measurements to determine uneven leg length and may observe the patient walking to note spine curvature.

TESTS AND PROCEDURES

X-ray study of the spine

 ## TREATMENT

GENERAL MEASURES

- Physical therapy and back exercises aimed at strengthening back muscles
- Back brace (sometimes worn for several years)
- If legs are of unequal length, a shoe lift for the shorter leg
- Surgery to correct the deformity (severe cases only).

Scoliosis

Doctor
Office
Phone
Pager

Special notes to patient:

Seasonal Affective Disorder

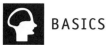 ## BASICS

DESCRIPTION
Seasonal affective disorder (SAD) is depression caused by disturbance of circadian rhythms, occurring most often in the winter months. It is believed to be the result from a decrease in exposure to sunlight.

SIGNS AND SYMPTOMS
In addition to feelings of sadness and anxiety, symptoms include excessive sleepiness, lethargy, carbohydrate craving, and weight gain.

CAUSES
Decreased exposure to sunlight; exact cause is unknown

MOST OFTEN AFFECTED
More common in women and in individuals living in the northern latitudes

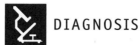 ## DIAGNOSIS

WHAT THE DOCTOR LOOKS FOR
The doctor will take a medical history, with particular attention to symptoms of depression.

TESTS AND PROCEDURES
The individual may be asked to chart symptoms.

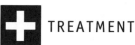 ## TREATMENT

GENERAL MEASURES
- Phototherapy (light therapy)
- Monoamine oxidase (MAO) inhibitor or fluoxetine (Prozac)
- Psychotherapy

Seasonal Affective Disorder

Doctor
Office
Phone
Pager

Special notes to patient:

Seizure Disorders

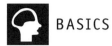 ## BASICS

DESCRIPTION
A seizure is a sudden change in behavior, characterized by a sensory perception or motor activity with or without a change in awareness or consciousness. Seizures can involve convulsions. "Epilepsy" is the name given to a particular group of seizure disorders.

SIGNS AND SYMPTOMS
- Generalized seizures
  - Absence: loss of consciousness or posture
  - Myoclonic: repetitive muscle contractions
  - Tonic-clonic: sustained muscle contraction followed by rhythmic contractions of all four extremities
- Partial seizures
- Febrile seizures (see separate entry on febrile seizures)
  - Most common in children between 3 months and 5 years of age
  - Fever without evidence of any other defined cause for seizures

CAUSES
- Brain tumor
- Insufficient oxygen in blood (breath-holding, carbon monoxide poisoning, anesthesia)
- Stroke
- Poisoning (lead, alcohol, strychnine)
- Eclampsia
- Other factors (e.g., sound, light, cutaneous stimulation)
- Fever (see entry on febrile seizures)
- Head injury
- Heat stroke
- Infection
- Metabolic disorders
- Withdrawal from, or intolerance of, alcohol

SCOPE
About 1.5 million people in the United States have epilepsy.

MOST OFTEN AFFECTED
All ages; males and females affected equally; family history increases risk

RISK FACTORS
Multiple factors

 ## DIAGNOSIS

WHAT THE DOCTOR LOOKS FOR
The doctor will perform a physical examination to identify the cause of seizures.

TESTS AND PROCEDURES
- Blood tests
- Computed tomography (CT) scan or magnetic resonance imaging (MRI) can be done to assist in the diagnosis.
- An electroencephalogram (EEG) can be done to assess brain function.

GENERAL MEASURES
- Protect the person's airway, keeping it free of saliva and other fluids.
- Do not try to restrain person; let seizure run its course.
- Protect person from injury, particularly the head.
- Do not put fingers or any other item between the person's teeth.

ACTIVITY
As tolerated

DIET
Regular

 ## MEDICATIONS

COMMONLY PRESCRIBED DRUGS
- Phenytoin (Dilantin)
- Phenobarbital
- Carbamazepine (Tegretol)
- Valproic acid (Depakene)
- Divalproex sodium
- Ethosuximide (Zarontin)
- Clonazepam (Klonopin)

CONTRAINDICATIONS
Read drug product information.

PRECAUTIONS
Read drug product information.

DRUG INTERACTIONS
Read drug product information.

OTHER DRUGS
- Felbamate (Felbatol)
- Gabapentin (Neurontin)
- Lamotrigine (Lamictal)
- Primidone (Mysoline)
- Tiagabine (Gabitril)
- Several additional drugs awaiting U.S. Food and Drug Administration approval

 ## FOLLOW-UP

PATIENT MONITORING
See the doctor regularly.

COMPLICATIONS
Drug toxicity

WHAT TO EXPECT
- The outcome depends on the individual circumstances.
- Seizure activity may become less frequent. If a patient has been seizure-free for 2 years, withdrawal of therapy may be considered. Relapse rate after 3 years of being off medications is 33%.

 ## MISCELLANEOUS

PREGNANCY
Antiseizure medication can cause birth defects.

FURTHER INFORMATION
Epilepsy Foundation of America, 4351 Garden City Drive, Landover, MD 20785, (800) EFA-1000

Seizure Disorders

Doctor
Office
Phone
Pager

Special notes to patient:

Seizures, Febrile

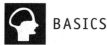 ## BASICS

DESCRIPTION

A febrile seizure is a seizure occurring with fever in infancy or childhood, without evidence of other underlying cause.

- Simple: single episode in 24 hours, lasting less than 15 minutes, accounts for 85% of febrile seizures.
- Complex: multiple episodes in 24 hours and lasting more than 15 minutes, accounts for 15% of febrile seizures.

SIGNS AND SYMPTOMS

- Fever usually 102.2°F (39°C) or greater
- Convulsions
  - Usually occur within hours of fever onset
  - The seizure is the initial sign of illness in 25% of cases.
  - Duration is less than 15 minutes with simple seizures; longer with complex episodes.
  - Average frequency is once in 24 hours with simple seizures; more with complex

CAUSES

- Fever may lower seizure threshold in susceptible children.
- Temperature usually greater than 102.2°F (39°C), but rate of change may be more important than temperature
- Viral illnesses
- Bacterial infections
- Mumps, measles, rubella immunization (MMR) within prior 7 to 10 days or diphtheria, pertussis, tetanus immunization (DPT) within prior 48 hours

SCOPE

Febrile seizures, which affect 2% to 5% of all children, comprise 30% of all childhood seizures.

MOST OFTEN AFFECTED

Of febrile seizures, 95% occur in children under 5 years of age; peak incidence is at 2 years of age; males affected slightly more frequently than females

RISK FACTORS

Febrile seizure in a sibling raises risk two- to threefold.

 ## DIAGNOSIS

WHAT THE DOCTOR LOOKS FOR

- The doctor will perform a physical examination to identify the cause of seizures.
- Seizures can be caused by many disorders.

TESTS AND PROCEDURES

- Blood tests
- Urinalysis
- Spinal fluids can be sampled by lumbar puncture (spinal tap).
- An electroencephalogram (EEG) can be done to evaluate brain function.
- Computed tomography (CT) scan of brain

 ## TREATMENT

GENERAL MEASURES

- Febrile seizures require emergency department treatment or extended observation based on health status, seizure type, and other factors.
- Supportive care
- Tepid sponge bath to lower temperature
- If seizure lasts less than 10 minutes, institute supportive measures such as laying individual on side, protecting from injury, and maintaining airway.

ACTIVITY

Bedrest during observation interval

DIET

Nothing by mouth

 ## MEDICATIONS

COMMONLY PRESCRIBED DRUGS

- Rectal or oral acetaminophen, ibuprofen
- Oxygen

CONTRAINDICATIONS

Allergy to drug

PRECAUTIONS

Read drug product information.

OTHER DRUGS

- Phenobarbital
- Phenytoin
- Valproic acid
- Paraldehyde

 ## FOLLOW-UP

PATIENT MONITORING

The doctor should see the patient as often as needed, based on the severity and origin of the fever.

PREVENTION

Acetaminophen, ibuprofen for rectal temperature greater than 100.5°F (38°C)

COMPLICATIONS

- Febrile seizures do not cause death, retardation, behavioral problems, or developmental delays.
- Children with febrile seizures are at greater than average risk to develop epilepsy later in life.

WHAT TO EXPECT

- About 30% develop recurrent febrile seizures; 50% if first episode occurs before 12 months of age and 45% if two siblings have had febrile seizures.
- Of recurrences, 95% occur within 1 year.
- Epilepsy occurs in 0.5% of the general population but in 3% to 4% of the population who have had febrile seizure.

 ## MISCELLANEOUS

PEDIATRIC

Range is 3 months to 5 years of age; peak incidence occurs at 2 years of age. Of febrile seizures, 95% occur in children 5 years of age or younger.

Seizures, Febrile

Doctor
Office
Phone
Pager

Special notes to patient:

Shingles

 ## BASICS

DESCRIPTION

Herpes zoster, also called "shingles," is a disease usually presenting as a painful eruption of skin blisters on one side of the body. It is caused by the reactivation of varicella zoster (chickenpox) virus that has been dormant in nerves.

SIGNS AND SYMPTOMS

- Prior to rash:
  - Tingling
  - Itching
  - Sharp or knifelike pain
- Acute phase:
  - Constitutional symptoms
  - Fatigue
  - Malaise
  - Headache
  - Low-grade fever
  - Skin rash
  - Weakness
  - Red bumps that evolve into groups of blisters
  - Vesicles weep pus, blood, or both in 3 to 4 days
  - Rash resolves in 14 to 21 days
- Chronic phase:
  - Persistent nerve pain
  - Weakness of specific nerves (e.g., facial nerves)

CAUSES

Reactivation of dormant varicella zoster (chicken pox) virus

SCOPE

Herpes zoster affects 10% to 20% of the population at some time.

MOST OFTEN AFFECTED

The incidence of herpes zoster increases with age. Of cases, 80% occur in persons above 20 years of age; males and females are affected equally.

RISK FACTORS

- Increasing age
- Immune system disorder
- Spinal surgery
- Spinal cord radiation

 ## DIAGNOSIS

WHAT THE DOCTOR LOOKS FOR

- The doctor will perform a physical examination to identify the signs of herpes zoster.
- Other conditions that can cause similar symptoms include skin disorders, gallbladder inflammation, and heart attack.

TESTS AND PROCEDURES

- Blood tests and other procedures are rarely necessary.
- Fluid from a blister can be sampled for laboratory analysis.
- A sample of affected skin can be obtained by biopsy to assist in the diagnosis.

GENERAL MEASURES

- Herpes zoster is managed in the outpatient setting, except for severe or complicated cases.
- Wet dressings applied for 30 to 60 minutes, four to six times per day
- Lotions (e.g., calamine)

ACTIVITY

No restrictions

DIET

No special diet

 ## MEDICATIONS

COMMONLY PRESCRIBED DRUGS

- Antiviral
  - Acyclovir (Zovirax)
  - Famciclovir
  - Valacyclovir
- Pain relievers
  - Acetaminophen
  - Codeine
  - Nonsteroidal antiinflammatory drugs (NSAIDs)
- Silver sulfadiazine (Silvadene)
- Tricyclic antidepressants
- Lidocaine
- Gabapentin
- Capsaicin cream
- Amitriptyline

CONTRAINDICATIONS

Read drug product information.

PRECAUTIONS

Read drug product information.

DRUG INTERACTIONS

Read drug product information.

OTHER DRUGS

- Vidarabine
- Idoxuridine in dimethyl sulfoxide (DMSO)

 ## FOLLOW-UP

PATIENT MONITORING

See the doctor as often as needed, based on symptoms.

PREVENTION

- None at present
- Individuals with shingles can transmit herpes zoster virus to susceptible persons.
- Chickenpox vaccine does not eliminate virus.

COMPLICATIONS

- Persistent pain
- Eye involvement
- Brain infection
- Severe skin infection
- Hepatitis
- Inflammation of lungs
- Other nerve disorders

WHAT TO EXPECT

- Resolution of rash within 14 to 21 days
- The incidence of persistent pain (at least 1 month after rash has healed) increases dramatically with age.

 ## MISCELLANEOUS

PEDIATRIC

Occurs rarely in children

GERIATRIC

- Increased incidence of herpes zoster
- Increased incidence of persistent pain

PREGNANCY

Can occur during pregnancy

Shingles

Doctor
Office
Phone
Pager

Special notes to patient:

Sinusitis

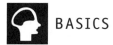 ## BASICS

DESCRIPTION

Sinusitis is an inflammation of the nasal sinuses. It can be acute (brief) or chronic (long-lasting), depending on duration of the infection. It occurs when pus accumulates in the sinus area.

SIGNS AND SYMPTOMS

- Nasal congestion
- Gradual buildup of a feeling of pressure in the sinus area, with tenderness
- Nasal discharge
- Malaise
- Sore throat (sometimes)
- Headache
- Fever
- Pain over cheeks and upper teeth, worse with bending
- Pain over eyebrows
- Pain over eyes
- Pain behind eyes
- Cough (occasional)
- Postnasal drip
- Swelling around eyes
- Symptoms aggravated by air travel

CAUSES

- Bacterial, viral, or fungal infections
- Precedes an upper respiratory infection
- Predisposing factors: chronic nasal swelling, thick mucus, nasal polyps, allergies, sudden temperature changes

SCOPE

Common

MOST OFTEN AFFECTED

All ages; males and females affected equally

RISK FACTORS

- Allergies
- Immune system suppression
- Continuous positive airway pressure
- Air travel during upper respiratory infection
- Tooth abscess
- Swimming in contaminated water

 ## DIAGNOSIS

WHAT THE DOCTOR LOOKS FOR

The doctor will perform a physical examination to identify sinusitis; numerous other conditions can cause similar signs and symptoms.

TESTS AND PROCEDURES

- Blood tests
- The sinus can be swabbed for laboratory analysis.
- The sinus can be examined by endoscopy.
- Tissue or fluid from the sinus can be obtained to assist in diagnosis.
- X-ray study and computed tomography (CT) scan can be used to assess the sinuses.

 ## TREATMENT

GENERAL MEASURES

- Steam inhalations can provide comfort and aid draining.
- Avoid smoke and other environmental pollutants if possible.
- Avoid smoking cigarettes.
- Surgery may be required.

ACTIVITY

No restrictions. May need additional rest during the acute phase.

DIET

No special diet. Drink plenty of fluids.

 ## MEDICATIONS

COMMONLY PRESCRIBED DRUGS

- Antibiotics: amoxicillin, trimethoprim-sulfamethoxazole
- Pain relievers
- Decongestants
- Antihistamines

CONTRAINDICATIONS

Read drug product information.

PRECAUTIONS

Read drug product information.

DRUG INTERACTIONS

Read drug product information.

OTHER DRUGS

Decongestant spray

 ## FOLLOW-UP

PATIENT MONITORING

See the doctor until symptoms completely resolve.

PREVENTION

Treat nasal congestion before sinusitis develops.

COMPLICATIONS

- Inflammation of the covering of the brain and spinal cord
- Abscess of brain or related structures
- Bone infection
- Infection around eye
- Unnecessary dental work because of confusion cause of pain

WHAT TO EXPECT

- Acute: favorable prognosis with timely treatment and avoidance of complications
- Chronic: may improve if cause is removed or drainage is feasible

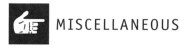 ## MISCELLANEOUS

GERIATRIC

- Incidence of sinusitis increases up to 75 years of age and then decreases.
- Sinusitis is more difficult to heal when it occurs among the elderly.

FURTHER INFORMATION

Asthma & Allergy Foundation of America, 1717 Massachusetts Ave., Suite 305, Washington, DC 20036, (800) 7-Asthma

Sinusitis

Doctor
Office
Phone
Pager

Special notes to patient:

Sleep Apnea, Obstructive

BASICS

DESCRIPTION

Sleep apnea consists of episodes of upper airway obstruction during sleep, often depriving the body of oxygen. It is nearly always associated with snoring. Periods of nonbreathing (apnea) often terminate with a snort or gasp. Repeated episodes of apnea disrupt sleep, leading to excessive daytime sleepiness. The usual course is chronic (long-lasting).

SIGNS AND SYMPTOMS

- Excessive daytime sleepiness
- Loud snoring
- Disrupted sleep
- Repeated awakenings with a transient feeling of shortness of breath
- Feeling tired and not refreshed on awakening in the morning
- Sleeping partner reports periods of stopped breathing
- Complaints of poor concentration, memory problems, irritability
- Morning headaches
- Short-temperedness
- Decreased libido (common)
- Depression
- High blood pressure

CAUSES

Upper airway narrowing can be caused by obesity, enlarged tonsils and uvula, low soft palate, excess tissue in soft palate, large tongue, skull or facial abnormalities, and abnormal control of upper airway muscle or breathing during sleep.

SCOPE

Obstructive sleep apnea affects 4% to 8% of the adult population in the United States.

MOST OFTEN AFFECTED

Middle-aged individuals; men more frequently than women

RISK FACTORS

- Obesity
- Nasal obstruction
- Hypothyroidism
- Large tongue
- Small jaw
- Acromegaly
- High blood pressure, cardiovascular disease, lung disease

DIAGNOSIS

WHAT THE DOCTOR LOOKS FOR

- The doctor will obtain a history and perform a physical examination to develop a diagnosis of obstructive sleep apnea.
- Other causes of excessive daytime sleepiness should be investigated, including narcolepsy, inadequate sleep, or depression.
- Other conditions that can be associated with sleep apnea should be assessed (e.g., asthma, heart failure, lung disease, panic attacks, seizures, or gastroesophageal reflux).

TESTS AND PROCEDURES

- Blood tests
- X-ray study of the head and neck
- Echocardiography
- Polysomnogram (nighttime sleep study)
- Magnetic resonance imaging (MRI), computed tomography (CT) scan, or fiberoptic evaluation of upper airway

TREATMENT

GENERAL MEASURES

- Obstructive sleep apnea is managed in the outpatient setting, except for surgery that involves hospitalization.
- If sleep apnea only occurs when sleeping on the back, then avoid sleeping on the back. Use a tennis ball sewn onto a nightshirt or wear a fanny-pack with tennis balls on the back while sleeping.
- Surgery may be required for mild to severe obstructive sleep apnea.
- Dental appliances may be of benefit.
- Continuous positive-airway pressure (CPAP) or biphasic positive-airway pressure (BiPAP) may be of benefit.
- Avoid driving if daytime sleepiness is significant.
- No alcohol within 6 hours of bedtime
- Avoid sedatives and sleeping pills.

ACTIVITY

Significantly sleepy patients should not drive motor vehicles or operate heavy equipment until treated.

DIET

Obese patients must lose weight. All patients must avoid weight gain and alcohol.

MEDICATIONS

COMMONLY PRESCRIBED DRUGS

- Protriptyline
- Fluoxetine (Prozac)

CONTRAINDICATIONS

None

PRECAUTIONS

Can cause or worsen narrow-angle glaucoma or urinary retention. Use cautiously with rapid heart rate conditions.

DRUG INTERACTIONS

Read drug product information.

OTHER DRUGS

- Medroxyprogesterone
- Acetazolamide (Diamox)

Sleep Apnea, Obstructive

Doctor
Office
Phone
Pager

Special notes to patient:

Sleep Apnea, Obstructive

 ## FOLLOW-UP

PATIENT MONITORING

See the doctor as often as needed for the management of snoring, excessive daytime sleepiness, or sleep disruption.

PREVENTION

- Excess weight is one of the most common causes of obstructive sleep apnea; in many cases, losing weight is the best cure.
- Avoid the use of alcohol, sedatives, or depressants.

COMPLICATIONS

- Untreated, obstructive sleep apnea is associated with high blood pressure, irregular heart rhythms, and heart failure.
- Excessive daytime sleepiness is a significant cause of death and injury.

WHAT TO EXPECT

- With appropriate control of apnea, excessive daytime sleepiness quickly improves dramatically.
- All therapy, other than surgery and weight loss in obese patients, involves methods of control, rather than cure. Lifelong compliance with weight loss or nasal CPAP is necessary.
- Untreated, obstructive sleep apnea will worsen.

 ## MISCELLANEOUS

PEDIATRIC

- Obstructive sleep apnea is not common in pediatric age group.
- If present, it is often caused by enlarged tonsils, craniofacial abnormalities, or diseases such as cerebral palsy or spinal muscular atrophy. Response to tonsil removal is often good.

GERIATRIC

Obstructive sleep apnea appears to increase in frequency after middle age and after menopause in women. It often coexists with other health problems in the elderly.

PREGNANCY

Rare

Sleep Apnea, Obstructive

Doctor
Office
Phone
Pager

Special notes to patient:

Snakebite

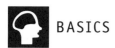 ## BASICS

DESCRIPTION

Two types of poisonous snakes are found in the United States: coral snakes and pit vipers, the latter of which includes rattlesnakes and water moccasins. Many other varieties of poisonous snakes are maintained as pets.

- Coral snakes have a characteristic rounded head with round pupils. Coloration is important. In the United States, poisonous coral snakes have broad rings of red and black that are separated by narrow rings of yellow. ("Red on yellow, kill a fellow; red on black, venom lack.") Coral snakes are found in Arizona, Texas, Arkansas, Louisiana, and southeastern United States.
- Rattlesnakes and water moccasins characteristically have triangular-shaped heads, eyes with elliptical pupils, and small, heat-sensing facial pits located between the nostril and the eye. They are most commonly found in southeastern and southwestern United States.

SIGNS AND SYMPTOMS

- Signs and symptoms vary by species.
- Fang marks: one or two punctures; may be shallow or appear as a scratch
- Pain out of proportion to size of puncture wound
- Swelling of site: swelling progresses up the extremity
- Weakness, dizziness
- Numbness or tingling in extremity, mouth, tongue
- Bruising of skin
- Rapid heart rate
- Double vision
- Nausea and vomiting
- Muscle twitching, spasms
- Mental status changes, including coma

CAUSES

- Contact with poisonous snake
- Coral snakes are nocturnal and timid; therefore, they rarely bite humans. They must be deliberately provoked to bite.

SCOPE

At least 8,000 snakebites occur annually in the United States; 20% to 25% of these bites do not result in envenomation (injection of venom).

MOST OFTEN AFFECTED

Individuals 19 to 30 years of age; males affected more often than females

RISK FACTORS

- Risk-taking behaviors
- Judgment impaired by alcohol or drug intoxication

 ## DIAGNOSIS

WHAT THE DOCTOR LOOKS FOR

The doctor will perform a physical examination to determine whether the wound is actually caused by a snakebite. The doctor will determine whether the snake was a venomous and identify the species of snake involved.

TESTS AND PROCEDURES

- Blood tests
- Urinalysis

 ## TREATMENT

GENERAL MEASURES

- True envenomations and resulting signs and symptoms demand immediate emergency department evaluation, with hospital admission, if necessary.
- Provide emergency first aid as needed, including rescue breathing and cardiopulmonary resuscitation (CPR).
- Provide reassurance to victim.
- Remove rings and constrictive items between site of envenomation and body.
- Place affected injured part at level of heart.
- Do NOT attempt to cut the snakebite wound and suck out the venom.

ACTIVITY

Bedrest with elevation of extremity. Physical therapy may be needed in severe cases of envenomation.

DIET

Nothing by mouth initially

 ## MEDICATIONS

COMMONLY PRESCRIBED DRUGS

- Antivenin is not available for all poisonous snakes.
- Polyvalent *Crotalidae* antivenin: pit vipers (rattlesnakes, water moccasins)
- *Micrurus fulvius* antivenin: North American coral snake

CONTRAINDICATIONS

History of allergy to horse serum

 ## FOLLOW-UP

PATIENT MONITORING

- See the doctor within 48 hours, then as needed.
- Physical therapy referral should be made early for optimal outcome.

PREVENTION

- Use preventive measures if handling snakes
- In snake-infested areas:
  - Wear protective shoes and clothing when walking
  - Do not insert hands or feet into cracks or crevices or hollow logs
  - Carry a flashlight if walking at night

COMPLICATIONS

- Serum sickness from antivenin therapy
- Local wound infection
- Pneumonia

WHAT TO EXPECT

- If properly treated, death is rare.
- Death can occur even with antivenin therapy.
- Deterioration can occur, despite antivenin treatment; complete paralysis can occur.
- Muscle strength may not return to normal for 4 to 6 weeks.
- Long-term illness is rare.

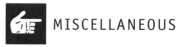 ## MISCELLANEOUS

PEDIATRIC

Course may be more severe.

GERIATRIC

Course may be more severe.

Snakebite

_____	Doctor
_____	Office
_____	Phone
_____	Pager

Special notes to patient:

Sore Throat

BASICS

DESCRIPTION
Sore throat, or pharyngitis, is an inflammation most commonly caused by acute infection.

SIGNS AND SYMPTOMS
- Sore throat
- Enlarged tonsils
- Enlarged lymph nodes in neck
- Absence of cough, hoarseness, or lower respiratory symptoms
- Fever above 102.5°F (39.1°C)
- Rash
- Loss of appetite
- Chills
- Malaise
- Headache
- Reddened eyes

CAUSES
- Bacterial or viral infection
- Chronic (long-lasting): noninfectious; chemical irritation; smoking; cancer

SCOPE
An estimated 30 million cases of sore throat are diagnosed yearly in the United States.

MOST OFTEN AFFECTED
Pharyngitis occurs in all age groups; males and females affected equally

RISK FACTORS
- Epidemics
- Age (young are more susceptible)
- Family history
- Close quarters (e.g., military barracks)
- Immune system disorders
- Fatigue
- Smoking
- Excess alcohol consumption
- Oral sex
- Diabetes mellitus
- Recent illness

DIAGNOSIS

WHAT THE DOCTOR LOOKS FOR
- The doctor will evaluate the status of the throat.
- The cause of sore throat should be identified and treated.

TESTS AND PROCEDURES
The throat can be swabbed for laboratory analysis.

TREATMENT

GENERAL MEASURES
- Salt-water gargles
- Acetaminophen
- Dyclonine lozenges
- Cool-mist humidifier

ACTIVITY
As tolerated

DIET
No restrictions. Extra fluids are encouraged.

MEDICATIONS

COMMONLY PRESCRIBED DRUGS
- Penicillin
- Erythromycin
- Cephalexin

CONTRAINDICATIONS
Allergy to specific antibiotic

PRECAUTIONS
Read drug product information.

DRUG INTERACTIONS
Read drug product information.

FOLLOW-UP

PATIENT MONITORING
Contact the doctor by telephone, as needed, while ill.

PREVENTION
Avoid contact with infected people.

COMPLICATIONS
- Rheumatic fever
- Kidney inflammation
- Abscess of tonsil
- Systemic infection
- Ear infection
- Rhinitis
- Sinusitis
- Pneumonia

WHAT TO EXPECT
- Sore throat often lasts 5 to 7 days; fever peaks at 2 to 3 days.
- Symptoms will resolve spontaneously without treatment, but complications are possible.
- Severe complications may require surgery.

Sore Throat

	Doctor
	Office
	Phone
	Pager

Special notes to patient:

Sprains and Strains

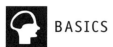 ## BASICS

DESCRIPTION
A sprain is an injury to a ligament. A strain is a partial or complete disruption of the muscle or tendon. Strains usually are associated with overuse injuries, whereas sprains usually result from trauma (falls, twisting injuries, or motor vehicle accidents).

SIGNS AND SYMPTOMS
- Swelling
- Pain
- Reddening or bruising
- Tenderness
- Gait disturbances, if severe
- Decreased range of motion of joint and joint instability

CAUSES
- Falls
- Motor vehicle accident
- Trauma
- Excessive exercise or inadequate warm-up and stretching before activity
- Poor conditioning

SCOPE
At one time or another, almost 80% of persons experience a sprain or strain.

MOST OFTEN AFFECTED
- Sprains: any age in which patient is physically active
- Strains: usually in individuals 15 to 40 years of age
- Males are affected more frequently than females.

RISK FACTORS
- Change in or improper shoe gear, protective gear, or environment (e.g., surface)
- Inappropriate increase in training schedule

 ## DIAGNOSIS

WHAT THE DOCTOR LOOKS FOR
- The doctor will perform a physical examination to assess for the presence of sprain or strain.
- Other musculoskeletal disorders should be ruled out, including fractures, tendonitis, bursitis, and other conditions (e.g., tendonitis, bursitis, bony injuries).
- Muscle hematomas account for some of the signs and symptoms of strains (rare).

TESTS AND PROCEDURES
- X-ray study
- Computed tomography (CT) scan or magnetic resonance imaging (MRI) can be done.
- The joint can be examined by arthroscopy in some cases.

 ## TREATMENT

GENERAL MEASURES
- **R**est, **I**ce, **C**ompression, **E**levation (RICE) therapy
- Elastic bandage wrap (Ace) increases comfort.
- Splint for pain relief and stability
- Crutches and gait training
- After initial treatment, rehabilitation may be recommended.

ACTIVITY
- Bedrest for acute injuries
- Physical therapy for more severe injuries
- Elevate joint while sleeping.

DIET
Weight loss, if obese

 ## MEDICATIONS

COMMONLY PRESCRIBED DRUGS
- Nonsteroidal antiinflammatory drugs (NSAIDs)
- Narcotics for severe pain

CONTRAINDICATIONS
Read drug product information.

PRECAUTIONS
Read drug product information.

DRUG INTERACTIONS
Read drug product information.

OTHER DRUGS
- Pain relievers
- Analgesic balms
- Capsaicin cream

 ## FOLLOW-UP

PATIENT MONITORING
See the doctor as often as necessary.

PREVENTION
- Maintain a reasonable level of physical fitness.
- Avoid excessive physical stresses.
- Wear exercise gear (particularly shoes).
- Use proper equipment for the activity.
- Know the risks associated with the intended activity.
- Appropriate conditioning and warm-up and cool-down exercises

COMPLICATIONS
- Chronic joint instability
- Arthritis

WHAT TO EXPECT
With appropriate treatment and rest, recovery takes 6 to 8 weeks or longer, depending on injury severity.

 ## MISCELLANEOUS

GERIATRIC
More likely to see associated bone injuries because of decreased joint flexibility and prevalence of osteoporosis

Sprains and Strains

Doctor
Office
Phone
Pager

Special notes to patient:

Stroke (Brain Attack)

BASICS

DESCRIPTION

Stroke, or cerebrovascular accident (CVA), is the sudden onset of a neurologic deficit caused by a loss of blood circulation to a portion of the brain, either by blood clot (infarction) or bleeding (hemorrhage). Stroke rehabilitation involves restoration of function after both medical and neurologic stability have been achieved.

SIGNS AND SYMPTOMS

- The signs and symptoms of stroke vary, depending on the part of the brain affected.
- Paralysis or loss of sensation on one side of the body
- Visual disturbances
- Paralysis of the facial muscles on one side
- Dizziness, difficulty walking or moving
- Difficulty speaking, understanding language
- Altered level of consciousness
- Sudden headache, nausea, vomiting, and incoordination

CAUSES

- Coronary artery disease
- High blood pressure
- Blockage of arteries in brain
- Formation of clots within the heart or blood vessels
- Foreign body in bloodstream
- Frequently, the combination of gout, diabetes, and hypertension that has been untreated for 5 to 10 years can contribute to the onset of a stroke.
- Blood vessel disorders
- Blood-clotting disorders
- Other causes: trauma, drug use, other diseases

SCOPE

About 160 cases of stroke per 100,000 persons occur in the United States annually.

MOST OFTEN AFFECTED

The risk of stroke increases in people above 45 years of age and is highest in individuals 60 to 80 years of age; more common in males than females

RISK FACTORS

Among the risk factors, many are lifestyle-oriented and preventable (e.g., coffee consumption, obesity, inactivity, hyperactivity to the point of exhaustion, mood swings, sexual hyperactivity, starvation, antidepressant or diet reduction medication, alcohol or recreational drug habituation, and unusual stress states). Risk factors include the following:

- Increasing age
- High blood pressure
- Heart disease
- Smoking
- Diabetes
- Family history

DIAGNOSIS

WHAT THE DOCTOR LOOKS FOR

- The doctor will perform a physical examination to determine the severity and extent of damage caused by stroke.
- Conditions that can appear similar to stroke include epilepsy, migraine headache, tumor, diabetes, infection, and trauma.
- The doctor should also identify and treat conditions known to be associated with stroke (e.g., heart disease, high blood pressure, bleeding disorders, and other diseases).
- Different types of stroke disorders can occur in one person.

TESTS AND PROCEDURES

- Blood tests
- Urinalysis
- The carotid arteries can be evaluated by ultrasound.
- Cerebral angiography
- An electrocardiogram (ECG) and echocardiogram can be done.
- Computed tomography (CT), magnetic resonance imaging (MRI), and positron emission tomography (PET) can be done to assist in diagnosis.
- A sample of spinal fluid can be obtained by lumbar puncture (spinal tap).
- Special sensory and neurologic tests can be done to assess recovery.

TREATMENT

GENERAL MEASURES

- Immediately after stroke:
  - Provide emergency first aid as needed, including rescue breathing and cardiopulmonary resuscitation (CPR)
  - Call 911
  - Seek medical attention as soon as possible
- In many cases, thrombolytic (clot-busting) therapy may restore circulation, if given promptly after stroke.
- During the acute phase, management of stroke requires hospitalization.
- Recovery of stroke may require care at a rehabilitation center or special care facility; or, stroke may be managed on an outpatient basis.
- A full-service rehabilitation center and rehabilitation medicine team can have an effect on the patient's independence and dependency
- Full-service rehabilitation center characteristics include closed units; regular team meetings to discuss long- and short-term objectives; quality assurance system in place; accreditation by Commission on Accreditation of Rehabilitation Facilities.
- Surgery may be recommended.

ACTIVITY

- Walking as soon as possible
- Physical therapy, occupational therapy, speech pathology, psychology, and nursing therapy should be provided for at least 3 hours/day during hospitalization.
- Whereas most rehabilitative efforts take place within a very short time after stroke, successful rehabilitative efforts have taken as long as 5 years.

DIET

- Depends on other medical conditions
- Diet as tolerated (no added salt if hypertensive)

MEDICATIONS

COMMONLY PRESCRIBED DRUGS

- Thrombolytics (clot-bursting drugs)
- Enteric-coated aspirin (EC ASA)
- Ticlopidine (Ticlid)
- Clopidogrel (Plavix)

CONTRAINDICATIONS

- EC ASA: peptic ulcer disease, allergy to aspirin or other nonsteroidal antiinflammatory drugs (NSAIDs)
- Ticlopidine: known hypersensitivity to the drug, blood disorders, severe liver failure

PRECAUTIONS

EC ASA therapy can aggravate peptic ulcer disease, and can worsen asthma.

DRUG INTERACTIONS

Read drug product information.

OTHER DRUGS

Nimodipine, nicardipine, dipyridamole

Stroke (Brain Attack)

Doctor
Office
Phone
Pager

Special notes to patient:

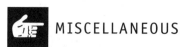
Stroke (Brain Attack)

FOLLOW-UP

PATIENT MONITORING
See the doctor 1 month after stroke, every 3 months for first year, then annually.

PREVENTION
Stroke is usually an unnecessary illness; major risk factors are nearly all preventable.
- Stop smoking.
- Control blood pressure, diabetes, and dietary fats.
- Daily aspirin to reduce clots (only with doctor's permission)
- Use alcohol in moderation, if at all.
- Regular exercise
- Maintain positive psychological outlook.
- Maintain weight control.
- The progressive physical and mental deterioration noted with high blood pressure and heart disease is not inevitable.
- Family support may help the patient to become interested in his or her health and may assist the patient in maintaining health
- Disuse will add subsequent complications and long-term effects.
- Surgery (endarterectomy) may prevent stroke.

COMPLICATIONS
- Muscle and joint disorders
- Depression

WHAT TO EXPECT
- The outcome varies depending on severity and location of stroke.
- Overall, the outcome is generally good, although pneumonia, respiratory failure, heart failure, and heart attack occur more frequently after stroke.

MISCELLANEOUS

PREGNANCY
Hypertension in pregnancy can lead to stroke.

FURTHER INFORMATION
National Stroke Association, 300 East Hampden Ave., Suite 240, Englewood, CO, 80110-2622

Stroke (Brain Attack)

Doctor
Office
Phone
Pager

Special notes to patient:

Stye

 ## BASICS

DESCRIPTION
A stye, or hordeolum, is an inflammation or infection of the eyelid margin, often involving the hair follicles of the eyelashes.

SIGNS AND SYMPTOMS
- Redness of the edge of the eyelid with peeling and weeping
- Inflammation of the eyelashes
- Itching or peeling of the eyelids, chronic redness, eye irritation leading to tenderness and pain

CAUSES
- The most common cause of stye is a staphylococcal infection, although other organisms may also be involved.
- Seborrhea can predispose to eyelid infections.

SCOPE
Extremely common

MOST OFTEN AFFECTED
Stye can affect all age groups; males and females with equal frequency

RISK FACTORS
- Predisposing eyelid infection
- Poor eyelid hygiene
- Contact lens wear
- Application of make-up may "clog pores" and predispose to a stye

 ## DIAGNOSIS

WHAT THE DOCTOR LOOKS FOR
The doctor will perform a physical examination to identify the presence of a stye.

 ## TREATMENT

GENERAL MEASURES
- Warm compresses to the area of inflammation can help increase blood supply and promote healing.
- Clean the eyelids using a solution of tap water and baby shampoo or a commercially prepared hypoallergenic cleanser.
- The stye should not be squeezed.
- Good personal hygiene should be maintained, with attention to cleansing the eyelids on a daily basis to prevent recurrent infections.
- Apply an antibiotic ointment (e.g., erythromycin) to the margin of the eyelid after proper cleansing (except children under 12 years of age or in cases wherein is seen a risk of vision problems). The antibiotic helps reduce bacterial growth.
- Minor surgery may be required to drain infection.

ACTIVITY
No restrictions

DIET
No special diet

MEDICATIONS

COMMONLY PRESCRIBED DRUGS
- Erythromycin ophthalmic ointment
- Aminoglycoside ophthalmic ointment (gentamicin)

CONTRAINDICATIONS
None

PRECAUTIONS
None

DRUG INTERACTIONS
None

OTHER DRUGS
None

 ## FOLLOW-UP

PATIENT MONITORING
See the doctor within several weeks to assess the effectiveness of therapy.

PREVENTION
Eyelid hygiene

COMPLICATIONS
None expected.

WHAT TO EXPECT
Styes usually resolve with treatment but tend to recur in some patients.

Stye

Doctor
Office
Phone
Pager

Special notes to patient:

Sudden Infant Death Syndrome (SIDS)

BASICS

DESCRIPTION

Sudden infant death syndrome is defined as the sudden death of an infant under 1 year of age that remains unexplained after a thorough case investigation, including a complete autopsy, examination of the death scene, and review of the clinical history.

- Apparent life-threatening event (ALTE) (e.g., apnea that sometimes but not always precedes SIDS) is a related entity.

SIGNS AND SYMPTOMS

Infants dying from SIDS generally appeared healthy or may have had a minor upper respiratory or gastrointestinal infection in the last 2 weeks of life.

CAUSES

- Many theories abound about the cause of SIDS. Subtle developmental abnormalities may have resulted from brain injury.
- Possible causes:
  - Abnormal respiratory control
  - Upper airway obstruction
  - Nervous system abnormalities
  - Irregular heart rhythms
  - Carbon dioxide rebreathing in face-down position on soft surface
  - SIDS may occur when a combination of factors coincide; such triggers may include infectious agents, climatic changes, or environmental factors.

SCOPE

About 4,700 cases of SIDS are reported annually in the United States.

MOST OFTEN AFFECTED

SIDS is rare in the first month of life. Peak incidence occurs in infants between 2 and 4 months of age; 90% of deaths occur by 6 months of age; more common in males than females

RISK FACTORS

- Most SIDS deaths occur in children who are "low-risk." However, several risk factors are associated with SIDS:
  - Race: Native-Americans and African-Americans have highest incidence.
  - Season: late fall and winter months
  - Time of day: between midnight and 6 AM
  - Activity: during sleep
  - Low birthweight
  - Poverty

- Maternal factors:
  - Teenage mothers
  - Maternal use of cigarettes or drugs (cocaine, opiates) during pregnancy
  - Large number of children; maternal anemia during pregnancy
- Respiratory or gastrointestinal infection in recent past
- Sleep practices:
  - Prone sleep position
  - Heavier clothing and bedding, soft bedding
- Lack of breast-feeding
- Passive cigarette smoke exposure after birth

DIAGNOSIS

WHAT THE DOCTOR LOOKS FOR

The doctor will perform a physical examination to rule out an identifiable cause of distress or death, including suffocation, metabolic disorders, child abuse, homicide, or other conditions.

TESTS AND PROCEDURES

- For apparent life-threatening events:
  - Arterial blood can be drawn for laboratory analysis.
  - X-ray study
  - An electrocardiogram (ECG) can be done.
  - A electroencephalogram (EEG) can be done to monitor brain activity.
  - Other tests can be done to assist in diagnosis.

TREATMENT

GENERAL MEASURES

- Because a death from SIDS is sudden and the cause is unknown, no way exits to "treat" SIDS. However, some measures may be effective in preventing SIDS:
  - Maternal avoidance of cigarette and illicit drug use during pregnancy
  - Breast-feeding
  - Avoid letting the baby sleep on the stomach.
  - Avoid excessive bed clothing and soft bedding.
  - Avoid passive cigarette smoke exposure.
- Recent studies suggest significant risk reduction when baby is placed on the back or side for sleep. Because infants placed on their side can turn over during sleep onto their stomach, it is now believed that back position is best.

FOLLOW-UP

PATIENT MONITORING

Some authorities recommend monitoring of siblings of prior SIDS victims.

PREVENTION

See *General Measures*

WHAT TO EXPECT

- SIDS deaths have a powerful impact on families and their functioning. Healthcare providers can play an important role in providing immediate information about SIDS and sensitive counseling to limit parents' misinformation and feelings of guilt.
- Counseling needs of families vary from short-term to long-term; support groups are helpful to many couples. Providers should be familiar with resources available in their communities to help families mourning a SIDS death. Parents need to be counseled about subsequent pregnancies.
- Follow-up counseling, including a review of the autopsy report with the family after some time has passed, is important to help with understanding this condition and to clear the tremendous guilt these families experience.

MISCELLANEOUS

PEDIATRIC

Occurs in infants only

FURTHER INFORMATION

- American Sudden Infant Death Syndrome Institute, Atlanta, GA, (800) 232-SIDS
- National SIDS Alliance/National SIDS Foundation, Columbia, MD, (800) 221-SIDS
- Back to Sleep Information Line, (800) 505-CRIB (sponsored by the U.S. Public Health Service)
- National SIDS Resource Center, (703) 821-8955, ext. 249

Sudden Infant Death Syndrome (SIDS)

Doctor
Office
Phone
Pager

Special notes to patient:

Sunburn

BASICS

DESCRIPTION
A sunburn is an acute reaction to the toxic effects of ultraviolet (UV) in sunlight.

SIGNS AND SYMPTOMS
- Mild reddening with subsequent peeling
- Pain
- Swelling
- Skin tenderness
- Blisters
- Fever, chills, weakness
- Shock
- Secondary infections

CAUSES
- Exposure to sunlight (or other UV light source) following administration of photosensitivity-producing drugs.
- Overexposure to UV rays; danger increases proportionately with higher altitudes

SCOPE
Common

MOST OFTEN AFFECTED
All ages

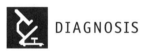 DIAGNOSIS

TESTS AND PROCEDURES
None required

TREATMENT

GENERAL MEASURES
- Avoid additional exposure until well.
- Use tap-water compresses.
- Avoid topical anesthetic lotions and ointments.

MEDICATIONS

COMMONLY PRESCRIBED DRUGS
Prednisone

CONTRAINDICATIONS
Read drug product information.

PRECAUTIONS
Read drug product information.

DRUG INTERACTIONS
Read drug product information.

FOLLOW-UP

PREVENTION
- Prevention with sunscreens rated SPF (sun protection factor) 15 or higher
- Avoid sun exposure during "peak tanning hours," approximately 11:00 AM to 2:00 PM.

COMPLICATIONS
Usually none

WHAT TO EXPECT
- Long-term risks include:
  - Melanoma and other skin cancers
  - Skin aging

MISCELLANEOUS

PEDIATRIC
Children at high risk

Sunburn

Doctor
Office
Phone
Pager

Special notes to patient:

Swimmer's Ear

 ## BASICS

DESCRIPTION
Otitis externa, called "swimmer's ear," is an inflammation of the external ear canal. It can be caused by infection with bacteria or fungus.

SIGNS AND SYMPTOMS
- Itching
- Plugging of the ear
- Pain
- Reddening
- Discharge of pus
- Eczema of ear

CAUSES
- Trauma
- Infection (bacterial, fungal)
- Skin disorders (e.g. eczema, seborrhea)

SCOPE
Unknown; incidence is higher in the summer months

MOST OFTEN AFFECTED
All ages; males and females affected equally

RISK FACTORS
- Trauma of external ear canal
- Swimming
- Hot, humid weather
- Use of a hearing aid
- Advancing age
- Diabetes
- Debilitating disease

 ## DIAGNOSIS

WHAT THE DOCTOR LOOKS FOR
The doctor will evaluate the ear and identify the cause of inflammation.

TESTS AND PROCEDURES
- Fluid from the ear can be sampled for laboratory analysis.
- X-ray study of the head (rarely)

 ## TREATMENT

GENERAL MEASURES
- Otitis externa is managed in the outpatient setting, except for severe cases that require hospitalization.
- The external ear canal should be thoroughly cleaned.
- Pain relievers
- Antiitch and antihistamine medication

ACTIVITY
No restrictions

DIET
No restrictions

MEDICATIONS

COMMONLY PRESCRIBED DRUGS
- Topical therapy for approximately 10 days
- Pain relievers
- Acetic acid (2%)
- Antibiotics, antifungal medications

CONTRAINDICATIONS
Allergies to prescribed drugs; read drug product information.

PRECAUTIONS
Read drug product information.

DRUG INTERACTIONS
Read drug product information.

 ## FOLLOW-UP

PATIENT MONITORING
- See the doctor 48 hours after treatment begins to assess improvement and at the end of therapy.
- For chronic otitis externa, see the doctor every 2 to 3 weeks for repeated cleansing of ear canal.

PREVENTION
- Avoid prolonged exposure to moisture.
- Use preventive antiseptics.
- Treat skin conditions.
- Eliminate trauma to canal.
- Diagnose and treat underlying medical conditions.

COMPLICATIONS
Inflammation may spread.

WHAT TO EXPECT
- Acute otitis externa rapidly responds to therapy with total resolution.
- In the case of chronic otitis externa, most cases resolve with repeated cleansing and antibiotic therapy. Occasionally, surgery is required.

Swimmer's Ear

Doctor
Office
Phone
Pager

Special notes to patient:

Syphilis

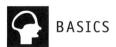 ## BASICS

DESCRIPTION
Syphilis is a sexually transmitted disease that is characterized by sequential stages. After the initial period of symptoms, the disease can remain latent, flaring up years later. Syphilis can also occur congenitally, passed from mother to baby during pregnancy.

SIGNS AND SYMPTOMS
- A chancre or lesion usually found on genitalia, which heals in 3 to 6 weeks; 75% have no further symptoms.
- Latent phase may be marked by rash, frequently on palms and soles; bald patches on scalp, eyebrows, and beard; moist lesions on genital area; generalized flulike symptoms of aches and malaise; may be accompanied by more severe symptoms
- Tertiary syphilis: symptoms involving cardiovascular and bone disease, dementia, and other severe symptoms

CAUSES
- Exposure through sexual contact
- Exposure to infected body fluids
- Congenital (passed to fetus during pregnancy)

SCOPE
About 20 cases of syphilis per 100,000 persons are reported annually in the United States. In some groups, the rate is six times higher; reported cases are rising rapidly.

MOST OFTEN AFFECTED
Sexually active individuals; males affected more frequently than females

RISK FACTORS
- Multiple sexual partners
- Intravenous (IV) drug use
- Male homosexuality
- Infants can be exposed through the birth canal.
- Exposure to infected body fluids

 ## DIAGNOSIS

WHAT THE DOCTOR LOOKS FOR
The doctor will perform a physical examination to identify the presence of syphilis.

TESTS AND PROCEDURES
- Blood tests
- A sample of spinal fluids can be obtained by lumbar puncture (spinal tap).
- A sample of skin can be obtained by biopsy for laboratory analysis.

 ## TREATMENT

GENERAL MEASURES
- Syphilis is usually managed in the outpatient setting.
- All sexual contacts must be traced and treated.
- Keep follow-up appointments to monitor success of therapy.
- Avoid intercourse until treatment is complete.
- Local health department can provide literature and contact tracing.

ACTIVITY
Full activity, but no sexual contacts until cured

DIET
No special diet

 ## MEDICATIONS

COMMONLY PRESCRIBED DRUGS
Penicillin

CONTRAINDICATIONS
Allergy to penicillin

PRECAUTIONS
Read drug product information.

DRUG INTERACTIONS
None

OTHER DRUGS
- Erythromycin
- Tetracycline
- Ceftriaxone (Rocephin)

 ## FOLLOW-UP

PATIENT MONITORING
Blood tests should be repeated for 3 months, then annually. Blood tests may done be more frequently for individuals also infected with the human immunodeficiency virus (HIV).

PREVENTION
- Safe sex practices
- Mutually monogamous relationship
- Use of condoms

COMPLICATIONS
- Cardiovascular disease
- Central nervous system disease
- Kidney disease
- Irreversible organ damage
- Many other disorders

WHAT TO EXPECT
The prognosis is excellent in all cases, except late syphilis complications and a few HIV-infected patients.

 ## MISCELLANEOUS

PEDIATRIC
Must consider possible child abuse

PREGNANCY
Early detection is imperative; all expectant mothers should have testing as part of routine prenatal care.

Syphilis

Doctor
Office
Phone
Pager

Special notes to patient:

Systemic Lupus Erythematosus (SLE)

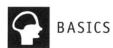

BASICS

DESCRIPTION

Systemic lupus erythematosus (SLE), an autoimmune disorder involving the inflammation of many body systems, is characterized by a fluctuating, chronic course. SLE varies from mild to severe and can be lethal.

SIGNS AND SYMPTOMS

- Arthritis
- Fever
- Loss of appetite
- Malaise
- Weight loss
- Skin lesions
- Mouth ulcers
- Eye pain, redness
- Chest pain, shortness of breath
- Pallor
- Nausea, vomiting, diarrhea
- Muscle tenderness, aching, stiffness
- Headaches, visual problems
- Psychosis, delirium

CAUSES

- Most cases have unknown causes.
- Drugs

SCOPE

SLE affects about 20 of 100,000 persons annually in the United States.

MOST OFTEN AFFECTED

All ages; most common in individuals 30 to 50 years of age; females affected about 10 times more often than males

RISK FACTORS

- Race: African-Americans, Hispanics, Asians, and Native-Americans have a higher prevalence than whites.
- Genetic factors

DIAGNOSIS

WHAT THE DOCTOR LOOKS FOR

- The doctor will perform a physical examination to identify the signs and symptoms of SLE.
- Many other disorders mimic SLE (e.g., rheumatoid arthritis, connective tissue diseases, scleroderma, cancer, fever, and many skin rashes).

TESTS AND PROCEDURES

- Blood tests
- Urinalysis
- Chest x-ray study
- Echocardiography
- Samples of skin, kidney, or nerves can be obtained by biopsy for laboratory analysis.
- Blood vessels of the brain can be examined by a radiologic procedure called "cerebral angiography."
- Magnetic resonance imaging (MRI) can be done to assist with diagnosis.

TREATMENT

GENERAL MEASURES

- Protect skin from ultraviolet light by using sunscreens, hats, and so forth.
- Early intervention, when infections occur
- Conserve energy.
- Stress avoidance or management

ACTIVITY

- As active as possible
- Individuals with arthritis may be limited by their pain, but active exercises are encouraged.

DIET

No special diet, unless complications (e.g., kidney failure) are present

MEDICATIONS

COMMONLY PRESCRIBED DRUGS

- No one drug of choice available. Treatment is aimed at symptom relief.
- Immunosuppressants
- Nonsteroidal antiinflammatory drugs (NSAIDs)
- Hydroxychloroquine
- Prednisone
- Cyclophosphamide
- Methotrexate
- Immune globulin, intravenous (IVIG)

CONTRAINDICATIONS

Read drug product information.

PRECAUTIONS

Read drug product information.

DRUG INTERACTIONS

Read drug product information.

FOLLOW-UP

PATIENT MONITORING

- Individuals with acute flares should see the doctor frequently (weekly to monthly) for medication adjustment.
- In the absence of acute attack, see the doctor as often as necessary.

PREVENTION

- Avoiding sun exposure is only necessary for approximately one sixth of SLE patients (those who self-report such sensitivity).
- Routine vaccinations are safe and appropriate for patients with SLE.
- Drugs known to induce SLE in normal individuals are not necessarily contraindicated in patients who have idiopathic SLE.

Systemic Lupus Erythematosus (SLE)

Doctor
Office
Phone
Pager

Special notes to patient:

Systemic Lupus Erythematosus (SLE)

COMPLICATIONS

Fever, inflammation of blood vessels, muscle disorders, bone disorders, lung disease, heart disease, nerve disorders, blood-clotting disorders, and numerous other conditions.

WHAT TO EXPECT

- Most patients with SLE follow a course of remissions and acute episodes. Many experience spontaneous permanent remission.
- Treatment of kidney lupus (the most serious form) has increased the 5-year life expectancy to more than 90%. For patients surviving the first 2 years of disease, life expectancy is essentially normal.
- In patients with drug-induced SLE, symptoms should gradually decrease when the suspected agent is discontinued.

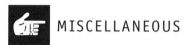 MISCELLANEOUS

GERIATRIC

Higher percentage of males affected by SLE among the elderly

PREGNANCY

- Onset of SLE and flares are more common during pregnancy.
- Fetal loss is increased for mothers with SLE.
- Newborns of mothers who have SLE are more likely to have irregular heart rhythms.
- Consultation with a specialist during pregnancy is recommended.

FURTHER INFORMATION

- Arthritis Foundation, 1314 Spring St. N.W., Atlanta, GA 30309, (404) 872-7100
- Lupus Foundation of America, 1717 Massachusetts Ave., NW, Suite 203, Washington, DC 20036, (800) 558-0121

Systemic Lupus Erythematosus (SLE)

Doctor
Office
Phone
Pager

Special notes to patient:

Temporomandibular Joint (TMJ) Syndrome

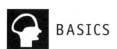
BASICS

DESCRIPTION
Temporomandibular joint (TMJ) syndrome is characterized by pain and tenderness in the jaw muscles and sound, pain, or both over the joint, with limitation of jaw movement.

SIGNS AND SYMPTOMS
- Facial pain
- Pain of the TMJ (in the jaw)
- Locking or catching of the jaw
- Jaw clicking, grinding, popping
- Headache
- Earache
- Neck pain

CAUSES
- TMJ disorders
- Grinding of the teeth
- Chewing muscle spasm
- Trauma
- Poorly fitting dentures

SCOPE
Up to half the population in the United States has symptoms or signs of TMJ syndrome, but only 5% to 25% seek treatment.

MOST OFTEN AFFECTED
More common among individuals 30 to 50 years of age; more common in females than males

RISK FACTORS
- Chronic habits, such as clenching or grinding of the teeth
- Osteoarthritis, rheumatoid arthritis
- Dental problems
- Psychosocial stress

DIAGNOSIS

WHAT THE DOCTOR LOOKS FOR
- The doctor will perform a physical examination to identify TMJ syndrome.
- Other conditions that can cause similar signs and symptoms should be investigated (e.g., fracture or dislocation, nerve disorders, dental disorders, or cancer).

TESTS AND PROCEDURES
- Tests can be done to assess jaw function.
- X-ray study, magnetic resonance imaging (MRI), and other radiology procedures can be done to assist in the diagnosis.
- The jaw can be examined by arthroscopy.

TREATMENT

GENERAL MEASURES
- Jaw rest
- Local heat therapy
- Antiinflammatory medications
- Muscle relaxants
- Pain relievers
- Correction of dental problems
- Stress reduction
- Behavior modification to eliminate oral habits that may contribute to TMJ syndrome

ACTIVITY
Jaw rest

DIET
Soft diet to reduce chewing

MEDICATIONS

COMMONLY PRESCRIBED DRUGS
- Nonsteroidal antiinflammatory drugs (NSAIDs).
- No single drug is more effective than another.

CONTRAINDICATIONS
- History of severe allergy to aspirin
- Peptic ulcer disease
- Renal insufficiency

PRECAUTIONS
- Peptic ulcers, gastritis, or gastrointestinal bleeding can occur with chronic use of NSAIDs.
- Kidney disorders

DRUG INTERACTIONS
Numerous interactions; read drug product information.

OTHER DRUGS
- Analgesic agents
- Muscle relaxants

FOLLOW-UP

PATIENT MONITORING
See the doctor as often as needed to assess the level of discomfort and the effect of therapy.

PREVENTION
- Be aware of any teeth-clenching or grinding habits, and relax the jaw by disengaging the teeth.
- Avoid wide, uncontrolled opening of the mouth (e.g., yawning).
- Stress management; behavioral modification counseling may be helpful

COMPLICATIONS
- Degenerative joint disease
- Chronic TMJ dislocation
- Loss of joint range of motion
- Depression and chronic pain syndromes

WHAT TO EXPECT
- With conservative therapy, symptoms resolve within 3 months in 75% of the cases.
- The most benefit is received from a comprehensive treatment approach, including correction of dental problems, restoration of normal muscle function, pain control, stress management, and behavior modification.

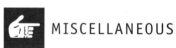

PREGNANCY
No association

Temporomandibular Joint (TMJ) Syndrome

	Doctor
	Office
	Phone
	Pager

Special notes to patient:

Tendinitis

 ## BASICS

DESCRIPTION
Tendinitis is an inflammation of a tendon—a fibrous cord that connects muscle to bone—that can affect adjacent areas.

SIGNS AND SYMPTOMS
- Pain over the point of inflammation. Tendinitis is usually worsened by active motion, but can present at rest.
- Tenderness over the affected tendon
- Mild reddening and increased heat of overlying skin

CAUSES
Usually related to repetitive activity or trauma, but can be without obvious cause

SCOPE
Common

MOST OFTEN AFFECTED
All ages; males affected slightly more frequently than females

RISK FACTORS
Professional athletes and manual laborers are especially susceptible to tendinitis because of repetitive use of a particular joint.

 ## DIAGNOSIS

WHAT THE DOCTOR LOOKS FOR
- The doctor will perform a physical examination to identify the presence and severity of tendinitis.
- Other conditions can cause symptoms similar to tendinitis (e.g., tendon injury, bursitis, arthritis, or infection).

TESTS AND PROCEDURES
Ultrasound, computed tomography (CT) scan, and magnetic resonance imaging (MRI) can be done to assist with diagnosis.

 ## TREATMENT

GENERAL MEASURES
Treatment goals are to relieve pain, reduce inflammation, and rest the joint.

ACTIVITY
- In acute phases, the involved muscle and tendon should be rested. Use slings and splints for the upper extremity. Use braces, canes, or crutches for the lower limbs.
- Physical therapy, once patient is free of pain

DIET
No special diet

 ## MEDICATIONS

COMMONLY PRESCRIBED DRUGS
- Nonsteroidal antiinflammatory drugs (NSAIDs)
- Corticosteroids: injected

CONTRAINDICATIONS
Read drug product information.

PRECAUTIONS
Read drug product information.

DRUG INTERACTIONS
Read drug product information.

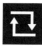 ## FOLLOW-UP

PATIENT MONITORING
Symptoms will usually subside within a few days after treatment.

PREVENTION
After adequate rest and treatment, it is important to prevent recurrences. Circular bands for forearm extension tendinitis or knee tendinitis may be useful.

COMPLICATIONS
- Tendon rupture, fractures
- Repeated bouts of pain

WHAT TO EXPECT
Most cases subside without complications.

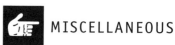

PEDIATRIC
Osgood-Schlatter disease is seen in adolescents, especially during a growth spurt.

Tendinitis

Doctor
Office
Phone
Pager

Special notes to patient:

Tinea

BASICS

DESCRIPTION
Tinea is a fungal infection of the skin. It can cause bright red, sharply defined rings of dry skin on the face, trunk, or extremities (ringworm). It can affect the head (tinea capitis), the groin (tinea cruris, or jock itch), or the feet (tinea pedis, or athlete's foot).

SIGNS AND SYMPTOMS
- Rash
- Itching
- Bright red, sharply defined circular areas of dry skin
- Patient may experience intense itching
- May affect groin (jock itch)
- May affect area between toes (athlete's foot)
- Changes in skin pigmentation

CAUSES
Fungal infection

SCOPE
Fairly common

MOST OFTEN AFFECTED
All ages; males and females affected equally

RISK FACTORS
- Warm climates
- Daycare centers or schools
- Institutionalization
- Poor hygiene
- Wearing wet clothing or socks
- Obesity
- Direct contact with an active lesion on a human, an animal, or from soil (rarely)
- Working with animals
- Immune system suppression

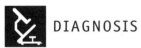
DIAGNOSIS

WHAT THE DOCTOR LOOKS FOR
The doctor will perform a physical examination to identify the presence of tinea.

TESTS AND PROCEDURES
The affected area can be swabbed for laboratory analysis.

TREATMENT

GENERAL MEASURES
- Proper hygiene
- Careful handwashing
- Launder towel, clothing, and head wear of infected individual.
- Check other family members.
- Topical medications

ACTIVITY
Avoid contact sports (e.g., wrestling) for 2 days after starting treatment

DIET
Unrestricted diet

MEDICATIONS

COMMONLY PRESCRIBED DRUGS
- Miconazole (Monistat-Derm, Micatin)
- Clotrimazole (Lotrimin, Mycelex)
- Ketoconazole (Nizoral, Nizoral shampoo)
- Econazole (Spectazole)
- Naftifine (Naftin, Lamisil)
- Griseofulvin (Gris-PEG)
- Itraconazole, itraconazole (Sporanox)
- Ciclopirox (Loprox)
- Haloprogin (Halotex)
- Tolnaftate (Tinactin)
- Undecylenic acid (Desenex)

CONTRAINDICATIONS
Known allergy to agent

PRECAUTIONS
Read drug product information.

DRUG INTERACTIONS
Numerous interactions; read drug product information.

FOLLOW-UP

PATIENT MONITORING
See the doctor as often as necessary.

PREVENTION
- Avoid items in *Risk Factors*.
- Avoid contact with suspicious lesions.
- Good personal hygiene
- Do not share head wear, brushes, or combs.
- Wear rubber or wooden sandals in community showers or bathing places.
- Carefully dry between the toes after showering or bathing
- Change socks frequently.
- Apply drying or dusting powder.

COMPLICATIONS
- Bacterial superinfection
- Generalized, invasive infection
- Scarring
- Hair loss
- Spread of disease

WHAT TO EXPECT
Resolution without complications, within 1 to 2 weeks of therapy

Tinea

Doctor
Office
Phone
Pager

Special notes to patient:

Toxic Shock Syndrome

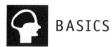 ## BASICS

DESCRIPTION

- Toxic shock syndrome (TSS) is an acute, multisystem illness caused by the bacterium *Staphylococcus aureus*. TSS is characterized by the sudden onset of high fever, peculiar skin rash, and shock.
- Menstrual TSS: associated with menstruation and tampon use
- Nonmenstrual TSS: more common than the menstrual form; associated with surgical wounds, barrier contraception, and so on. Can occur in children, men, and women.

SIGNS AND SYMPTOMS

- Almost always present:
  - Temperature above 102°F (38.9°C)
  - Reddened skin
  - Rash
  - Peeling skin a few days after rash appears
  - Shock, fainting
  - Nausea or vomiting
- Commonly present:
  - Headache
  - Confusion or agitation
  - Acute respiratory distress syndrome
  - Sore throat
  - Vaginitis or vaginal discharge
  - Reddened eyes
  - Swelling around the eyes
  - Edema or swelling of the body
  - Muscle and joint ache
  - Scant urine production
  - Diarrhea
- Rarely present:
  - Arthritis
  - Enlarged lymph glands
  - Heart disease
  - Visual sensitivity to light
  - Seizure

CAUSES

Toxins produced by *S. aureus*

SCOPE

Annually, 0.22 to 1.23 cases of toxic shock syndrome per 100,000 persons are reported in the United States.

MOST OFTEN AFFECTED

All ages, but especially individuals 30 to 60 years of age; women affected more frequently than men

RISK FACTORS

- Infection with *S. aureus*
- Continuous use of super-absorbency tampons during menstruation
- Use of regular-absorbency tampons during menstruation
- Use of contraceptive sponge

 ## DIAGNOSIS

WHAT THE DOCTOR LOOKS FOR

- The doctor will perform an examination to identify the presence of TSS.
- Other conditions that can appear similar to TSS (e.g., scarlet fever, drug reactions, Rocky Mountain spotted fever, Kawasaki disease, and other infections) should be investigated.

TESTS AND PROCEDURES

- Blood tests
- Blood, nose, vagina, wound, or other body areas can be swabbed for laboratory analysis.

 ## TREATMENT

GENERAL MEASURES

- Treatment of TSS requires hospitalization.
- Removal of tampon or other vaginal foreign bodies
- Intravenous (IV) fluids
- Management of kidney or heart failure
- Mechanical ventilation may be necessary.
- Surgery may be required.

ACTIVITY

Bedrest throughout acute illness

DIET

As tolerated

 ## MEDICATIONS

COMMONLY PRESCRIBED DRUGS

- Fluid replacement
- Dopamine
- Oxacillin, nafcillin

CONTRAINDICATIONS

Penicillin allergy

PRECAUTIONS

Read drug product information.

DRUG INTERACTIONS

Read drug product information.

OTHER DRUGS

- Clindamycin
- Vancomycin
- Immune globulin, intravenous (IVIG)

 ## FOLLOW-UP

PATIENT MONITORING

See the doctor and other healthcare professionals continuously during hospitalization.

PREVENTION

- Avoid continuous tampon use during menstruation.
- Avoid super-absorbency tampons.
- Change tampon frequently during the day.
- Use sanitary napkins at night.
- Early medical attention to infected wounds

COMPLICATIONS

- Acute kidney failure
- Adult respiratory distress syndrome
- Excessively heavy menstrual flow
- Loss of hair
- Nail loss
- Other complications

WHAT TO EXPECT

- Death rate is 3% to 9%.
- Recurs in 10% to 15% of cases

 ## MISCELLANEOUS

PEDIATRIC

Can occur as a complication of chickenpox

GERIATRIC

Can result from cellulitis or surgical wound infections

OTHERS

None

PREGNANCY

Can result from infections after birth, especially cesarean section wound infection or episiotomy infections

Toxic Shock Syndrome

	Doctor
	Office
	Phone
	Pager

Special notes to patient:

Toxoplasmosis

 ## BASICS

DESCRIPTION

Toxoplasmosis is an infection with the protozoan *Toxoplasma gondii*. Four types of infection are seen:

- Congenital toxoplasmosis: acute infection of mother during gestation that is passed to fetus.
- Ocular toxoplasmosis: eye infection, usually resulting from congenital exposure but remaining latent until the second or third decade of life
- Acute toxoplasmosis in person with normal immune system: acute, self-limiting infection in normal host
- Acute toxoplasmosis in person with immune deficiency: a life-threatening infection involving many organ systems (e.g. heart, lung, liver), especially the central nervous system

SIGNS AND SYMPTOMS

- No symptoms in 80% to 90% of cases
- Fever, malaise, night sweats, muscle ache
- Sore throat
- Rash
- Brain inflammation
- Paralysis of half the body, seizures, mental status changes
- Visual changes
- Heart, lung inflammation

CAUSES

- *T. gondii*
- Congenital disease is passed from newly infected mother to fetus during pregnancy.
- Other syndromes may result from newly acquired infection or reactivation of latent infection.
- Ingestion of meats or foods containing eggs present in cat feces
- Infection can be transmitted by blood transfusion or organ transplantation.

SCOPE

- Up to 70% of healthy adults in the United States have been exposed to *T. gondii*.
- Toxoplasmosis affects more than 3,500 newborns in the United States annually.

MOST OFTEN AFFECTED

All ages; males and females affected equally

RISK FACTORS

- Immune system disorders (e.g., acquired immunodeficiency syndrome [AIDS])
- Risk of transmission to fetus is greatest during third trimester.

 ## DIAGNOSIS

WHAT THE DOCTOR LOOKS FOR

The doctor will perform a physical examination to identify the presence of toxoplasmosis.

TESTS AND PROCEDURES

- *T. gondii* can be isolated from blood, body fluids, or tissue.
- Blood tests
- Spinal fluid can be obtained by lumbar puncture (spinal tap).
- If pregnancy is involved, amniocentesis and fetal ultrasound can be done.
- Computed tomography (CT) scan or magnetic resonance imaging (MRI) of head can be performed.
- A sample of lymph node or brain tissue can be obtained by biopsy for laboratory analysis.

 ## TREATMENT

GENERAL MEASURES

- Toxoplasmosis is managed in the outpatient setting, except for severe disease, which requires hospitalization.
- Usually no treatment in individuals without symptoms, except a child under 5 years of age
- Symptomatic patients should be treated until immunity is assured.

ACTIVITY

Level of activity depends on severity of disease and organ systems involved.

DIET

No special diet

 ## MEDICATIONS

COMMONLY PRESCRIBED DRUGS

- Sulfadiazine (Microsulfon)
- Pyrimethamine (Daraprim)
- Leucovorin (folinic acid)

CONTRAINDICATIONS

- Pyrimethamine should not be used in the first trimester of pregnancy.
- Known hypersensitivity to pyrimethamine or sulfadiazine

PRECAUTIONS

Numerous precautions; read drug product information.

DRUG INTERACTIONS

Read drug product information.

OTHER DRUGS

- Spiramycin
- Clindamycin
- Corticosteroids
- Atovaquone (Mepron), azithromycin (Zithromax), clarithromycin (Biaxin)

Toxoplasmosis

	Doctor
	Office
	Phone
	Pager

Special notes to patient:

Toxoplasmosis

 ## FOLLOW-UP

PATIENT MONITORING

- See the doctor every 2 weeks until stable, then monthly during therapy.
- Repeat blood tests monthly.

PREVENTION

- Avoid eating raw meat, unpasteurized milk, and uncooked eggs.
- Avoid contact with cat feces.
- Pregnant women should not empty animal litter boxes.

COMPLICATIONS

- Seizure disorder
- Brain damage
- Partial or complete blindness
- Many complications can occur with congenital toxoplasmosis, including mental retardation, seizures, deafness, and blindness.

WHAT TO EXPECT

- Individuals with immune system disorders often experience relapse if treatment is stopped.
- Treatment may prevent the development of complications in infants with congenital toxoplasmosis.

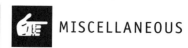

OTHERS

None

PREGNANCY

- Take extra precautions to avoid contact with cats.
- Do not eat raw meat; wash all fruits and vegetables carefully.
- See a specialist when toxoplasmosis infection occurs during pregnancy.

FURTHER INFORMATION

National Institute of Allergy and Infectious Disease, Department of Health and Human Services, Bldg. 31, Room 7A-32,
9000 Rockville Pike, Bethesda, MD 20892, (301) 496-5717

Toxoplasmosis

Doctor
Office
Phone
Pager

Special notes to patient:

Transient Ischemic Attack (TIA)

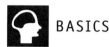 ## BASICS

DESCRIPTION

Transient ischemic attack, called "TIA" or "mini stroke," is the sudden onset of a neurologic deficit caused by a lack of oxygenated blood being delivered to the brain. A TIA lasts less than 24 hours.

SCOPE

About 160 new cases of TIA per 100,000 persons occur annually in the United States.

MOST OFTEN AFFECTED

Risk increases above 45 years of age and is highest among individuals 60 to 70 years of age; men affected more often than women

SIGNS AND SYMPTOMS

- Paralysis of one side of the body, loss of sensation on one side of the body, difficulty speaking, visual disturbances
- Double vision, vertigo, incoordination, paralysis of facial muscles, difficulty swallowing, difficulty moving
- Less often: headaches, seizures, amnesia, confusion

CAUSES

- Atherosclerotic plaques in the carotid artery that lead to formation of blood clots
- High blood pressure
- Heart disease: valve disorders, heart attack, irregular heart rhythm (atrial fibrillation)
- Blood-clotting disorders
- Other causes: spontaneous TIA, trauma

RISK FACTORS

- Age
- High blood pressure
- Heart disease
- Smoking
- Diabetes
- Family history

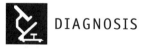 ## DIAGNOSIS

WHAT THE DOCTOR LOOKS FOR

- The doctor will perform a physical examination to identify TIA.
- Other possible causes of similar signs and symptoms (e.g., migraine, seizures, and other disorders) should be investigated.

TESTS AND PROCEDURES

- Blood tests
- Ultrasound can be used to assess carotid arteries.
- Blood vessels in the brain can be imaged with a radiology procedure, called "cerebral angiography."
- The electrocardiogram (ECG) will be monitored.
- Computed tomography (CT) scan can be used to assist in diagnosis.

 ## TREATMENT

GENERAL MEASURES

- TIA is managed in the outpatient setting, except for surgery or procedures requiring hospitalization.
- Strict control of medical risk factors (e.g., diabetes, hypertension, hyperlipidemia, cardiac disease)
- Cessation of smoking
- Surgery (endarterectomy) may be required.

ACTIVITY

No restrictions

DIET

As appropriate to underlying medical problems (e.g., diabetic diet, low-fat diet, low-salt diet)

 ## MEDICATIONS

COMMONLY PRESCRIBED DRUGS

- Enteric-coated aspirin
- Ticlopidine

CONTRAINDICATIONS

Many contraindications; read drug product information.

PRECAUTIONS

Aspirin may worsen peptic ulcer or asthma.

SIGNIFICANT POSSIBLE INTERACTIONS

Read drug product information.

 ## FOLLOW-UP

PATIENT MONITORING

See the doctor every 3 months for first year, then annually.

PREVENTION

- Stop smoking
- Control blood pressure, diabetes; reduce lipids in bloodstream.
- Aspirin, ticlopidine
- Low fat diet

COMPLICATIONS

- Stroke
- Seizure
- Trauma, if patient experiences sudden fall because of weakness

WHAT TO EXPECT

Individuals with TIA have a 5% to 20% risk of stroke within 1 year. Risk is cumulative thereafter. Risk increases with number of multiple risk factors and severity of carotid narrowing.

 ## MISCELLANEOUS

GERIATRIC

Atrial fibrillation is a frequent cause of TIA among the elderly.

PREGNANCY

Clotting disorders leading to mini-strokes are associated with pregnancy and birth.

FURTHER INFORMATION

National Stroke Association, 300 East Hampden Ave., Suite 240, Englewood, CO 80110-2622

Transient Ischemic Attack (TIA)

	Doctor
	Office
	Phone
	Pager

Special notes to patient:

Tuberculosis

 ## BASICS

DESCRIPTION

Tuberculosis (TB) is an increasingly common bacterial infection. After organisms take residence in the lung, TB can lead to involvement of multiple areas of the body, including middle ear, bones, joints, brain, heart, and skin. Organisms can survive many years in the body. The highest risk for active disease occurs within the first 2 years after exposure.

SCOPE

The incidence of TB varies greatly; approximately 32 to 100 cases per 100,000 persons occur annually in the United States.

MOST OFTEN AFFECTED

TB can affect all ages; more common in males than females

SIGNS AND SYMPTOMS

- Cough
- Spitting of blood
- Fever and night sweats
- Weight loss
- Decreased activity
- Enlarged lymph glands
- Chest pain

CAUSES

Mycobacterium tuberculosis, *Mycobacterium bovis*, and *Mycobacterium africanum*.

RISK FACTORS

- Urban, homeless, minority
- Institutionalization (e.g., correctional facility)
- Immune system disorders
- Cancer
- Diabetes
- Chronic kidney failure
- Malnutrition
- Chronic high dose steroids
- Close contact with an infected individual

 ## DIAGNOSIS

WHAT THE DOCTOR LOOKS FOR

- The doctor will perform a physical examination to identify the presence of tuberculosis.
- Conditions that can appear similar to TB should be ruled out, including pneumonia, cancer, and fungal infections.

TESTS AND PROCEDURES

- Blood tests
- Special tests for tuberculosis, including sputum culture
- Chest x-ray study
- Spinal fluid can be sampled by lumbar puncture (spinal tap).
- A sample of bone marrow can be obtained by biopsy for laboratory analysis.

 ## TREATMENT

GENERAL MEASURES

- TB is managed in the outpatient setting.
- TB requires careful evaluation and monitoring to make sure medication is taken properly.
- Public health authorities are notified.

ACTIVITY

- As tolerated
- Coughing children may be contagious.
- After a few days of treatment, coughing persons are usually not contagious.

DIET

No restrictions

 ## MEDICATIONS

COMMONLY PRESCRIBED DRUGS

- Isoniazid
- Rifampin
- Pyrazinamide
- Streptomycin
- Rifapentine
- Rifabutin

CONTRAINDICATIONS

Read drug product information.

PRECAUTIONS

Read drug product information.

DRUG INTERACTIONS

- Rifampin: colors urine, tears, and secretions orange and can permanently stain contact lenses. May inactivate birth control pills.
- Isoniazid: peripheral nerve inflammation and allergy are possible

OTHER DRUGS

- Ethambutol
- Steroids

 ## FOLLOW-UP

PATIENT MONITORING

- See the doctor every 2 to 3 months for duration of treatment.
- Repeat x-ray study at 2- to 3-month intervals.

PREVENTION

- TB screening at 15 months of age and annually for individuals who are in close contact with people with TB
- Careful tracking to identify and treat contagious persons is mandatory. The public health department should be notified of all confirmed cases.

COMPLICATIONS

- Progression of disease outside the lungs to other systems
- Spread of disease
- Drug resistance

WHAT TO EXPECT

Generally, few complications and full resolution, if drugs are taken regularly as prescribed for full course

MISCELLANEOUS

GERIATRIC

Symptoms can be more subtle in the elderly and may be attributed to aging or other health problems.

Tuberculosis

Doctor
Office
Phone
Pager

Special notes to patient:

Ulcerative Colitis

 ## BASICS

DESCRIPTION

Ulcerative colitis, also called "idiopathic proctocolitis," is one of a group of inflammatory bowel diseases of unknown cause characterized by periodic acute episodes of rectal bleeding and various constitutional symptoms.

SIGNS AND SYMPTOMS

- Bloody diarrhea
- Abdominal pain
- Fever
- Weight loss
- Joint pain
- Inflammation of the backbone
- Eye diseases
- Painful nodes on the lower extremities
- Chronic ulcers of the skin
- Mouth ulcers
- Liver and gallbladder disease
- Blood-clotting disorders

CAUSES

The basic cause of ulcerative colitis is unknown. Genetic, infectious, immunologic, and psychological factors have been suggested.

SCOPE

Ulcerative colitis affects 70 to 150 per 100,000 persons; six to eight new cases per 100,000 population occur annually in the United States.

MOST OFTEN AFFECTED

Ulcerative colitis most often affects those between 15 and 35 years of age. It also affects individuals in their 80s. The disease occurs with equal frequency in males and females. Ulcerative colitis tends to run in families; about 8% to 11% have a family history of the disease. It is more common in Jews than other ethnic groups.

RISK FACTORS

- None known
- Higher incidence in Jews and those with a family history
- Lower risk associated with smoking

 ## DIAGNOSIS

WHAT THE DOCTOR LOOKS FOR

- Other sources of rectal bleeding, including hemorrhoids, Crohn's disease, diverticula, cancer, infection, antibiotic usage
- The colon can be visually inspected by sigmoidoscopy or colonoscopy.

TESTS AND PROCEDURES

- Blood tests to detect inflammation and anemia, and to assess liver function
- A barium enema can be performed to evaluate the large colon.
- A sample of intestinal tissue can be obtained by biopsy for examination.

 ## TREATMENT

GENERAL MEASURES

- The overall goal of treatment is to control inflammation, prevent complications, and replace nutritional losses and blood volume.
- Ulcerative colitis is usually managed on an outpatient basis, except for severe episodes, which may require hospitalization.
- Complications or disease that does not respond to medical treatment may require surgery.

ACTIVITY

Full activity, as tolerated

DIET

No specific diet; milk products do not need to be avoided unless the person is lactose intolerant.

MEDICATIONS

COMMONLY PRESCRIBED DRUGS

- Sulfasalazine is the treatment of choice for mild flare-ups and management of ulcerative colitis.
- Limited disease can be treated with enemas and suppositories.
- Oral or parenteral corticosteroids are used for more severe flare-ups.
- Approximately 10% of patients have chronic disease activity and require continuous steroid doses.
- Immunomodulators (e.g. azathioprine, mercaptopurine, methotrexate, levamisole, and cyclosporine) are controversial in a disease potentially curable by surgery. However, these drugs have been shown to be effective in patients for whom surgery is not an option.
- Antimicrobial agents are sometimes useful in Crohn's disease, but not in ulcerative colitis.
- Antidiarrheal agents: diphenoxylate-atropine and loperamide can be used to help control diarrhea.

CONTRAINDICATIONS

- Allergy to any of the aforementioned medications
- Read drug product information.

PRECAUTIONS

Use of antidiarrheal agents in severe disease could cause a serious colon condition.

DRUG INTERACTIONS

Read drug product information.

Ulcerative Colitis

Doctor

Office

Phone

Pager

Special notes to patient:

Ulcerative Colitis

 FOLLOW-UP

PATIENT MONITORING

- Regularly scheduled appointments are important to evaluate for disease activity, appearance of complications, and psychological and social well-being.
- Colonoscopy should be performed every 1 to 2 years after the disease has been present for 7 to 8 years.
- The liver should be evaluated annually.
- The gallbladder can be evaluated by cholangiography to assess the flow of bile.

PREVENTION

Regular checkups with primary care provider for physical examination and colonoscopy

COMPLICATIONS

- Perforation of the intestine
- Other intestinal disorders
- Liver disease
- Colon cancer. Cancer can affect up to 30% of those who have had colitis for 25 years.

WHAT TO EXPECT

- The course of the disorder is extremely variable. About 75% to 85% of patients have a repeat episode of acute illness, and up to 20% may eventually require surgery.
- The risk of death from an initial attack is relatively low (about 5% of patients).
- Colon cancer risk is the single most important risk factor affecting long-term prognosis.

 MISCELLANEOUS

PEDIATRIC

- Approximately 20% of patients are 21 years of age or younger.
- Cancer surveillance is important.

GERIATRIC

Having an initial attack above 60 years of age is linked with a higher risk of death.

PREGNANCY

- Outcome of pregnancy is similar to general population.
- Treatment with sulfasalazine does not seem to affect pregnancy.
- Person with ulcerative colitis should delay pregnancy until time when disease is inactive.

FURTHER INFORMATION

National Foundation for Ileitis and Colitis, 444 Park Avenue S., 11th Floor, New York, NY 10016-7374, (800)343-3637

Ulcerative Colitis

Doctor
Office
Phone
Pager

Special notes to patient:

Urinary Incontinence

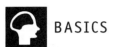

BASICS

DESCRIPTION

Urinary incontinence is the involuntary loss of urine from the bladder. It can occur while asleep or awake. The amount of urine lost can vary greatly. The condition becomes a medical issue when it is perceived to be a social or health problem by the patient or family.

SIGNS AND SYMPTOMS

- Involuntary loss of urine
- Urinary urgency
- Burning with urination
- Irritation of the perineal region

CAUSES

- Pelvic muscle weakness
- Urethral sphincter weakness
- Bladder irritation (e.g., cystitis, tumors, stones)
- Neurologic disorders (e.g., stroke, dementia, spinal injury, multiple sclerosis)
- Anatomic obstruction (e.g., prostate disorders, scarring)

SCOPE

- About 10 million persons in the United States have urinary incontinence.
- Affects 5% to 15% elderly living at home, 50% of nursing home residents

MOST OFTEN AFFECTED

Urinary incontinence primarily affects the elderly (65 years of age or older). Incidence increases with age. Women are affected more often than men.

RISK FACTORS

- Increasing age
- Estrogen deficiency (women)
- Prostatic hypertrophy (men)
- Multiple births (women)
- Dementia
- Diabetes
- Spinal cord injury
- Multiple sclerosis
- General debilitated condition
- Stroke

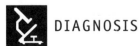

DIAGNOSIS

WHAT THE DOCTOR LOOKS FOR

- The diagnosis of urinary incontinence is generally made on the basis of the patient history.
- Physical examination of men should include examination of the abdomen, digital rectal examination to assess the prostate, and a neurologic examination.
- Physical examination of women should include examination of the abdomen, pelvic examination, and neurologic examination.
- The doctor may ask the patient to reproduce the activities (e.g., coughing, sneezing, laughing) that result in loss of urine.
- The doctor should seek causes of loss of bladder control (e.g., urinary tract infection or a side effect of diuretics or other medication).

TESTS AND PROCEDURES

- Urinalysis and culture
- Blood test for prostate-specific antigen (PSA)
- The urinary system can be visually assessed by a radiology procedure called "intravenous pyelogram" (IVP).
- Special procedures can be done to assess bladder function (e.g., cystometry, voiding cystourethrogram, and cystometrogram).
- Ultrasound can be used to assess the urinary system or prostate.

TREATMENT

GENERAL MEASURES

- Urinary incontinence is usually managed on an outpatient basis.
- All conditions relating to urinary incontinence (e.g., urinary tract infection, bladder tumors, prostatic hypertrophy) should be identified and treated.
- Patient should be taught proper toilet hygiene.
- Patient may be taught pelvic floor (Kegel) exercises or biofeedback, or have behavioral training.
- Some patients may require catheterization or incontinence pads. Some patients with incontinence caused by prostatic hypertrophy may benefit from transurethral resection of the prostate (TURP).
- Some patients with stress incontinence may benefit from bladder surgery.

ACTIVITY

Full activities should be encouraged.

DIET

- No special diet
- In situations where access to bathroom facilities is limited, a person with incontinence may want to avoid high-volume fluid intake and reduce intake of caffeine or alcohol-containing beverages.

MEDICATIONS

COMMONLY PRESCRIBED DRUGS

- Detrusor instability: oxybutynin, propantheline (Pro-Banthine), dicyclomine (Bentyl), flavoxate (Urispas), imipramine (Tofranil)
- Sphincter incompetence: pseudoephedrine (Sudafed), phenylpropanolamine, imipramine (Tofranil)
- Overflow or atonic bladder: bethanechol (Urecholine)
- Overflow or prostatic enlargement: prazosin (Minipress), finasteride (Proscar), Tamsulosin (Flomax)

CONTRAINDICATIONS

- Read drug product information.
- May be contraindicated in patients with glaucoma or prostatic hypertrophy

PRECAUTIONS

- The smallest dose possible should be used in elderly patients.
- Common side effects include dry mouth, blurred vision, constipation, low blood pressure on standing, and mental confusion.

DRUG INTERACTIONS

Varies for each drug; read drug product information.

OTHER DRUGS

- Oral or topical estrogens for stress incontinence associated with vaginitis
- Prostaglandin inhibitors (experimental)
- Calcium antagonists (experimental)
- Desmopressin (DDAVP) nasal spray for bed-wetting

Urinary Incontinence

Doctor
Office
Phone
Pager

Special notes to patient:

Urinary Incontinence

 FOLLOW-UP

PATIENT MONITORING

- Patient should be seen every other week while learning exercises and medication dosage is being adjusted.
- Patient should be seen every 3 months once incontinence is under control and medication doses are stable.
- Patient should be evaluated for side effects of medication.
- Intraocular pressure can be tested for patients at high risk.
- Patient should have periodic urinalysis to detect early urinary tract infection.

PREVENTION

- Women should routinely use Kegel exercises following childbirth.
- Women should have regular pelvic examinations to detect disease early.
- Men should have regular rectal examinations to identify prostatic disease early and receive treatment for hypertrophy.

COMPLICATIONS

- Urinary tract infection
- Kidney disease
- Adverse drug reactions

WHAT TO EXPECT

Prognosis is generally good. Most patients can achieve an increase in bladder control with appropriate medical management.

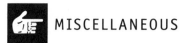 MISCELLANEOUS

GERIATRIC

Urinary incontinence is most common in the aging population.

PREGNANCY

Stress incontinence can occur during pregnancy.

Urinary Incontinence

	Doctor
	Office
	Phone
	Pager

Special notes to patient:

Urinary Tract Infection in Men

 ## BASICS

DESCRIPTION
Lower urinary tract infection (UTI), also called "cystitis," is usually caused by bacteria.

SIGNS AND SYMPTOMS
- Frequent urination
- Difficult urination
- Urinary urgency
- Hesitancy
- Slow urinary stream
- Dribbling of urine
- Frequent urination during sleep hours
- Discomfort in the lower abdomen
- Low back pain
- Blood in the urine
- Systemic symptoms (chills, fever) present with coexisting kidney or prostate disease

CAUSES
Bacterial infection

SCOPE
UTI is not commonly found in men in the United States.

MOST OFTEN AFFECTED
UTI is uncommon in men under 50 years of age, with about 8 infections per 10,000 men aged 21 to 50 years. Incidence increases with age.

RISK FACTORS
- Benign prostatic hypertrophy (BPH)
- Cognitive impairment
- Fecal incontinence
- Urinary incontinence
- Anal intercourse
- Recent urologic surgery, catheterization, or other procedures
- Infection of the prostate or kidney
- Immune system disorders
- Outlet obstruction

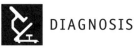 ## DIAGNOSIS

WHAT THE DOCTOR LOOKS FOR
- Anatomic or functional conditions that may be causing symptoms
- Other infections of the genitourinary system
- Patients with UTI often have associated conditions, including kidney and prostate disease.

TESTS AND PROCEDURES
- Urinalysis and culture for microbiologic evaluation
- A radiologic procedure called "intravenous pyelography" can be done to assess the urinary tract.
- Ultrasound can be used to evaluate the urinary system.
- The bladder can be visually examined by the doctor with a cystoscope.

 ## TREATMENT

GENERAL MEASURES
- UTI is managed on an outpatient basis, except for acute illness with toxicity or kidney failure.
- The patient should be given fluids and pain relief, as required.
- Discontinue sexual activity until cured.

ACTIVITY
Activity as tolerated

DIET
No special diet

 ## MEDICATIONS

COMMONLY PRESCRIBED DRUGS
- For acute UTI, first infection, no risk factors for treatment: 7 to 10 days of oral antibiotics
- For complicated or repeated UTI: 14 to 21 days of antibiotics

CONTRAINDICATIONS
Read drug product information.

PRECAUTIONS
Read drug product information.

SIGNIFICANT POSSIBLE INTERACTIONS
Read drug product information.

 ## FOLLOW-UP

PATIENT MONITORING
- Individuals with UTI should be closely followed by the doctor until the infection is cured.
- Urinalysis should be periodically repeated.

PREVENTION
Predisposing factors should be promptly treated.

COMPLICATIONS
- Kidney disorders
- Infection may get worse
- Recurring infection

WHAT TO EXPECT
Infections usually clear up with appropriate antibiotic treatment.

 ## MISCELLANEOUS

PEDIATRIC
UTI is usually associated with obstruction to normal flow of urine.

GERIATRIC
Bacteria are commonly found in the urine of an elderly person. If no symptoms are present, treatment is not necessary. Giving antibiotics may allow the growth of resistant microbes.

FURTHER INFORMATION
National Kidney Foundation, 30 E. 33rd St., Suite 1100, New York, NY 10016, (212) 889-2210

Urinary Tract Infection in Men

Doctor
Office
Phone
Pager

Special notes to patient:

Urinary Tract Infection in Women

BASICS

DESCRIPTION
Urinary tract infection (UTI) is also called "cystitis." UTI causes inflammation of the bladder.
UTI is caused by bacteria.

SIGNS AND SYMPTOMS
- Any or all of the following may be present:
  - Burning during urination
  - Pain during urination
  - Urgency (sensation of need to urinate frequently)
  - Sensation of incomplete bladder emptying
  - Blood in urine
  - Lower abdominal pain or cramping
  - Offensive odor of urine

CAUSES
Bacterial infection

SCOPE
Between 3% and 8% of women have bacteria in their urine at any given time. About 43% of women between 14 and 61 years of age have had at least one episode of UTI. It is the cause of 7 million visits to the doctor annually.

MOST OFTEN AFFECTED
Young adult and older females

RISK FACTORS
- Previous UTI
- Diabetes mellitus
- Pregnancy
- More frequent or vigorous sexual activity than usual
- Use of spermicide or diaphragm
- Underlying condition of the urinary tract (e.g., tumors or stones)

DIAGNOSIS

WHAT THE DOCTOR LOOKS FOR
- Vaginitis
- Sexually transmitted diseases
- Other causes of blood in the urine (e.g., kidney stones or cancer)
- Psychological dysfunction
- Interstitial cystitis

TESTS AND PROCEDURES
- Urinalysis and culture for microbiologic evaluation
- Urine can be obtained by bladder catheterization.
- X-ray study, ultrasound, or endoscopic imaging can be done to assess the urinary tract.
- Special procedures (e.g., voiding cystourethrogram) can be done.

TREATMENT

GENERAL MEASURES
- UTI is managed on an outpatient basis, except for complicated or upper urinary tract infections.
- The patient should maintain good fluid intake.
- One fourth of women with UTI have another infection within 6 months. Women with repeated UTI and no underlying urinary tract abnormality may receive long-term antibiotic treatment.
- Patients with chronic indwelling urinary catheters always have infections. UTI should not be treated unless the patient has fever, sepsis, or other systemic symptoms.

ACTIVITY
Avoid sexual intercourse when symptoms are present.

DIET
No special diet

MEDICATIONS

COMMONLY PRESCRIBED DRUGS
- Antibiotics
  - Sulfamethaxazols-trimethoprim (Septra, Bactrim)
  - Ampicillin
  - Nitrofurantoin (Macrodantin)
- Urinary analgesics
  - Phenazopyridize (Pyridium)

CONTRAINDICATIONS
Read drug product information. Some drugs should not be used during pregnancy.

PRECAUTIONS
Read drug product information.

DRUG INTERACTIONS
Read drug product information.

OTHER DRUGS
Antibiotic therapy can be changed, based on microbiologic assessment.

Urinary Tract Infection in Women

Doctor
Office
Phone
Pager

Special notes to patient:

Urinary Tract Infection in Women

 FOLLOW-UP

PATIENT MONITORING

- Return to the doctor if symptoms are not resolved or markedly improved within 48 hours.
- Return to the doctor if fever, chills, or flank pain develops.
- First or rare UTI: A young or middle-aged, nonpregnant adult woman requires no follow-up if a single dose of antibiotic clears the infection.
- If UTI is not resolved within 2 to 3 days after single dose therapy, urine should be cultured for microbiologic evaluation. Antibiotic therapy can be changed.
- All other patients should have urine culture repeated after treatment to make sure the infection has been cleared.

PREVENTION

- Maintain good fluid intake.
- Women with frequent or intercourse-related UTI should empty bladder immediately before and following intercourse and consider postcoital antibiotic treatment.

COMPLICATIONS

Kidney disease

WHAT TO EXPECT

For most patients, symptoms resolve within 2 to 3 days after starting treatment.

 MISCELLANEOUS

PEDIATRIC

Infants and young children at higher risk of kidney disease

GERIATRIC

- The elderly may have bacteria in their urine but may not have symptoms. This condition generally does not require treatment if the urinary tract is otherwise normal.
- The elderly are more likely to have an underlying urinary tract abnormality.
- Acute UTI is often associated with incontinence in the elderly.

PREGNANCY

UTI during pregnancy always requires culture and usually requires 10 to 14 days of antibiotic treatment. After treatment of acute infection, pregnant women often receive antibiotics for the remainder of pregnancy.

Urinary Tract Infection in Women

Doctor
Office
Phone
Pager

Special notes to patient:

Vaginal Bleeding During Pregnancy

 ## BASICS

DESCRIPTION

Vaginal bleeding during pregnancy has many causes. The bleeding can range in severity from mild (with normal pregnancy outcome) to life threatening for both infant and mother. It can vary from light to heavy, from brown to bright red, and can be painless or painful.

SIGNS AND SYMPTOMS

- Bleeding can vary from light to heavy.
- Color of blood varies from brown to bright red.
- May be painless or painful

CAUSES

- Vaginal infection or trauma
- Disorders of the cervix
- Complications of pregnancy
- "Bloody show" (bloody discharge that normally precedes labor)
- Unknown: No cause is found in 50% of first trimester bleeding.

SCOPE

Vaginal bleeding is common in the United States.

MOST OFTEN AFFECTED

Women of childbearing age

RISK FACTORS

Varies, based on individual causes

 ## DIAGNOSIS

WHAT THE DOCTOR LOOKS FOR

- Vaginal or cervical causes of bleeding can occur throughout pregnancy.
- The doctor will perform a thorough pelvic examination.
- A sample of fluid can be withdrawn from the womb.
- An internal examination can be performed by minimally invasive laparoscopy (to look inside the abdomen).

LABORATORY

- Blood tests, including clotting studies and hormone tests
- Ultrasound: Several ultrasound studies may be required in early pregnancy to make diagnosis.

 ## TREATMENT

GENERAL MEASURES

- During the first trimester, most patients with bleeding can be managed on an outpatient basis.
- During late pregnancy, most patients with bleeding need to be hospitalized for observation.
- In late pregnancy bleeding, the amount of bleeding and the status of mother and baby indicate whether urgent cesarean section is needed or whether conservative measures are appropriate.
- Threatened abortion: bedrest and nothing by vagina (no intercourse or douching). If bleeding is severe, hospitalization and close observation are needed.
- Surgery may be necessary for ectopic pregnancy, incomplete miscarriage, and the like.
- Grief counseling is appropriate if pregnancy loss is inevitable.

ACTIVITY

Bedrest, no intercourse, no douching

DIET

No restrictions

 ## MEDICATIONS

COMMONLY PRESCRIBED DRUGS

None

 ## FOLLOW-UP

PATIENT MONITORING

- See the doctor daily to weekly, depending on diagnosis and bleeding severity.
- Report any increase in the amount or frequency of bleeding to the doctor.
- Seek immediate care if abdominal pain occurs or bleeding suddenly increases.
- Bring any tissue that is passed vaginally for examination.

COMPLICATIONS

- Anemia
- Shock
- Fetal or maternal death
- Infection
- Premature delivery of baby, with associated complications
- Bleeding disorders

WHAT TO EXPECT

The outcome depends on the cause of the vaginal bleeding, its severity and how promptly it is diagnosed and treated. About 1 of 826 ectopic pregnancies (pregnancy in which the embryo implants in the fallopian tube instead of the uterus) results in the death of the mother.

MISCELLANEOUS

PREGNANCY

A complication of pregnancy

FURTHER INFORMATION

American College of Obstetricians & Gynecologists (ACOG), 409 12th St., SW, Washington, DC 20024-2188, (800) 762-ACOG

Vaginal Bleeding During Pregnancy

Doctor
Office
Phone
Pager

Special notes to patient:

Vaginal Yeast Infection

 ## BASICS

DESCRIPTION
Candidal vulvovaginitis is a vaginal infection caused by a yeast (*Candida*). It can cause itching and burning of the vulva, often with abnormal vaginal discharge.

SCOPE
- Of nonpregnant, premenopausal women, 16% are carriers of infection without symptoms.
- Of vaginal infections, 40% are caused by *Candida*.

MOST OFTEN AFFECTED
Women: from their first menstrual period until menopause

SIGNS AND SYMPTOMS
- Intense itching of the vulva
- Thick, curdlike vaginal discharge
- Painful or difficult urination
- Reddened, inflamed skin on vulva
- Reddening, pain, and itching of perineal area or upper thigh
- Thick, white patches on vaginal skin

CAUSES
Overgrowth of *Candida* in vagina

RISK FACTORS
- Pregnancy
- Diabetes mellitus
- Antibiotic therapy
- Steroid therapy
- Immune system disorders
- Synthetic underpants and undergarments
- Hypothyroidism
- Oral contraceptive medications (low-dose contraceptive pills usually do not increase infection risk)
- Anemia
- Zinc deficiency

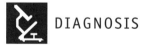 ## DIAGNOSIS

WHAT THE DOCTOR LOOKS FOR
- Other possible genitourinary infections (e.g., trichomonas or gonorrhea)
- Possible allergic reactions

TESTS AND PROCEDURES
- Culture for microbiologic analysis
- Pap smear

 ## TREATMENT

GENERAL MEASURES
- Vulvovaginitis is managed on an outpatient basis.
- Any foreign body should be removed, if present.
- Consider povidone iodine douche for relief of symptoms until specific therapy is effective.
- If urination causes burning, urinate through a tubular device such as a toilet-paper roll or plastic cup with the end cut out; pour warm water over vaginal area while urinating.
- Diabetes must be strictly controlled if the patient is diabetic.

ACTIVITY
- Avoid overexertion, heat, and excessive sweating.
- Delay sexual intercourse until symptoms clear.

DIET
Limit sweets and dairy products in cases of recurrent infections.

 ## MEDICATIONS

COMMONLY PRESCRIBED DRUGS
- Fluconazole (Diflucan)
- Miconazole nitrate (Monistat)
- Butoconazole nitrate (Femstat)
- Terconazole (Terazol)
- Clotrimazole (Gyne-Lotrimin)

PRECAUTIONS
Read drug product information.

SIGNIFICANT POSSIBLE INTERACTIONS
Read drug product information.

OTHER DRUGS
- A different drug can be used if the infection recurs.
- Oral nystatin
- Topical gentian violet
- Boric acid

FOLLOW-UP

PATIENT MONITORING
- No specific follow-up is generally needed.
- See doctor if symptoms persist.
- If infection recurs, sexual partner(s) may require treatment as well.

PREVENTION
- Keep the genital area clean. Use plain, unscented soap.
- Take showers rather than tub baths.
- Wear cotton underpants with a cotton crotch.
- Avoid clothing made from nonventilating materials, including most synthetic underclothing.
- Avoid tight-fitting jeans or slacks.
- Sleep in loose gown without underpants.
- Do not sit around in wet clothing, especially a wet bathing suit.
- Avoid frequent douches.
- After urinating or bowel movements, cleanse by wiping or washing from front to back.
- Lose weight, if obese.

COMPLICATIONS
Bacterial infections of the vagina or vulva

WHAT TO EXPECT
- Vigorous treatment usually results in a complete cure.
- Infections often recur.

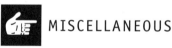 ## MISCELLANEOUS

PEDIATRIC
Less common before puberty

PREGNANCY
Common during pregnancy

FURTHER INFORMATION
American College of Obstetricians & Gynecologists (ACOG), 409 12th St., SW, Washington, DC 20024-2188, (800) 762-ACOG

Vaginal Yeast Infection

Doctor
Office
Phone
Pager

Special notes to patient:

Varicose Veins

 ## BASICS

DESCRIPTION
Varicose veins are elongated, enlarged veins that primarily affect the legs wherein blood flow is restricted.

SIGNS AND SYMPTOMS
- Sometimes, no symptoms
- Leg muscular cramps, aches
- Enlarged, tortuous superficial veins, mostly in the legs
- Swelling of affected Limb
- Fatigue
- Symptoms worsen during menstruation
- Pain, if varicose ulcer develops

CAUSES
- Faulty valves in one or more lower leg vein
- Deep thrombophlebitis
- Increased pressure in the veins
- In many individuals, no cause is identified.

SCOPE
Varicose veins affect about 20% of adults in the United States.

MOST OFTEN AFFECTED
Persons of middle age. Varicose veins are five times more common in women than in men.

RISK FACTORS
- Pregnancy
- Occupations requiring prolonged standing or restrictive clothing (e.g., tight girdles)

 ## DIAGNOSIS

WHAT THE DOCTOR LOOKS FOR
- Diagnosis of varicose usually is made by physical examination.
- The doctor should consider other conditions that may appear similar (e.g., nerve disorders or arthritis).

TESTS AND PROCEDURES
The patient can be evaluated on a tilting table or bed.

TREATMENT

GENERAL MEASURES
- Varicose veins are usually managed on an outpatient basis.
- Conservative methods:
  - Frequent rest periods with legs elevated
  - Lightweight, elastic compression hosiery. Best put on before getting out of bed.
  - Avoidance of girdles and other restrictive clothing
  - If ulcers develop, use warm, wet dressings.
- Spider veins can be treated by injection.
- Surgery and other methods:
  - Surgery may be done if pain, recurrent phlebitis, or skin changes are present or for cosmetic improvement in severe cases.
  - Ligation and stripping
  - Injections
  - For extensive scarring: The entire area can be surgically removed, followed by skin graft.

ACTIVITY
- Avoid long periods of standing.
- Appropriate exercise routine as part of conservative treatment
- Walking regimen after therapy is important to help promote healing.
- Apply elastic stockings before lowering legs from the bed.
- Never sit with legs hanging down.

DIET
- No special diet
- Weight loss diet recommended, if obesity is a problem.

 ## MEDICATIONS

OTHER DRUGS
Antibiotics for infected ulcers

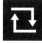 ## FOLLOW-UP

PATIENT MONITORING
- The doctor should follow the patient doctor until surgery or conservative therapy brings maximal benefit.
- Treatment or surgery may not prevent development of varicose veins. Procedures may need to be repeated in later years.

PREVENTION/AVOIDANCE
See *Activity*

COMPLICATIONS
- Bleeding
- Chronic swelling
- Infection
- Varicose ulcers
- Skin color changes
- Eczema
- Recurrence after surgical treatment
- Scarring or nerve damage from stripping technique

WHAT TO EXPECT
- Varicose veins usually become chronic.
- The outcome can be favorable with appropriate treatment.

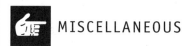 ## MISCELLANEOUS

PEDIATRIC
Varicose veins are uncommon in children.

GERIATRIC
Recommended therapy is elastic support hose and frequent rest with legs elevated rather than stripping.

PREGNANCY
Varicose veins are a frequent problem of pregnancy. Use of elastic stockings is recommended for women who have a history of varicose veins or when activities involve extensive standing.

FURTHER INFORMATION
National Heart, Lung, and Blood Institute, Communications & Public Information Branch, National Institutes of Health, Building 31, Room 41-21, 9000 Rockville Pike, Bethesda, MD 20892, (301) 496-4236

Varicose Veins

Doctor
Office
Phone
Pager

Special notes to patient:

Vitamin Deficiency

 ## BASICS

DESCRIPTION

Vitamin deficiency develops slowly and is difficult to diagnose. Multiple deficiencies of vitamins occur more frequently than deficiency of a single vitamin.

SIGNS AND SYMPTOMS

- Vitamin A (retinol)
  - Night blindness
  - Dandruff, dry scaly skin
  - Dry eyes
  - Growth retardation, loss of appetite, and anemia commonly found in children
- Vitamin B_1 (thiamine)
  - Beriberi
  - Wernicke-Korsakoff syndrome
- Vitamin B_2 (riboflavin)
  - Inflammation at the corners of the mouth
  - Dry, peeling lips
  - Corneal disease
  - Diminished vision in one eye
  - Dermatitis
  - During pregnancy, deficiency leads to fetal skeletal abnormalities (e.g., shortened bones and deformed growth).
- Vitamin B_3 (niacin [nicotinic acid], niacinamide)
  - Pellagra
- Vitamin B_6 (pyridoxine)
  - Convulsions in infants
  - Anemia
  - Nerve disorders
  - Seborrhealike skin lesions
- Vitamin B_{12} (cobalamin)
  - Nerve disorders
  - Anemia
  - Some psychiatric syndromes
- Vitamin C (ascorbic acid)
  - Scurvy (loose teeth, gingivitis, hemorrhages)
- Vitamin D
  - Rickets
  - Softening of the bone
- Vitamin E (alpha-tocopherol)
  - Blood disorders
- Vitamin K
  - Bleeding

SCOPE
Unknown

MOST OFTEN AFFECTED
The elderly are most often affected. Men and women are affected equally. Some forms of vitamin deficiency are inheritable.

CAUSES
- Inadequate dietary intake
- Impaired absorption or storage of vitamins

RISK FACTORS
- Alcoholism
- Malabsorption
- Gallbladder disease
- Dialysis
- Chronic malnutrition
- Deficiencies of other vitamins
- Drug interactions
- Infants
- Elderly
- Lower socioeconomic status
- Laxative abuse
- Genetic disorder
- Prolonged lactation (vitamin C)
- Intestinal parasites
- Drug abuse
- Food faddism or bizarre nutritional practices
- Gastrointestinal surgery

 ## DIAGNOSIS

WHAT THE DOCTOR LOOKS FOR
- The doctor will take a history and perform a thorough physical examination of the patient.
- The doctor should consider other causes of similar signs and symptoms (e.g., as neurologic, intestinal, or skin diseases).

TESTS AND PROCEDURES
Blood test to measure vitamin levels

 ## TREATMENT

GENERAL MEASURES
- The patient with vitamin deficiency is usually managed on an outpatient basis.
- Severe cases may require hospitalization for observation.
- Any underlying causes should be treated.
- Therapy involves replacing vitamins.
- Maintenance vitamin supplement, as required
- For vitamin D deficiency: adequate exposure to sunlight
- The doctor may refer the patient to social service agencies if socioeconomic factors contribute to vitamin deficiency.
- The patient may need help with alcohol or smoking cessation.

ACTIVITY
As tolerated

DIET
- For dietary deficiencies: nutritional counseling with emphasis on appropriate foods and the proper methods for preparation
- Abstain from alcohol.

 ## MEDICATIONS

COMMONLY PRESCRIBED DRUGS
Appropriate vitamins as needed

CONTRAINDICATIONS
Read drug product information.

PRECAUTIONS
Read drug product information.

DRUG INTERACTIONS
Read drug product information.

Vitamin Deficiency

Doctor
Office
Phone
Pager

Special notes to patient:

Vitamin Deficiency

 FOLLOW-UP

PATIENT MONITORING

See the doctor as needed, depending on severity of problem.

PREVENTION

- Proper nutrition
- Supplemental vitamins if needed
- Compliance with vitamin supplementation regimens is important to health.
- Reduce risk factors that lead to deficiency, where possible.
- Vitamin D deficiency: adequate exposure to sunlight (30 minutes several times a week)

COMPLICATIONS

- Vitamin A deficiency: Risk of death is high in advanced cases; eye lesions are a threat to vision.
- Vitamin B_1 deficiency: can be fatal if untreated
- Vitamin B_6 deficiency: Chronic deficiency can increase risk of kidney stones.
- Vitamin D deficiency: skeletal deformities, greenstick fractures, bone pain
- Excessive synthetic vitamin K can lead to anemia and jaundice in infants

WHAT TO EXPECT

With proper diagnosis and therapy, full recovery without complications can be expected.

 MISCELLANEOUS

PEDIATRIC

- Vitamin D deficiency rickets is now rare in the United States, but can occur in breast-fed infants who do not receive a vitamin D supplement, or in infants fed a nonfortified milk-based formula.
- Vitamin E deficiency in infants usually results from formulas high in polyunsaturated fatty acids that are fortified with iron but not vitamin E.
- Vitamin K deficiency is common among newborns

GERIATRIC

The elderly are more likely to have multiple risk factors that can lead to vitamin deficiencies.

PREGNANCY

Pregnant women should take a supplemental multivitamin tablet that contains at least 60 mg of elemental iron and 1.0 mg of folic acid.

Vitamin Deficiency

	Doctor
	Office
	Phone
	Pager

Special notes to patient:

Vulvovaginitis, Estrogen Deficient

 ## BASICS

DESCRIPTION
Estrogen-deficient vulvovaginitis is a thinning and atrophy of female genital tissue, caused by decreased blood flow from changes in estrogen levels. It is often associated with urinary incontinence.

SIGNS AND SYMPTOMS
- Vaginal dryness
- Decreased vaginal secretions
- Difficult or painful urination
- Itching

CAUSES
- Menopause (surgical or natural)
- Ovarian surgery
- Radiation of the pelvis

SCOPE
Without estrogen replacement therapy (ERT), it will affect all women, to some degree.

MOST OFTEN AFFECTED
Predominantly a problem of the postmenopausal woman

RISK FACTORS
- Metabolic disorders caused by estrogen deficiency
- Vaginal infections with bacteria and fungi

 ## DIAGNOSIS

WHAT THE DOCTOR LOOKS FOR
The doctor will look for other conditions that may be causing symptoms (e.g., cancer)

TESTS AND PROCEDURES
- Blood tests, including hormone levels
- Urinalysis and culture
- Cells from urine or vaginal swab can be microscopically analyzed.

 ## TREATMENT

GENERAL MEASURES
- Estrogen-deficient vulvovaginitis is managed in an outpatient setting.
- Symptoms can be relieved and reversed by ERT.
- Relief of symptoms as needed (e.g., cool baths or compresses)

ACTIVITY
No restriction

DIET
No special diet

 ## MEDICATIONS

COMMONLY PRESCRIBED DRUGS
A wide variety of estrogen preparations are available.

CONTRAINDICATIONS
- ERT should not be given to those with a history of breast cancer or estrogen-positive tumor receptors.
- ERT may not be given if the patient has a history of uterine malignancy.

PRECAUTIONS
Read drug product information.

SIGNIFICANT POSSIBLE INTERACTIONS
Read drug product information.

 ## FOLLOW-UP

PATIENT MONITORING
Symptoms should resolve within 30 to 60 days. See the doctor if symptoms do not resolve.

COMPLICATIONS
Complications are those associated with ERT (e.g., bleeding, nausea, headache, libido changes, clotting disorders).

WHAT TO EXPECT
The outcome of estrogen-deficient vulvovaginitis is excellent. Most symptoms are relieved with ERT.

PREGNANCY
The lactating mother of a newborn may have low levels of estrogen. Lubrication may help relieve symptoms of difficult urination. Symptoms will resolve when breast-feeding is stopped.

FURTHER INFORMATION
American College of Obstetricians & Gynecologists (ACOG), 409 12th St., SW, Washington, DC 20024-2188, (800) 762-ACOG

Vulvovaginitis, Estrogen Deficient

	Doctor
	Office
	Phone
	Pager

Special notes to patient:

Warts

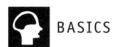 BASICS

DESCRIPTION

Warts are painless, benign skin tumors characterized by an area of well-defined thickening of the skin. They are caused by a virus passed by direct contact with an infected person or from recently shed virus kept intact in a moist, warm environment. Many types of warts are seen, with different appearances and growth patterns. Plantar warts are individual or groups of warts that occur on the sole of the foot.

SIGNS AND SYMPTOMS

- Rough-surfaced, raised, skin-colored bumps 1 to 10 ml in diameter
- Warts can occur individually, in a line, or in a cluster.
- Some warts appear as a taller, flexible mass of skin resembling cauliflower.
- Some warts are flat and reddish.
- Signs and symptoms of plantar warts include:
  - Individual or grouped warts on the sole of the foot
  - Foot pain
  - Formation of callus
  - Pain in the foot, leg, or back caused by distortion of normal posture

SCOPE

Warts affect 7% to 10% of the population in the United States, primarily young adults and children. Plantar warts are widespread, affecting about 2% of the population.

MOST AFFECTED

Warts can affect persons of any age, but are more common among children and young adults. They are more common among women than men.

CAUSES

Human papillomavirus (HPV)

RISK FACTORS

- Acquired immunodeficiency syndrome (AIDS) or other immune system disorder
- Immunosuppressive drug use
- Dermatitis
- Locker room use
- Skin trauma

 DIAGNOSIS

WHAT THE DOCTOR LOOKS FOR

- The doctor will consider other conditions that appear similar (e.g., corns, calluses, or scar tissue).
- Visual inspection usually confirms the diagnosis of warts.

TESTS AND PROCEDURES

A biopsy of tissue can be obtained for pathologic examination.

 TREATMENT

GENERAL MEASURES

- Warts are managed on an outpatient basis.
- Spontaneous remissions are common and are probably related to the normal immune response.
- If warts cause no symptoms, no treatment is necessary. However, warts can spread.
- Conservative, nonscarring treatments are preferred.
- Treatment is associated with a 60% to 70% cure rate.
- Repeated warm soaks followed by peeling the top layer of skin may speed disappearance.
- Over-the-counter remedies containing salicylic acid may help. Read and follow directions carefully.
- Other measures include use of a heel bar or appropriate padding to relieve pressure points where warts tend to aggregate.
- Occlusion: the easiest and least expensive treatment. The wart is covered with a waterproof tape for a week. The tape is removed and left open for 12 hours, then retaped if the wart is still present. The environment under the tape hinders viral growth.
- Surgical measures include:
  - Cryotherapy: Freezing of warts is often preferred because scar formation is minimized; usually requires several treatments.
  - Excision with electrocautery, laser, or curettage
  - Blunt dissection: a simple surgical procedure that is effective and usually nonscarring; involves separating wart from normal skin with a blunt instrument

ACTIVITY

Plantar warts occasionally cause discomfort, requiring a decrease in activity.

 MEDICATIONS

COMMONLY PRESCRIBED DRUGS

- No effective antiviral wart medications currently exist.
- All treatments begin by paring the wart as closely as possible, then soaking the area in warm water to moisten the wart.
- Chemotherapy: topical retinoids: tretinoin (retinoic acid, Retin-A) Salicylic acid (Trans-Ver-Sal, Mediplast, Duofilm, Keralyt)

CONTRAINDICATIONS

Read product information for specific drugs. A vascular disorder may be a contraindication for some treatments. Infection may be a contraindication.

Warts

Doctor
Office
Phone
Pager

Special notes to patient:

Warts

PRECAUTIONS

Avoid normal skin when using topical chemicals. Treatment can cause the formation of scars.

OTHER DRUGS

- Chemotherapy:
- Benzoyl peroxide
  - Other chemotherapy: dichloroacetic acid, trichloroacetic acid, podophyllin, 5-fluorouracil, silver nitrate, idoxuridine (Herplex Liquifilm)
  - Bleomycin: expensive and causes severe pain, but has a 75% cure rate
- Vesicants containing cantharidin (Cantharone)
- Immunotherapy:
  - Dinitrochlorobenzene (DNCB)
  - Interferon

FOLLOW-UP

PATIENT MONITORING

Close observation for recurrence when treatment may be better.

PREVENTION

- Warts are infectious and can be transmitted to others. Warts should be covered during treatment to avoid being transmitted to healthy skin or to other people.
- Avoid the wound fluid after cryotherapy.
- Use personal footwear in locker room settings.

POSSIBLE COMPLICATIONS

- Warts can spread to healthy skin.
- Removal of plantar warts can cause chronic pain and formation of scar.
- Warts of the nail bed can cause deformity of fingernails.
- Some warts can become malignant—watch for rapid growth, easy bleeding, discoloration.

WHAT TO EXPECT

The outcome of warts varies. Many times, warts completely resolve with or without treatment. The course of plantar warts is highly variable. Most resolve spontaneously in weeks to months.

MISCELLANEOUS

PEDIATRIC

Warts are more common in children. The duration of plantar warts is generally shorter in children than in adults.

GERIATRIC

Less common in non-immunocompromised adults

FURTHER INFORMATION

American Academy of Dermatology, (708) 330-0230.

Warts

Doctor
Office
Phone
Pager

Special notes to patient:

Index

-A-

Abdominal pain
  in appendicitis, 41
  and migraine in children, 343
  in pancreatitis, 379
Abortion, spontaneous (miscarriage), 345–346, 515
Abscess, gastrointestinal, 171
Abuse
  of child (see Child abuse)
  sexual (see Sexual abuse and assault)
  of substances (see Substance abuse)
ABVD chemotherapy in Hodgkin's disease, 251
ACE inhibitors
  in heart attack, 231
  in heart failure, 121
  in hypertension, 255
Acebutolol (see Beta blockers)
Acetaminophen (Tylenol and others)
  in fever and seizures, 451
  in influenza, 273, 275
  in insect bites and stings, 281
  in meningitis, viral, 331
  in migraine, 341
  poisoning from, 1–4
  in shingles, 453
Acetazolamide in glaucoma, 213
Acetylcysteine in acetaminophen poisoning, 1
Acne, 5–6
Acquired immunodeficiency syndrome (AIDS), 247–250
  Kaposi's sarcoma in, 247, 295
  toxoplasmosis in, 493
Acute appendicitis, 41–42
Acute bronchitis, 77–78
Acute diarrhea, 165–166
Acute epiglottitis, 183
Acute glaucoma, angle-closure, 213
Acute glomerulonephritis (kidney inflammation), 215–216
Acute lymphoblastic leukemia (ALL) in adults, 309–310
Acute pancreatitis, 379
Acute renal (kidney) failure (ARF), 425–426
Acute situational anxiety, 37
Acyclovir. see also Antiviral drugs
  in chickenpox, 97
  in herpes simplex virus infections, 241, 243
  in pneumonia, 395
  in shingles, 453
ADA (American Diabetes Association), 159
Adenovirus infection, 7–8
ADHD (attention deficit hyperactivity disorder), 55–58
Adjustment disorder with anxious mood, 37
Adolescents
  acne in, 5
  alcohol abuse in, 9, 11
  attention deficit hyperactivity disorder in, 55, 57
  bed wetting (nocturnal enuresis) in, 63
  common cold in, 117
  German measles (rubella) in, 209
  gonorrhea in, 217
  mononucleosis in, 351
  mumps in, 359
  obsessive-compulsive disorder in, 369
  pelvic inflammatory disease (PID) in, 217, 385
  sexually transmitted diseases (STDs) in, 217, 385
alpha-Adrenergic agents in hypertension, 255
beta-Adrenergic agonists in asthma, 51, 53

beta-Adrenergic blockers (see Beta blockers)
Adult-onset (non-insulin-dependent) diabetes mellitus (NIDDM), 159–162
Affective disorder, seasonal (SAD), 447–448
Age-related conditions. see also Adolescents; Children; Elderly; Infants
  macular degeneration (ARMD), 323–324
AIDS/HIV, 247–250
  Kaposi's sarcoma in, 247, 295
  toxoplasmosis in, 493
Airway obstruction
  in asthma, 51
  in epiglottitis, 183
  sleep apnea in, 457
Alcohol use and alcoholism, 9–12
  acetaminophen poisoning in, 1
  cirrhosis in, 113
  hepatitis in, 239
  pancreatitis in, 379
  pernicious anemia in, 27
  vitamin deficiency in, 521
Aleve (see Naproxen sodium (Aleve, Anaprox))
ALL (acute lymphoblastic leukemia), 309–310
Allergy
  anaphylaxis in, 25
    in food allergy, 25, 193
    in insect bites and stings, 25 (see also Insect bites and stings)
  asthma in, 51 (see also Asthma)
  balanitis in, 59
  dermatitis in, 153
  to drugs
    anaphylaxis in, 25
    cutaneous reactions in, 139
  to foods, 193–194
    anaphylaxis in, 25, 193
    rash in, 193, 419
  to insect bites and stings, 279, 281
    anaphylaxis in, 25
  pink eye (conjunctivitis) in, 389
  rhinitis in (hay fever), 429–432
  sinusitis in, 455 (see also Sinusitis)
  urticaria (hives) in, 419
Allopurinol in gout, 219
Alopecia (hair loss), 13–14
Alpha-adrenergic agents in hypertension, 255
Alpha-tocopherol (vitamin E) deficiency, 521, 523
Alteplase (tissue plasminogen activator) in heart attack, 231
ALTEs (Apparent Life-Threatening Events), 473
  sudden infant death syndrome in, 473 (see also Sudden infant death syndrome)
Altitude illness, 15–18
Alzheimer's disease, 19–22, 147
  insomnia in, 19, 283
Amantadine
  in hepatitis, 239
  in influenza, 77, 273, 275
  in pneumonia, 395
Amblyopia (lazy eye), 303–304
Amenorrhea (absence of menstrual periods), 23–24
American Diabetes Association (ADA), 159
Amitriptyline (Elavil, Endep)
  in depression, 149 (see also Antidepressant drugs)
  in headache, 225
    migraine, 343
  in insomnia, 283

Amlodipine (*see* Calcium channel blockers)
Amnesia, dissociative, 167
Amphetamine diet drugs, 365
Amphotericin B. *see also* Antifungal drugs
   in candidiasis, 87
Ampligen in chronic fatigue syndrome, 107
Anal problems
   in hemorrhoids (piles), 237–238
   in pinworms (Enterobius vermicularis), 391
   in rectal prolapse, 237
Anaphylaxis (allergic shock), 25–26
   in food allergy, 25, 193
   in insect bites and stings, 25 (*see also* Insect bites and stings)
Anemia, 27–32
   iron deficiency, 287–288
   in parvovirus B19 infection, 383
   pernicious (vitamin B12 deficiency), 27–28
   sickle cell, 29–32
Angina, 33–34
   in arteriosclerosis, 43
Angiotensin-converting enzyme inhibitors
   in heart attack, 231
   in heart failure, 121
   in hypertension, 255
Angiotensin II receptor blockers in hypertension, 255
Animal bites, 35–36
   rabies in, 413–414
   from snakes, 461–462
Antacids
   in gastritis, 201
   in gastroesophageal reflux disease, 203, 205
   in peptic ulcer disease, 387
Anthelminthics (vermifuges) in pinworms, 391
Anti-anxiety drugs. *see also* Benzodiazepines
   in anxiety, 37, 39
   in irritable bowel syndrome, 289
Anti-asthma drugs, 51, 53
Antibiotics
   in acne, 5
   in animal bites, 35
   in appendicitis, 41
   in balanitis (penile inflammation), 59
   in blepharitis, 67
   in bronchitis, acute, 77
   in chlamydial infections, 103
   in cholera, 105
   in contact dermatitis, 153
   in cystic fibrosis, 141
   in diverticular disease, 171
   in epididymitis, 181
   in epiglottitis, 183
   in gastritis, 201
   in gingivitis, 211
   in gonorrhea, 217
   in impetigo, 269
   in laryngitis, 301
   in Lyme disease, 317
   in meningitis, 329
   in otitis media, 339
   in paronychia, 361
   in peptic ulcer disease and Helicobacter pylori infection, 387
   in pink eye (conjunctivitis), 389
   in pneumonia, 393
   in Rocky Mountain spotted fever, 433
   in rosacea, 435
   in Salmonella infection, 437
   in sinusitis, 455
   in sore throat, 463
   in stye, 471
   in syphilis, 479
   in tick-borne infections, 317, 433
   in toxic shock syndrome, 491
   in tuberculosis, 499
   in ulcerative colitis, 501
   in urinary tract infections, 509, 511, 513
Anticholinergics
   in asthma, 51 (*see also* Anti-asthma drugs)
   in irritable bowel syndrome, 289
Anticoagulants (blood thinners)
   in angina pectoris, 33
   in claudication, 115
   in heart attack, 231
   interaction with antidiarrheal drugs, 165
Anticonvulsant drugs, 449, 451
Antidepressant drugs. *see also* specific drugs
   in anxiety disorders, 37, 39
   in bulimia nervosa, 79
   in dementia, 147
   in depression, 149
   in dissociative disorders, 167
   in insomnia, 283
   in nocturnal enuresis, 63
   in posttraumatic stress disorder, 397
   in tension headache, 225
Antidiarrheal drugs, 165
   in ulcerative colitis, 501
Anti-fever drugs (antipyretics) in influenza, 273
Antiflatulent drugs in irritable bowel syndrome, 289
Antifungal drugs
   in balanitis, 59
   in candidal infections, 87, 517
   in diaper rash, 163
   in tinea infections, 489
Antihistamines
   in anaphylaxis, 25
   in common cold, 117, 119
   in contact dermatitis, 153
   in cutaneous drug reactions, 139
   in hay fever (allergic rhinitis), 429
   in insect bites and stings, 279, 281
   in insomnia, 283
   in sinusitis, 455
   in urticaria (hives), 419
Anti-inflammatory drugs, non-steroidal (*see* NSAIDs)
Antipsychotic drugs in dementia, 147
Anti-retroviral drugs in HIV infection and AIDS, 247
Antispasmodics
   in diverticular disease, 171
   in irritable bowel syndrome, 289
Antivenin
   in snake bites, 461
   in spider bites, 281
Antiviral drugs
   in chickenpox, 97
   in croup, 137
   in herpes simplex virus infections, 241, 243
   in HIV infection and AIDS, 247
   in influenza, 273, 275
   in pneumonia, 395
   in shingles, 453
Anxiety, 37–40
   in Alzheimer's disease, 19

and depression, 149
and mood disorders, 37 (see also Mood disorders)
and obsessive-compulsive disorder, 37, 39, 369 (see also
  Obsessive-compulsive disorder)
Apnea
  apparent life-threatening events in, 473
  in sleep, 457-460
Apparent life-threatening events, 473
Appendicitis, acute, 41-42
Appetite suppressants in obesity, 365
ARF (acute renal [kidney] failure), 425-426
ARMD (age-related macular degeneration), 323-324
Arteriosclerosis, 43-45. see also Cardiovascular problems
  angina pectoris in, 33
  claudication in, 115
  dementia in, 147
  heart disease in, 43-45, 231
  transient ischemic attack in, 497
Arthritis, 47-50
  in Crohn's disease, 133
  in lupus erythematosus, 481
  in Lyme disease, 317
  osteoarthritis, 47-48
  in parvovirus B19 infection, 383
  in psoriasis, 411
  rheumatoid (RA), 49-50
Ascorbic acid (vitamin C)
  in common cold, 117
  deficiency of, 521
Aspirin. see also NSAIDs
  in arteriosclerotic heart disease, 43
  in chickenpox, 97
  in claudication, 115
  in common cold, 119
  in dysmenorrhea, 175
  in heart attack, 231
  in influenza, 273, 275
  in meningitis, viral, 331
  in migraine, 341
  in mononucleosis, 351
  in mumps, 359
  in osteoarthritis, 47
  and Reye's syndrome (see Reye's syndrome and aspirin use)
  in transient ischemic attack and stroke, 467, 497
Assault, sexual, 415-418
  of child, 415, 417
  posttraumatic stress disorder in, 417 (see also Posttraumatic
    stress disorder)
Asthma, 51-54
  and allergic rhinitis, 429 (see also Rhinitis, allergic)
Atenolol (see Beta blockers)
Atherosclerosis, 43-45. see also Cardiovascular problems
  angina pectoris in, 33
  claudication in, 115
  dementia in, 147
  heart attack in, 43, 231
  transient ischemic attack in, 497
Athlete's foot (tinea pedis), 489
Atropine in Meniere's disease, 325
Attention deficit hyperactivity disorder (ADHD), 55-58
Autoimmune disorders
  lupus erythematosus in, systemic (SLE), 481-484
  rheumatoid arthritis in, 49
  thyroid problems in, 259, 265
Axid (nizatidine) (see H2 blockers)
Azathioprine in ulcerative colitis, 501

-B-

B19 parvovirus infection, 383-384
  erythema infectiosum in, 383
Back pain, 313-316
  in lumbar disk disorders, 315-316
  in osteoporosis, 371
Bacterial food poisoning, 195-196
  diarrhea in, 165, 195
  in Salmonella contamination, 437-440
Bacterial infections
  balanitis in, 59
  blepharitis in, 67
  bronchitis in, acute, 77
  chlamydial, 103-104, 389
  cholera in, 105-106
  diarrhea in, 165
  epididymitis in, 181
  epiglottitis in, 183
  glomerulonephritis in, 216
  gonorrhea in, 217-218, 385
  impetigo in, 269
  meningitis (brain/spinal cord inflammation) in, 329-330
  otitis media in, 339
  pelvic inflammatory disease in, 385
  pink eye (conjunctivitis) in, 103, 389
  pneumococcal, vaccination against, 267, 393
  pneumonia in, 393-394
  Salmonella, 437-440
  sore throat in, 463
  stye in, 471
  toxic shock syndrome in (Staphylococcus aureus), 491-492
  tuberculosis in, 499-500
  of urinary tract, 509-514
Bad breath (halitosis), 221-222
  in gingivitis, 211 (see also Gingivitis)
Balanitis (penile inflammation), 59-60
Baldness (alopecia), 13-14
Basal cell carcinoma, 61-62
Bed wetting (nocturnal enuresis), 63-64, 505
Bellergal (ergotamine-belladonna-phenobarbital) in
    Meniere's disease, 325
Bell's palsy, 65-66
Benadryl (see Antihistamines)
Benazepril (see ACE inhibitors)
Benign breast disease, 191
Benign prostatic hypertrophy (BPH), 409-410
Benzodiazepines
  in alcoholism, 9
  in anxiety disorders, 37, 39
  in dissociative disorders, 167
  in insomnia, 283, 285
  in posttraumatic stress disorder, 397
  in schizophrenia, 443
Benzphetamine in obesity, 365
Beta blockers
  in angina pectoris, 33
  in glaucoma, 213
  in headache, 225
    migraine, 343
  in heart attack, 231
  in heart failure, 121
  in hypertension, 255
  in hyperthyroidism, 259
  in mitral valve prolapse, 347
Beta-agonists in asthma, 51, 53

Betaxolol (*see* Beta blockers)
Bile accumulation (jaundice), 291–292
Bismuth subsalicylate (Pepto-Bismol)
   in diarrhea, 165
   in gastritis, 201
Bisprolol (*see* Beta blockers)
Bites, 35–36
   insect, 279–282
     anaphylaxis in, 25
   rabies in, 413–414
   snake, 461–462
   tick, 279, 281
     Lyme disease in, 317–318
     Rocky Mountain spotted fever in, 433–434
Bladder problems
   in benign prostatic hypertrophy, 409
   inflammation (cystitis), 509, 511
   urinary incontinence in, 505, 507
Bleeding
   cerebral, stroke in, 467
   gastrointestinal
     in diverticular disease, 171
     in hemorrhoids, 237
     in peptic ulcer disease, 387
     in ulcerative colitis, 501
   iron deficiency anemia in, 287
   from nose (epistaxis), 363–364
   uterine, dysfunctional, 173–174
   vaginal, in pregnancy, 515–516
     miscarriage in, 345, 515 (*see also* Miscarriage)
   in vitamin K deficiency, 521
Blepharitis (eyelid inflammation), 67–68
Blindness from cataracts, 93
Blisters. *see also* Skin problems
   in herpes simplex virus infections, 241, 243
   in impetigo, 269
   in shingles, 453
Blood disorders in anemia (*see* Anemia)
Blood glucose disorders in diabetes mellitus, 155–162 (*see also* Diabetes mellitus)
Blood pressure
   high, 255–258 (*see also* Hypertension)
   low (hypotension), in heart failure, 121
Blood thinners (anticoagulants)
   in angina, 33
   in claudication, 115
   in heart attack, 231
   interaction with antidiarrheal drugs, 165
Blood vessel dilation (rosacea), 435–436
Bone and joint problems
   in bursitis, 85–86
   in carpal tunnel syndrome, 91–92
   in gout, 219–220
   low back pain in, 313–316
   in lumbar disk disorders, 315–316
   in menopause, 333, 335
   in osteoarthritis, 47–48
   in osteoporosis, 371–374
     in menopause, 333, 335
   in parvovirus B19 infection, 383
   in rheumatoid arthritis (RA), 49–50
   scoliosis (spinal curvature) in, 445–446
   in sprains and strains, 465–466
   temporomandibular joint (TMJ) syndrome in, 485–486
   in tendinitis, 487–488

Bone loss (osteoporosis), 371–374
   in menopause, 333, 335
Bowel problems. *see also* Gastrointestinal problems
   constipation in, 125–128 (*see also* Constipation)
   diarrhea in, 165–166 (*see also* Diarrhea)
BPH (benign prostatic hypertrophy), 409–410
"Brain attack" (stroke), 467–470
   dementia in, 147
   in hypertension, 467, 469, 497 (*see also* Hypertension)
   transient, 497–498
Brain disorders. *see also* Nervous system problems; Psychiatric/psychological problems
   edema at high altitude, 15
   in lead poisoning, 305, 307
   in meningitis, 329–332
Breast disease
   cancer, 69–72
   fibrocystic, 191–192
   infection (mastitis), 75
Breast feeding, 73–76
Breath, bad (halitosis), 221–222
   in gingivitis, 211 (*see also* Gingivitis)
Breathing problems (*see* Respiratory problems)
Bromocriptine in fertility problems, 189
Bronchitis
   acute, 77–78
   chronic, 109–112
Bronchodilators
   in anaphylaxis, 25
   in asthma, 51, 53
   in bronchitis, acute, 77
Bulimia nervosa, 79–82
Bupropion (Wellbutrin) in depression, 149. *see also* Antidepressant drugs
Burkitt's lymphoma, 319–320
Burns, 83–84
   in abused child, 83, 101
   in sun exposure, 61, 83, 475–476
Bursitis, 85–86
Buspirone in anxiety disorders, 37

-C-

Calcitonin, synthetic salmon (Calcimar, Miacalcin, Osteocalcin), in osteoporosis, 371
Calcium channel blockers
   in angina pectoris, 33
   in cluster headache, 223
   in hypertension, 255
Calcium supplements
   in endometriosis, 179
   in osteoporosis, 371, 373
Calculi
   cholelithiasis, 199–200
     pancreatitis in, 379
   nephrolithiasis, 297–300
Cancer
   acute lymphoblastic leukemia (ALL) in adults, 309–310
   of breast, 69–72
   cervical, in dysplasia of cervix, 95
   of colon, in ulcerative colitis, 503
   Hodgkin's disease (Hodgkin's lymphoma), 251–252
   Kaposi's sarcoma, 295–296
     in HIV infection and AIDS, 247, 295

lymphoma, 319–322
  Burkitt's, 319–320
  Hodgkin's, 251–252
  non-Hodgkin's, 321–322
ovarian, 375–376
  hirsutism in, 245
of prostate, 407–408
of skin
  in basal cell carcinoma, 61–62
  in Kaposi's sarcoma, 295
  in sunburn, 61, 83, 475
of stomach, in pernicious anemia, 27
Candidal infections (candidiasis), 87–88
  of nails, 87, 361
  of vagina, 87, 517–518
Capsaicin cream
  in bursitis, 85
  in osteoarthritis, 47
Captopril (see ACE inhibitors)
Carbon monoxide (CO) poisoning, 89–90
Carcinoma. see also Cancer
  basal cell, 61–62
Cardiovascular problems
  angina in, 33–34
  in arteriosclerosis, 43–45, 231
  claudication in, 115
  congestive heart failure in, 121–124
  heart attack (myocardial infarction) in, 43, 231–234
  in hypertension, 255–258
  in mitral valve prolapse, 347–348
  stroke and mini-stroke (cerebrovascular accidents, TIAs) in, 467–470, 497–498
  varicose veins in, 519
Carpal tunnel syndrome, 91–92
Cataracts, 93–94
Cathartics in constipation, 125
Cerebrovascular accident (stroke), 467–470
  dementia in, 147
  in hypertension, 467, 469, 497 (see also Hypertension)
  "mini-" (TIAs), 497–498
Cervix uteri
  cancer of, 95
  dysplasia of, 95–96
    in papilloma virus infections, 95, 207
Charcoal, activated, in acetaminophen poisoning, 1
Chemotherapy
  ABVD, in Hodgkin's disease, 251
  in breast cancer, 69, 71
  in Kaposi's sarcoma, 295
  in lymphoblastic leukemia of adult, acute, 309
  in lymphoma, 321
    Burkitt's, 319
    Hodgkin's, 251
  MOPP, in Hodgkin's disease, 251
  in ovarian cancer, 375
Chenodiol in gallstones, 199
Chest pain
  in angina pectoris, 33–34
  in arteriosclerotic heart disease, 43
  in asthma, 51
  in gastroesophageal reflux disease, 203, 205
  in heart attack, 231
  in mitral valve prolapse, 347
  in pneumonia, 393, 395
Chickenpox (varicella), 97–100
  immunization against, 97, 267

shingles after, 99, 453
Child abuse, 101–102
  burns in, 83, 101
  dissociative disorders in, 167, 169
  neglect in, 101
  posttraumatic stress disorder in, 399 (see also Posttraumatic stress disorder)
  sexual, 101, 415, 417
    gonorrhea in, 217
    herpes simplex virus infection in, 243
    syphilis in, 479
Children. see also Adolescents; Infants
  acetaminophen poisoning in, 1, 3
  acne in, 5
  adenovirus infections in, 7
  alcohol abuse in, 9, 11
  alopecia in, 13
  altitude sickness in, 17
  anemia in
    iron deficiency, 287
    pernicious (vitamin B12 deficiency), 27
    sickle cell, 29, 31
  animal bites in, 35
  anxiety disorders in, 39
  appendicitis in, 41
  asthma in, 51, 53
  attention deficit hyperactivity disorder in, 55–58
  balanitis in, 59
  bed wetting (nocturnal enuresis) in, 63–64
  bronchitis in, acute, 77
  burns in, 83
  bursitis in, 85
  cataracts in, 93
  chickenpox (varicella) in, 97, 99
  chlamydial infection in, 103
  cholera in, 105
  chronic fatigue syndrome in, 107
  common cold in, 117, 119
  croup in, 137
  cystic fibrosis in, 141–144
  depression in, 151
  diabetes mellitus in, 155, 157, 161
  diaper dermatitis in, 163
  diarrhea in, 165
  epiglottitis in, 183
  febrile seizures in, 451
  fecal incontinence in, 187
  food allergy in, 193
  food poisoning in, 195
    in Salmonella contamination, 439
  gallstones in, 199
  gastroesophageal reflux in, 203, 205
  German measles (rubella) in, 209
  gingivitis (gum inflammation) in, 211
  glomerulonephritis in, 215
  gonorrhea in, 217
  headaches in, 223
    migraine, 341, 343
  heart failure in, 123
  heat injury in, 235
  hemorrhoids in, 237
  herpes simplex virus infections in, 241, 243
  HIV infection and AIDS in, 247, 249
  hypertension in, 257
  hyperthyroidism in, 259
  hypothermia in, 263

Children. (*Continued*)
  immunization (vaccination) in, 267
  impetigo in, 269
  influenza in, 273, 275
  laryngitis in, 301
  lazy eye (amblyopia) in, 303
  lead poisoning in, 305, 307
  lice (pediculosis) in, 229
  Meniere's disease in, 325
  menorrhagia in, 337
  molluscum contagiosum in, 349
  motion sickness in, 353
  mumps in, 359
  nosebleed in, 363
  obesity in, 367
  otitis externa in, 477
  otitis media in, 339
  pica (eating of non-food items) in, 305, 307
    and lead poisoning, 305, 307 (*see also* Lead poisoning)
  pinworms in, 391
  pneumonia in, 393, 395
  posttraumatic stress disorder (PTSD) in, 397, 399
  psoriasis in, 411
  rash in, 419, 421
  Reye's syndrome and aspirin use in (*see* Reye's syndrome and aspirin use)
  rhinitis in, allergic, 429, 431
  scabies in, 441
  sexual assault of, 415, 417
  sleep apnea in, obstructive, 459
  syphilis in, 479
  tendinitis in, 487
  toxic shock syndrome in, 491
  ulcerative colitis in, 503
  urinary tract infections in, 509, 513
  vitamin deficiencies in, 27, 521, 523
  warts in, 529
Chlamydial infection
  conjunctivitis in, 103, 389
  sexually transmitted, 103–104
Chloral hydrate in insomnia, 283
Cholelithiasis (gallstones), 199–200
  pancreatitis in, 379
Cholera, 105–106
Cholesterol-lowering drugs
  in angina pectoris, 33
  in arteriosclerotic heart disease, 43
Chorea, Huntington's, 253–254
Chronic bronchitis, 109–112
Chronic fatigue syndrome, 107–108
Chronic glaucoma, open-angle, 213
Chronic obstructive pulmonary disease, 109–112
Chronic pancreatitis, 379
Chronic tension headaches, 225
Cimetidine (Tagamet) (*see* H2 blockers)
Ciprofloxacin (*see* Antibiotics)
Circadian dysrhythmia (jet lag), 293–294
Cirrhosis of liver, 113–114
"Clap" (gonorrhea), 217–218
  pelvic inflammatory disease in, 217, 385 (*see also* Pelvic inflammatory disease)
  as sexually transmitted disease, 217 (*see also* Sexually transmitted diseases)
Claudication, 115–116
Clemastine (Tavist) (*see* Antihistamines)
Climacteric (*see* Menopause)

Clomiphene citrate in fertility problems, 189
Clot-busting (thrombolytic) drugs
  in heart attack, 231
  in stroke, 467
Clotrimazole (*see* Antifungal drugs)
Cluster headaches, 223–224
CO (carbon monoxide) poisoning, 89–90
Cobalamin (vitamin B12) deficiency, 27, 521
  pernicious anemia in, 27 (*see also* Pernicious anemia)
Cold, common, 117–120. *see also* Laryngitis; Sore throat
Cold exposure
  frostbite in, 197–198
  hypothermia in, 261–264
  intolerance of (Raynaud's phenomenon), 423–424
  rash in, 419
Colic, renal, in nephrolithiasis, 297–300
Colitis, ulcerative, 501–504. *see also* Inflammatory bowel disease
Colon
  cancer of, in ulcerative colitis, 503
  Crohn's disease of, 133
  spastic, in irritable bowel syndrome, 289–290
  ulcerative colitis of, 501–504
Common cold, 117–120. *see also* Laryngitis; Sore throat
Compulsions, 369
Condoms, 129. *see also* Contraception
  female, 129
  male, 129
Condyloma acuminata (genital warts, venereal warts), 207–208
Congestive heart failure, 121–124
Conjunctivitis (pink eye), 389
  in chlamydial infection, 103, 389
Constipation, 125–128
  hemorrhoids (piles) in, 237
  in irritable bowel syndrome, 289 (*see also* Irritable bowel syndrome)
Contact dermatitis, 153–154
Continence problems (*see* Incontinence)
Contraception, 129–132
  oral agents in, 129, 131
    in dysmenorrhea, 175
    in endometriosis, 179
    in hirsutism, 245
Contraindications for drugs (*see* Drug precautions/interactions)
COPD (chronic obstructive pulmonary disease), 109–112
Coronary artery disease, 43–45
  angina pectoris in, 33
  heart attack in, 231
Corticosteroids (*see* Steroids)
Cough suppressants in common cold, 117
Cranial nerve disorders, Bell's palsy in, 65–66
Crib death (SIDS, sudden infant death syndrome), 473–474
Crohn's disease, 133–136
Cromolyn sodium in asthma, 51. *see also* Anti-asthma drugs
Croup, 137–138
Curvature of spine (scoliosis), 445–446
Cutaneous problems (*see* Skin problems)
Cyanocobalamin deficiency, 27–28, 521
Cystic fibrosis, 109, 141–144
  pancreatic disorders in, 141, 379
Cystitis, 509, 511

-D-

Deafness (*see* Ear problems)
Death of infant, sudden, 473–474

Decongestants. *see also* Antihistamines
  in allergic rhinitis, 429
  in common cold, 117, 119
  in sinusitis, 455
Degenerative disorders
  macular, age-related, 323–324
  osteoarthritis in, 47
Dehydration, 145–146
  in cholera, 105
  in diarrhea, 165
  in heat exposure, 235
Dementia, 147–148
  in Alzheimer's disease, 19–22, 147
  in Huntington's chorea, 253
  multi-infarct (in multiple strokes), 147
  in Parkinson's disease (parkinsonism), 381
Dental problems
  gingivitis (gum inflammation), 211–212 (*see also* Gingivitis)
  halitosis (bad breath) in, 221
  temporomandibular joint (TMJ) syndrome in, 485–486
Depersonalization disorder, 167
Depression, 149–152. *see also* Mood disorders
  and alcohol abuse, 9, 11
  in dementia, 147
    in Alzheimer's disease, 19, 21
  in seasonal affective disorder, 447
Dermatitis. *see also* Skin problems
  allergic, 153
  contact, 153–154
  diaper (diaper rash), 163–164
  primary, 153
Desipramine (Norpramin, Pertofrane)
  in dementia, 147
  in depression, 149 (*see also* Antidepressant drugs)
  in headache, 225
Dexfenfluramine (Redux) in obesity, 365
Diabetes mellitus, 155–162
  drug precautions in, 155, 159
  insulin-dependent (IDDM, type I diabetes, juvenile-onset diabetes), 155–158
  non-insulin-dependent (NIDDM, type II diabetes, adult-onset diabetes), 159–162
  in obesity, 159, 161, 367
Diaper rash, 153–164
Diaphragm, contraceptive, 129
Diarrhea, 165–166. *see also* Gastrointestinal problems
  in cholera, 105
  in food poisoning, 165, 195
  in irritable bowel syndrome, 289 (*see also* Irritable bowel syndrome)
  in protozoal infections, 165
  in travel, 165
  in ulcerative colitis, 501
  in viral infections, 165
Diazepam (*see* Benzodiazepines)
Didanosine in HIV infection and AIDS, 247
Diet
  in acne, 5
  in alcohol abuse, 9
  allergy to foods in, 193–194
    anaphylaxis in, 25, 193
    rash in, 193, 419
  in amenorrhea, 23
  in angina pectoris, 33
  in arteriosclerotic heart disease, 43
  in attention deficit hyperactivity disorder, 55
  in bulimia nervosa, 79, 81
  in cirrhosis, 113
  in cluster headache, 223
  in constipation, 125, 127
  in Crohn's disease, 133
  in diabetes mellitus, 155, 159
  in diarrhea, 165
  in diverticular disease, 171
  in dysmenorrhea, 175
  and eating disorders (*see* Eating disorders)
  in fecal incontinence, 187
  in fibrocystic breast disease, 191
  in gastroesophageal reflux disease, 203, 205
  in glomerulonephritis, 216
  in gout, 219
  in heart failure, 121
  in hemorrhoids, 237
  in hypertension, 255, 257
  in iron deficiency anemia, 287
  in macular degeneration, age-related, 323
  in obesity, 365, 367
  in osteoporosis, 371, 373
  in pernicious anemia, 27
  poisoning from food in, 195–196
    diarrhea in, 165, 195
    in Salmonella contamination, 437–440
  in sickle cell anemia, 29
  toxoplasmosis from food in, 493, 495
  in vitamin deficiency, 521, 523
Diethylpropion in obesity, 365
Digestive problems (*see* Gastrointestinal problems)
Dihydroergotamine mesylate in cluster headache, 223
Dilantin (phenytoin) in seizures, 449, 451. *see also* Seizures
Diltiazem (*see* Calcium channel blockers)
Diphenhydramine (Benadryl). *see also* Antihistamines
  in anaphylaxis, 25
  in insect bites and stings, 281
  in insomnia, 283
  in rash, 419
  in rhinitis, allergic, 429
Diphtheria, tetanus, pertussis (DPT) immunization, 267, 451
Disk (lumbar disk, spinal disk) disorders, 315–316
Dissociative amnesia, 167
Dissociative disorders, 167–170
Dissociative identity disorder, 167
Diuretics ("water pills")
  in glomerulonephritis (kidney inflammation), 215
  in heart failure, 121
  in hypertension, 255
  in renal failure, acute, 425
Diverticular disease, 171–172
Dizziness (vertigo)
  in inner ear infection, 277
  in Meniere's disease, 325
Doxepin (Adapin, Sinequan)
  in depression, 149 (*see also* Antidepressant drugs)
  in rash, 421
DPT (diphtheria, tetanus, pertussis) immunization, 267
  febrile seizures after, 451
Droperidol in Meniere's disease, 325
Drug allergy
  anaphylaxis in, 25
  cutaneous reactions in, 139, 419
Drug poisoning. *see also* Drug precautions/interactions
  from acetaminophen (Tylenol), 1–4
  from imipramine, 63

Drug precautions/interactions
  in acetaminophen poisoning, 1
  in acne, 5
  in alcohol detoxification, 9
  in allopurinol therapy, 219
  in alopecia, 13
  in Alzheimer's disease, 19
  in amantadine therapy, 273
  in amenorrhea, 23
  in angina pectoris, 33
  in antibiotic therapy
    in acne, 5
    in cholera, 105
    in diarrhea, 165
    in peptic ulcer disease, 387
    in Rocky Mountain spotted fever, 433
    in rosacea, 435
  in antidepressant drugs, 149
  in antidiarrheal drugs, 165
  in antifungal drugs, 87
  in antihistamines
    in common cold, 117
    in contact dermatitis, 153
  in antipsychotic drugs for dementia, 147
  in antiviral drugs, 241, 243, 273
  in anxiety disorders, 37
  in appendicitis, 41
  in aspirin use and Reye's syndrome (see Reye's syndrome and aspirin use)
  in asthma, 53
  in Bellergal (ergotamine-belladona-phenobarbital) for Meniere's disease, 325
  in benzodiazepines, 37
    in insomnia, 283
  in beta blockers for hypertension, 255
  in bismuth compounds (Pepto-Bismal)
    in diarrhea, 165
    in gastritis, 201
  in blepharitis, 67
  in calcium channel blockers for hypertension, 255
  in chemotherapy, 251
  in contraceptive methods, 129, 131
  in diabetes mellitus, 155, 159
  in expectorants for common cold, 117
  in fertility drugs, 189
  in glaucoma, 213
  in imipramine therapy, 63
  in immunizations (vaccinations), 267
  in ipecac therapy for acetaminophen poisoning, 1
  in isoniazid therapy, 499
  light sensitivity in, 311
  lupus erythematosus in, 481, 483
  in NSAID therapy, 47, 225
  in osteoarthritis, 47
  in penicillamine for kidney stones, 297
  in penile injection therapy, 271
  in phenothiazines in meningitis, 331
  in probenecid therapy, 219
  in rheumatoid arthritis, 49
  in rifampin therapy, 499
  in rimantadine therapy, 273
  in scopolamine
    in inner ear infections, 277
    in Meniere's disease, 325
    in motion sickness, 353
  in sedatives
    in insomnia, 283
    in Meniere's disease, 325
  in sickle cell anemia, 29
  skin (cutaneous) reactions in, 139, 419
  in steroid therapy for alopecia, 13
  in sulfasalazine for Crohn's disease, 133
  in tetracycline
    in cholera, 105
    in Rocky Mountain spotted fever, 433
    in rosacea, 435
  in weight loss drugs for obesity, 365
  in zolpidem for insomnia, 283
Dysmenorrhea, 175–176
  in endometriosis, 179
Dyspareunia, 377–378
  in menopause, 333, 377
Dysplasia, cervical, 95–96
  in papilloma virus infections, 95, 207

-E-

Ear problems
  infections
    inner (otitis interna, labyrinthitis), 277–278
    middle (otitis media), 339–340
    swimmer's ear (otitis externa), 477–478
  in Meniere's disease, 325–328
  tinnitus (ringing in ear)
    in inner ear infection, 277
    in Meniere's disease, 325
    in pernicious anemia, 27
Eating disorders
  bulimia nervosa in, 79–82
  obesity in, 365
  pica in, 305, 307
EBV (Epstein-Barr virus)
  and Burkitt's lymphoma, 319
  and lymphoblastic leukemia in adults, 309
  and mononucleosis, 351
Eclampsia (toxemia of pregnancy), 177–178
  in hypertension, 177, 401 (see also Hypertension)
  and preeclampsia, 177, 401 (see also Preeclampsia)
  seizures in, 177, 449
Econazole (see Antifungal drugs)
Edema (swelling)
  cerebral, in high altitude (HACE), 15
  pulmonary, in high altitude (HAPE), 15
Elavil (amitriptyline) (see Antianxiety drugs)
Elderly
  acetaminophen poisoning in, 3
  adenovirus infections in, 7
  alcohol abuse in, 11
  alopecia in, 13
  altitude sickness in, 17
  Alzheimer's disease in, 19–22
  anaphylaxis in, 25
  angina pectoris in, 33
  animal bites in, 35
  anxiety disorders in, 39
  appendicitis in, 41
  arteriosclerotic heart disease in, 45
  balanitis in, 59
  basal cell carcinoma in, 61

breast cancer in, 71
bronchitis in
   acute, 77
   chronic, 111
burns in, 83
bursitis in, 85
carbon monoxide poisoning in, 89
cataracts in, 93
chickenpox (varicella) in, 99
chronic fatigue syndrome in, 107
chronic obstructive pulmonary disease in, 111
cirrhosis in, 113
claudication in, 115
cold exposure in
   and frostbite, 197
   and hypothermia, 263
common cold in, 119
constipation in, 127
cutaneous drug reactions in, 139
dementia in, 19–22, 147
depression in, 151
dermatitis in, 153
   in incontinence, 163
diabetes mellitus in, 161
diarrhea in, 165
dissociative disorders in, 169
diverticular disease in, 171
ear infections in, 277
endometriosis in, 179
epididymitis in, 181
food poisoning in, 195
   in Salmonella contamination, 439
gallstones in, 199
gastroesophageal reflux disease in, 205
gingivitis (gum inflammation) in, 211
gout in, 219
headache in, 227
heart attack in, 233
heart failure in, 123
heat injury in, 235
hemorrhoids (piles) in, 237
herpes simplex virus infections in, 241
hirsutism in, 245
HIV infection and AIDS in, 249
hypertension in, 257
hyperthyroidism in, 259
hypothyroidism in, 265
immunization (vaccination) in, 267
impotence (erectile dysfunction) in, 271
influenza in, 273, 275
insomnia in, 285
iron deficiency anemia in, 287
Kaposi's sarcoma in, 295
laryngitis in, 301
lupus erythematosus in, 483
macular degeneration in, 323
Meniere's disease in, 325
menopause in, 333–336
menorrhagia in, 337
osteoarthritis in, 47
osteoporosis in, 371
painful intercourse (dyspareunia) in, 377
Parkinson's disease (parkinsonism) in, 381
pernicious anemia (vitamin B12 deficiency) in, 27
pneumonia in, 393, 395
posttraumatic stress disorder in, 397, 399

prostate hypertrophy in, benign, 409
psoriasis in, 411
Raynaud's phenomenon in, 423
renal failure in, acute, 425
rheumatoid arthritis in, 49
rhinitis in, allergic, 429, 431
scabies in, 441
sedatives for insomnia in, 285
shingles in, 453
sinusitis in, 455
skin rash in, 421
sleep apnea in, obstructive, 459
sprains and strains in, 465
toxic shock syndrome in, 491
transient ischemic attack in, 497
tuberculosis in, 499
ulcerative colitis in, 503
urinary incontinence in, 505, 507
urinary tract infections in, 509, 513
uterine bleeding in, 173
varicose veins in, 519
vitamin deficiency in, 523
   vitamin B12, 27
Emphysema, 109–112
Enalapril (*see* ACE inhibitors)
Encopresis (fecal incontinence), 187–188
Endocrine problems
   diabetes mellitus in, 155–162
   hyperthyroidism (goiter, Graves' disease) in, 259–260
   hypothyroidism (thyroid insufficiency, myxedema) in, 265–266
Endometriosis, 179–180
   fertility problems in, 179, 189
Enemas in constipation, 125
Engorgement of breasts in breast feeding, 75
Enterobius vermicularis (pinworms), 391–392
Enuresis (urinary incontinence), 505–508
   nocturnal (bed wetting), 63–64, 505
   in prostate problems, 409, 505, 507
   stress, 505, 507
   urinary tract infections in, 507, 509, 513
   and vulvovaginitis, estrogen deficient, 525
Epididymitis, 181–182
Epiglottitis, 183–184
Epilepsy, 449, 451
Epinephrine
   in allergic reactions, 25
      in insect bites and stings, 279, 281
   in glaucoma, 213
Episodic tension headaches, 225
Epistaxis (nosebleed), 363–364
Epstein-Barr virus (EBV)
   and Burkitt's lymphoma, 319
   and lymphoblastic leukemia in adults, 309
   and mononucleosis, 351
Erectile dysfunction (impotence), 271–272
   in multiple sclerosis, 355, 357
Ergotamine
   with belladonna and phenobarbital in Meniere's disease, 325
   in cluster headache, 223
   in migraine, 341, 343
ERT (estrogen replacement therapy) (*see* Estrogen replacement therapy)
Erythema infectiosum, 383
Erythromycin
   in acne, 5
   in impetigo, 269

Esophagus, in gastroesophageal reflux disease, 203–206
Essential hypertension, 255–258
Estrogen replacement therapy (ERT)
  in Alzheimer's disease, 19
  in amenorrhea (absence of menstrual periods), 23
  in menopause, 333, 335
  in menorrhagia (excessive flow), 337
  in osteoporosis, 333, 335, 371, 373
  in painful intercourse, 377
  in vulvovaginitis, estrogen deficient, 525
Exercise-induced rash, 419
Expectorants in common cold, 117
Eye/eyelid problems
  in age-related macular degeneration (ARMD), 323–324
  in blepharitis (eyelid inflammation), 67–68
  in cataracts, 93–94
  in conjunctivitis (pink eye), 389–390
    in chlamydial infection, 103, 389
  in eyelash lice, 229
  in glaucoma, 213
  in herpes simplex virus infections, 241
  in lazy eye (amblyopia), 303–304
  in retinal detachment, 427–428
  in stye (hordeolum), 471–472
  in toxoplasmosis, 493
Eyelash lice, 229

-F-

Facial nerve palsy, 65–66
Famciclovir
  in herpes simplex virus infections, 241, 243
  in shingles, 453
Famotidine (Pepcid) (see H2 blockers)
Fatigue, 185–186
  in chronic fatigue syndrome, 107–108
  in depression, 149
  in mononucleosis, 351
  of muscles, in claudication, 115
Febrile seizures, 449, 451–452
Feces (see Stool)
Fenfluramine in obesity, 365
Ferrous sulfate in iron deficiency anemia, 287
Fertility drugs, 189
Fertility problems (see Infertility)
Fever
  in influenza, 273
  in Rocky Mountain spotted fever, 433
  seizures in, 449, 451–452
"Fever blisters" (herpes simplex), 241
Fibrocystic breast disease, 191–192
Fibrosis, cystic, 109, 141–144
  pancreatic disorders in, 141, 379
Fifth disease, 383
Flu
  and common cold, 273 (see also Common cold)
  and influenza, 273–276 (see also Influenza)
  and pneumonia, 273 (see also Pneumonia)
  in viral infections, 273 (see also Viral infections)
Fluconazole. see also Antifungal drugs
  in candidal infections, 87, 517
Fluid problems
  cerebral edema (swelling in brain), 15
  dehydration in, 145–146
    in cholera, 105
    in heat exposure, 235
  pulmonary edema, 15
  in renal failure, acute, 425
Fluoxetine (Prozac) in depression, 149. see also Antidepressant drugs
Fluvastatin (see Cholesterol-lowering drugs)
Food. see also Diet
  allergy to, 193–194
    anaphylaxis in, 25, 193
    rash in, 193, 419
  poisoning from, bacterial, 195–196
    diarrhea in, 165, 195
    in Salmonella contamination, 437–440
  toxoplasmosis from, 493, 495
Foot
  plantar warts of, 527–530
  tinea infection of, 489
Fosinopril (see ACE inhibitors)
Frostbite, 197–198. see also Cold exposure
Fugue, dissociative, 167
Fungal infections
  balanitis in, 59
  candidal, 87–88
    of nails, 87, 361
    of vagina, 87, 517–518
  of nails, 87, 361
  tinea (ring worm, jock itch, athlete's foot), 13, 489–490
Furosemide (Lasix) (see Diuretics)

-G-

Gallstones (cholelithiasis), 199–200
  pancreatitis in, 379
Ganciclovir in pneumonia, 395
Gastritis (inflammation of stomach lining), 201–202
Gastroesophageal reflux disease (esophageal inflammation, heartburn), 203–206
Gastrointestinal problems
  in appendicitis, 41
  constipation in, 125–128
    and hemorrhoids, 237
    in irritable bowel syndrome, 289
  in cystic fibrosis, 141
  dehydration in, 145
  diarrhea in, 165–166 (see also Diarrhea)
  in diverticular disease, 171–172
  fecal incontinence (encopresis) in, 187–188
  in food allergy, 193
  in food poisoning, 165, 195
    in Salmonella contamination, 437, 439
  in gallstones (cholelithiasis), 199
  in gastritis (inflammation of stomach lining), 201–202
  in gastroesophageal reflux disease (esophageal inflammation, heartburn), 203–206
  in hemorrhoids (piles), 237–238
  in inflammatory bowel disease
    Crohn's disease (regional ileitis), 133–136
    ulcerative colitis (idiopathic proctocolitis), 501–504
  in irritable bowel syndrome (spastic colon), 289–290
  in motion sickness, 353
  in pancreatitis, 379
  in peptic ulcer disease, 387–388

and pernicious anemia, 27
in pinworms (Enterobius vermicularis), 391
Gemfibrozil (see Cholesterol-lowering drugs)
Genetic disorders (see Inherited conditions)
Genital herpes, 241, 243-244
Genitourinary problems, 505-518
  in acute renal failure (ARF), 425-426
  in cystitis, 509, 511
  in female (see Gynecologic problems)
  in glomerulonephritis, acute, 215
  in herpes simplex virus infections, 241, 243-244
  in infections, 509-514
    in men, 59, 407, 509-510
    sexually transmitted (see Sexually transmitted diseases)
    in urinary incontinence, 507, 509, 513
    in women, 511-514
  in kidney stones (urolithiasis, nephrolithiasis, renal colic), 297-300
  in male, 509-510
    balanitis, 59-60
    in candidal infections, 87
    in chlamydial infections, 103
    contraception, 129
    in epididymitis, 181-182
    fertility concerns in, 189
    in gonorrhea, 217
    in herpes simplex virus infection, 243
    impotence in, 271-272, 355, 357
    orchitis (testicular inflammation) in mumps, 359
    in papilloma virus infection and warts, 207
    in prostate cancer, 407-408
    in prostate hypertrophy, benign (BPH), 409-410
    in syphilis, 479
  in multiple sclerosis, 355, 357, 505
  painful intercourse in, 377
  urinary incontinence in, 505-508
    nocturnal, bed wetting in, 63-64, 505
    in prostate problems, 409, 505, 507
    stress, 505, 507
    and urinary infections, 507, 509, 513
    and vulvovaginitis, estrogen deficient, 525
  in warts (condyloma acuminata), 207-208
Geriatric problems (see Elderly)
German measles (rubella), 209-210
  vaccine, 209, 267, 451
Gingivitis (gum inflammation), 211-212
Glandular problems (see Endocrine problems)
Glaucoma, 213-214
  acute angle-closure, 213
  chronic open-angle, 213
Glomerulonephritis, acute (kidney inflammation), 215-216
Glucose disorders in diabetes mellitus, 155-162.
    see also Diabetes mellitus
Goiter (hyperthyroidism, Graves' disease), 259
Gonorrhea ("clap"), 217-218
  pelvic inflammatory disease in, 217, 385
Gout, 219-220
Graves' disease (hyperthyroidism, goiter), 259
"Grippe" (influenza), 273
Griseofulvin in tinea infections, 13, 489
Gum inflammation (gingivitis), 211-212
Gynecologic problems (women's problems)
  of breast
    cancer, 69-72
    fibrocystic disease, 191-192
  in cervical dysplasia, 95-96
  contraception, 129-132

  in cystitis (bladder inflammation), 511
  in dysfunctional uterine bleeding, 173-174
  in endometriosis, 179-180
    fertility problems in, 179, 189
  in estrogen deficiency
    painful intercourse in, 377
    vulvovaginitis in, 525-526
  fertility concerns in, 189
  hirsutism in, 245
  in menopause, 333-336
  menstrual (see Menstrual problems)
  in ovarian cancer, 375-376
  painful intercourse in, 377
  of pregnancy (see Pregnancy)
  in sexually transmitted diseases (STD) (see Sexually transmitted diseases)
  in urinary tract infections, 511-514
  in vulvovaginitis
    in estrogen deficiency, 525-526
    in yeast (candidal) infection, 87, 517-518

-H-

H2 blockers
  in gastritis, 201
  in gastroesophageal reflux disease (heartburn), 203, 205
  in peptic ulcer disease, 387
  in urticaria (hives), 421
HACE (high altitude cerebral edema), 15
Hair problems
  in alopecia (hair loss), 13-14
  in hirsutism (excessive growth), 245-246
Halitosis (bad breath), 221-222
  in gingivitis, 211 (see also Gingivitis)
Haloperidol. see also Antipsychotic drugs; Neuroleptics
  in dementia, 147
  in Huntington's chorea, 253
  in schizophrenia, 443
HAPE (high altitude pulmonary edema), 15
HAV (hepatitis A virus), 239, 267
Hay fever (allergic rhinitis), 429-432
HBV (hepatitis B virus), 239, 267
HCV (hepatitis C virus), 239
Head lice (pediculosis capitis), 229-230
Headache, 223-228
  in altitude illness, 15
  cluster, 223-224
  migraine, 341-344
  tension, 225-228
Hearing disorders (see Ear problems)
Heart attack (myocardial infarction), 231-234
  in atherosclerosis, 43, 231
Heart problems. see also Cardiovascular problems
  angina pectoris in, 33
  in arteriosclerosis (coronary artery disease, CAD), 43-45, 231
  congestive failure in, 121-124
  in mitral valve prolapse, 347-348
  in myocardial infarction, 43, 231-234
Heartburn (gastroesophageal reflux disease), 203-206
Heat exposure
  exhaustion and heat stroke in (hyperthermia), 235-236
  rash in, 419
  sunburn in, 61, 83, 475-476

Helicobacter pylori infections, 201
  and peptic ulcer disease, 387
Hemophilus influenza vaccine, 267
Hemorrhage (see Bleeding)
Hemorrhoids (piles), 237–238
Heparin (see Anticoagulants)
Hepatic conditions (see Liver problems)
Hepatitis, viral, 239–240
  A (HAV), 239, 267
  B (HBV), 239, 267
  C (HCV), 239
  vaccine, 239, 267
Herniated (ruptured) disk, 315
Herpes simplex virus infections, 241–244
  blisters in, 241
  genital, 241, 243–244 (see also Genital herpes)
Herpes zoster (shingles), 453–454
  after chickenpox, 99, 453 (see also Chickenpox)
High altitude, 15–18
  cerebral edema (HACE) in, 15
  pulmonary edema (HAPE) in, 15
High blood pressure (see Hypertension)
Hirsutism (excessive hair growth), 245–246
Histamine H2 blockers (see H2 blockers)
HIV infection and AIDS, 247–250
  Kaposi's sarcoma in, 247, 295
  toxoplasmosis in, 493
Hives (urticaria), 419–422. see also Rash; Skin problems
Hodgkin's disease (lymphoma), 251–252
Hordeolum (stye), 471–472
Hormone therapy
  in amenorrhea, 23
  in breast cancer, 69, 71
  estrogen in (see Estrogen replacement therapy)
  in osteoporosis, 333, 335, 371, 373
  progesterone (see Progesterone replacement therapy)
"Hot flashes" in menopause, 333. see also Menopause
HPV (human papilloma virus)
  and cervical dysplasia, 95, 207
  and genital warts, 207
Human immunodeficiency virus and AIDS (HIV/AIDS), 247–250
  Kaposi's sarcoma in, 247, 295
  toxoplasmosis in, 493
Human papilloma virus (HPV)
  and cervical dysplasia, 95, 207
  and genital warts, 207
Huntington's chorea, 253–254
Hydrocortisone (see Steroids)
Hyperactivity (attention deficit disorder, ADHD), 55–58
Hyperglycemia in diabetes mellitus, 155. see also Diabetes mellitus
Hypersensitivity (see Allergy; Anaphylaxis)
Hypertension
  essential, 255–258
  in kidney disorders, 215, 255
  in pregnancy, 257
    eclampsia and preeclampsia in, 177, 401–402
  transient ischemic attacks and stroke in, 467, 469, 497
Hyperthermia, 235–236. see also Heat exposure
Hyperthyroidism (Graves' disease, goiter), 259–260
Hypertrophy of prostate, benign, 409–410
Hypoglycemia in diabetes mellitus, 155. see also Diabetes mellitus
Hypotension in heart failure, 121
Hypothermia (cold exposure), 261–264
Hypothyroidism (thyroid insufficiency, myxedema), 265–266
Hypovolemic shock in cholera, 105

-I-

Ibuprofen
  in dysmenorrhea, 175
  in headache, 225
    migraine, 341
  in influenza, 273
Icterus (jaundice), 291–292
IDDM (insulin-dependent diabetes mellitus), 155–158
Identity disorder, dissociative, 167
Idiopathic proctocolitis (ulcerative colitis), 501–504. see also Inflammatory bowel disease
Ileitis, regional (Crohn's disease), 133–136
Imipramine
  in depression, 149 (see also Antidepressant drugs)
  in headache, 225
  in nocturnal enuresis, 63
Immune globulin
  rabies, 413
  varicella zoster, 97
Immunization (see Vaccination)
Immunodeficiency syndrome, acquired (AIDS), 247–250
  Kaposi's sarcoma in, 247, 295
  toxoplasmosis in, 493
Immunomodulator drugs in ulcerative colitis, 501
Imodium (loperamide)
  in diarrhea, 165 (see also Diarrhea)
  in irritable bowel syndrome, 289
Impetigo, 269–270
Implantable contraceptives, 129, 131
Impotence (erectile dysfunction), 271–272
  in multiple sclerosis, 355, 357
Incontinence
  diaper rash in, 163
  fecal (encopresis), 187–188
  urinary (enuresis), 505–508
    infections of urinary tract in, 507, 509, 513
    nocturnal, bed wetting in, 63–64, 505
    in prostate problems, 409, 505, 507
    stress, 505, 507
    and vulvovaginitis, estrogen deficient, 525
Indinavir in HIV infection and AIDS, 247
Infants. see also Children
  adenovirus infections in, 7
  breast feeding of, 73–76
  candidiasis in, 87
  cataracts in, 93
  chickenpox in newborn, 99
  chlamydial infection in, 103
  common cold in, 117
  croup in, 137
  cystic fibrosis in, 141, 143
  diaper rash (diaper dermatitis) in, 163
  febrile seizures in, 451
  gastroesophageal reflux disease in, 205
  German measles (rubella) in, 209
  gonorrhea in, 217
  herpes simplex virus infections in, 241
  HIV infection and AIDS in, 249
  hypothermia in, 263
  impetigo in, 269
  jaundice in, 291
  sickle cell anemia in, 29, 31
  sudden infant death syndrome (SIDS) in, 473–474
  toxoplasmosis in, 493, 495

Infarction
  cerebral, 467
    dementia in, 147
  myocardial (heart attack), 231–234
    in atherosclerosis, 43, 231
Infections. *see also* Infectious (contagious) diseases
  bacterial (*see* Bacterial infections)
  balanitis in, 59
  of breast (mastitis), 75
  chlamydial, 103–104, 389
  diarrhea in, 165
  of ear
    inner (otitis interna, labyrinthitis), 277–278
    middle (otitis media), 339–340
    swimmer's ear (otitis externa), 477–478
  fungal (*see* Fungal infections)
  laryngitis in, 301
  opportunistic, in HIV infection and AIDS, 247, 249
  parasitic (*see* Parasitic infections)
  pharyngitis in, 463
  pneumonia in, 7, 393–396
  protozoal
    diarrhea in, 165
    toxoplasmosis in, 493–496
  respiratory (*see* Respiratory problems, infections)
  sinusitis (inflammation/infection of sinuses) in, 455
  of skin
    candidal, 87
    tinea, 489–490
  sore throat in, 463–464
  of vagina, 87, 517–518
  viral (*see* Viral infections)
  yeast (candidal), 87–88
    of nails, 87, 361
    of vagina, 87, 517–518
Infectious (contagious) diseases. *see also* Infections
  chickenpox (varicella) in, 97–100
  cholera in, 105–106
  common cold in, 117–120
  German measles (rubella) in, 209
  HIV infection and AIDS in, 247–250
  meningitis (inflammation of brain and spinal cord) in, 329–332
  molluscum contagiosum in, 349
  mumps in, 359
  rabies in, 413–414
  scabies in, 441–442
  sexually transmitted (*see* Sexually transmitted diseases)
  tick-borne
    Lyme disease in, 317–318
    Rocky Mountain spotted fever in, 433–434
  tuberculosis in, 499–500
  warts in, 527–530
Infertility, 189–190
  in chlamydial infections, 103
  in endometriosis, 179, 189
  in epididymitis, 181
  in hirsutism, 245
Inflammation. *see also* Infections; Infectious (contagious) diseases
  acne in, 5–6
  of appendix vermiform, 41–42
  arthritis in
    osteoarthritis, 47
    rheumatoid, 49
  of brain and spinal cord (meningitis), 329–332
    bacterial, 329–330
    viral, 331–332
  bronchial (bronchitis), 77–78
  bursitis in, 85–86
  contact dermatitis in, 153–154
  of ear (*see* Ear problems, infections)
  of epiglottis, 183–184
  of esophagus (reflux disease, heartburn), 203–206
  of eyelid (blepharitis), 67–68
  gastrointestinal
    in Crohn's disease (regional ileitis), 133–136
    in diverticular disease, 171–172
    pancreatic (pancreatitis), 379–380
    of stomach lining (gastritis), 201–202
    in ulcerative colitis, 501–504
  genitourinary
    of bladder (cystitis), 509, 511
    epididymitis in, 181–182
    of kidneys (glomerulonephritis), 215–216
    pelvic inflammatory disease (PID) in, 217
    of penis (balanitis), 59–60
    in sexually transmitted diseases (*see* Sexually transmitted diseases)
    testicular (orchitis), in mumps, 359
  gout in, 219
  of gums (gingivitis), 211–212
  of larynx (laryngitis), 301–302
  nasal, in allergic rhinitis (hay fever), 429
  respiratory, in common cold, 117–120
  in sinusitis, 455
  of tendon (tendinitis), 487–488
  of uterus (endometriosis), 179–180
Inflammatory bowel disease
  Crohn's disease (regional ileitis), 133–136
  ulcerative colitis (idiopathic proctocolitis), 501–504
Influenza, 271–276
  bronchitis in, 77
  sore throat in, 273 (*see also* Sore throat)
  vaccine, 267, 275, 395
Inherited conditions
  cystic fibrosis in, 141
  diabetes mellitus in, 155, 159
  Huntington's chorea in, 253
  lazy eye (amblyopia) in, 303
  lupus erythematosus in, 481
  mitral valve prolapse in, 347
  sickle cell anemia in, 29–32
Injuries (*see* Trauma)
Insect bites and stings, 279–282
  anaphylaxis in, 25
Insomnia, 283–286
  in Alzheimer's disease, 19, 283
  in posttraumatic stress disorder, 397
Insulin-dependent diabetes mellitus (IDDM, type I diabetes, juvenile-onset diabetes), 155–158
Interactions of drugs (*see* Drug precautions/interactions)
Intercourse, painful (dyspareunia), 377–378
  in menopause, 333, 377
Interferon in hepatitis, 239
Intermittent claudication, 115
Intervertebral (spinal) disk disorders, 315–316
Intestinal problems (*see* Gastrointestinal problems)
Intrauterine devices (IUDs), 129, 131
Ipecac in acetaminophen poisoning, 1
Ipratropium in chronic obstructive pulmonary disease, 109
Iron deficiency anemia, 287–288
Irritable bowel syndrome (spastic colon), 289–290

Ischemia (lack of blood flow)
　of brain, 467–470, 497–498 (see also Stroke)
　of heart
　　in arteriosclerosis, 43–45
　　heart attack in, 43, 231–234 (see also Heart attack)
Isinopril (see ACE inhibitors)
Isoniazid. see also Antibiotics
　in tuberculosis, 499
Isotretinoin
　in acne, 5
　in rosacea, 435
Itching, 419. see also Rash; Skin problems
　in chickenpox, 97
　in contact dermatitis, 153
　in drug reactions, 139, 419
　in hemorrhoids, 237
　in lice (pediculosis), 229
　in pinworms, 391
　in psoriasis, 411
　in scabies, 441
　in shingles, 453
　in tinea infections (ring worm, jock itch, athlete's foot), 489
IUDs (intrauterine devices), 129, 131. see also Contraception

-J-

Jaundice (bile pigment accumulation, icterus), 291–292
Jaw problems in temporomandibular joint syndrome, 485–486
Jet lag (circadian dysrhythmia), 293–294
　insomnia in, 283
Jock itch (tinea cruris), 489
Joint problems (see Bone and joint problems)
Juvenile conditions. see also Children
　diabetes mellitus, 155–158
　pernicious anemia, 27

-K-

Kaposi's sarcoma, 295–296
　in HIV infection and AIDS, 247, 295
Ketoconazole. see also Antifungal drugs
　in tinea infections, 13, 489
Kidney problems. see also Genitourinary problems
　acute renal failure (ARF) in, 425–426
　in diabetes mellitus, 155, 159
　hypertension in, 215, 255
　inflammation (glomerulonephritis), 215–216
　kidney stone (urolithiasis, nephrolithiasis, renal colic), 297–300
　in lupus erythematosus, 481, 483

-L-

Labor, premature, 403–404
Labyrinthitis (inner ear infection), 277–278
Lactation and breast feeding, 73–76
Laryngitis, 301–302
Lasix (furosemide) (see Diuretics)

Laxatives in constipation, 125, 127
Lazy eye (amblyopia), 303–304
Lead poisoning, 305–308
　seizures in, 305, 307, 449
Leukemia, acute lymphoblastic (ALL), in adults, 309–310
Levothyroxine (Synthroid)
　in hypothermia, 261
　in hypothyroidism, 265
Lice, 279
　body (pediculosis corporis), 229
　eyelash (pediculosis capitis), 229
　head (pediculosis capitis), 229
　pubic (pediculosis pubis), 229
Light sensitivity (photosensitivity, sun poisoning), 311–312
　in lupus erythematosus, 481
Lithiasis
　cholelithiasis, 199–200
　　pancreatitis in, 379
　nephrolithiasis, 297–300
Lithium carbamate in cluster headaches, 223
Liver problems
　in cirrhosis, 113–114
　in hepatitis, 239, 267
　medication-related, from acetaminophen, 1, 3
Loperamide (Imodium)
　in diarrhea, 165
　in irritable bowel syndrome, 289
Lovastatin (see Cholesterol-lowering drugs)
Low back pain, 313–316
　in lumbar disk disorders, 315–316
Lumbar disk disorders, 315–316
Lung disease (see Respiratory problems)
Lupus erythematosus, systemic (SLE), 481–484
Lyme disease, 317–318
Lymphoma, 319–322
　Burkitt's, 319–320
　Hodgkin's (Hodgkin's disease), 251–252
　non-Hodgkin's, 321–322

-M-

Macular degeneration, age-related (ARMD), 323–324
Mammography
　in cancer of breast, 71
　in fibrocystic breast disease, 191
MAO inhibitors
　in bulimia nervosa, 79
　in depression, 149 (see also Antidepressant drugs)
Mastitis, 75
Mazindol in obesity, 365
Measles, 267
　German (rubella), 209–210
　　immunization against, 209, 267, 451
Median nerve compression in carpal tunnel, 91–92
Melatonin
　in insomnia, 285
　in jet lag, 293
Memory
　in dementia, 147
　　in Alzheimer's disease, 19
　in dissociative disorders, 167
Meniere's disease, 325–328
Meningitis (inflammation of brain and spinal cord), 329–332

bacterial, 329–330
viral, 331–332
Menopause, 333–336
  cluster headaches in, 223
  hirsutism in, 245
  painful intercourse (dyspareunia) in, 333, 377
  vulvovaginitis in, estrogen-deficient, 525–526
Menorrhagia (excessive flow), 337–338
Menstrual problems
  in amenorrhea (absence of menstrual periods), 23–24
  in dysmenorrhea (painful menstruation), 175–176
  in endometriosis (uterine inflammation), 179
  in menorrhagia (excessive flow), 337–338
  in premenstrual syndrome (PMS), 405–406
  and tampon-related toxic shock syndrome, 491
Mesalamine in Crohn's disease, 133
Metaproterenol in chronic obstructive pulmonary disease, 109
Methyl-butyl ether in gallstones, 199
Methylxanthines in asthma, 51. *see also* Anti-asthma drugs
Metoprolol (*see* Beta blockers)
Metronidazole. *see also* Antibiotics
  in Crohn's disease, 133
  in diarrhea, 165
Miacalcin in osteoporosis, 371
Miconazole (Monistat and others). *see also* Antifungal drugs
  in candidal infections, 517
  in tinea infections, 489
Middle ear infection (otitis media), 339–340
Migraine headache, 341–344
"Milk fever" (mastitis), 75
Mini-strokes (TIAs), 497–498. *see also* Stroke
  dementia in, 147
  in hypertension, 497 (*see also* Hypertension)
Minoxidil (Rogaine) in alopecia, 13
Miscarriage (spontaneous abortion), 345–346, 515. *see also* Premature labor
Mitral valve prolapse, 347–348
MMR (measles, mumps, rubella) vaccination, febrile seizures after, 451
Molluscum contagiosum, 349–350
Monoamine oxidase inhibitors
  in bulimia nervosa, 79
  in depression, 149
Mononucleosis (Epstein-Barr virus), 351–352
Mood disorders
  in alcohol abuse, 9, 11
  in Alzheimer's disease, 19, 21
  in anxiety disorders, 37
  in bulimia, 79
  in depression, 149–152
  in premenstrual syndrome, 405
  in seasonal affective disorder (SAD), 447
MOPP chemotherapy in Hodgkin's disease, 251
Motion sickness, 353–354
Mouth (*see* Dental problems)
Multi-infarct dementia, 147
Multiple sclerosis, 355–358
  urinary tract problems in, 355, 357, 505
Mumps, 359
  immunization against, 267, 359, 451
  orchitis in, 359
  pancreatitis in, 379
Muscle fatigue in claudication, 115
Musculoskeletal problems (*see* Bone and joint problems)
Mycostatin (*see* Antifungal drugs)

Myocardial infarction (heart attack, MI), 231–234
  in atherosclerosis, 43, 231
Myxedema (thyroid insufficiency, hypothyroidism), 265–266

-N-

Nadolol (*see* Beta blockers)
Nails, fungal infections of, 361–362
  candidal, 87, 361
Naproxen sodium (Aleve, Anaprox). *see also* NSAIDs
  in dysmenorrhea, 175
  in headache, 225
Nasal bleeding (epistaxis), 363–364
Nasal inflammation in allergic rhinitis (hay fever), 429–432
Nasal sprays. *see also* Antihistamines
  in allergic rhinitis, 429
  in common cold, 117
Neglect and child abuse, 101
Neonates (newborns) (*see* Infants)
Nephrolithiasis (renal colic, urolithiasis, kidney stones), 297–300
Nervous system problems
  Bell's palsy in, 65–66
  carpal tunnel syndrome in, 91–92
  in diabetes mellitus, 155, 159
  and headaches, 223 (*see also* Headache)
  in HIV infection and AIDS, 247
  Huntington's chorea in, 253
  in lead poisoning, 305, 307
  in Lyme disease, 317
  in meningitis, 329–332
  in multiple sclerosis, 355–358
  in Parkinson's disease (parkinsonism), 381–382
  in pernicious anemia (vitamin B12 deficiency), 27
  in rabies, 413
  seizure disorders in, 449
  in stroke and TIAs (transient ischemic attacks), 467–470, 497–498
  in syphilis, 479
  urinary incontinence in, 505
Neuroleptics in dissociative disorders, 167
Neurologic disorders (*see* Nervous system problems)
Nevirapine in HIV infection and AIDS, 247
Newborns (neonates) (*see* Infants)
Niacin (vitamin B3) deficiency, 521
NIDDM (non-insulin-dependent diabetes mellitus), 159–162
Nifedipine (*see* Calcium channel blockers)
Nipple problems in breast feeding, 75. *see also* Breast feeding
Nitroglycerin in angina pectoris, 33
Nizatidine (Axid) (*see* H2 blockers)
Nocturnal enuresis (bed wetting), 63–64, 505. *see also* Urinary incontinence
Non-Hodgkin's lymphoma, 321–322
Non-insulin-dependent diabetes mellitus (NIDDM), 159–162
Non-steroidal antiinflammatory drugs (*see* NSAIDs)
Nortriptyline (Pamelor, Aventyl)
  in depression, 149 (*see also* Antidepressant drugs)
  in headache, 225
    migraine, 343
Nosebleed (epistaxis), 363–364
NSAIDs
  in Alzheimer's disease, 19
  in back pain, 313, 315
  in bursitis, 85
  in carpal tunnel syndrome, 91

NSAIDs (*Continued*)
   in chronic fatigue syndrome, 107
   in dysmenorrhea, 175
   in epididymitis, 181
   in gout, 219
   in headache, 225
   in influenza, 273, 275
   in migraine, 341
   in osteoarthritis, 47
   precautions/interactions, 47, 225
   in rheumatoid arthritis, 49
   in shingles, 453
   in sprains and strains, 465
   in temporomandibular joint syndrome, 485
   in tendinitis, 487
Nutrition (*see* Diet)

-O-

Obesity, 365–368
   diabetes mellitus in, 159, 161, 367
   sleep apnea in, obstructive, 457, 459
Obsessive-compulsive disorder, 37, 39, 369–370
Obstructive pulmonary disease, chronic, 109–112
Obstructive sleep apnea, 457–460
Ocular disorders (*see* Eye/eyelid problems)
Opportunistic infections in HIV infection and AIDS, 247, 249
Oral contraceptives, 129, 131
   in dysmenorrhea, 175
   in endometriosis, 179
   in hirsutism, 245
Oral decongestants in common cold, 117
Oral hypoglycemic drugs, 159
Orchitis (testicular inflammation) in mumps, 359
Osgood-Schlatter disease, 487
Osteoarthritis, 47–48
Osteocalcin in osteoporosis, 371
Osteoporosis, 371–374
   in menopause, 333, 335
Otitis (ear inflammation/infection)
   externa (swimmer's ear), 477–478
   interna (inner ear, labyrinthitis), 277–278
   media (middle ear), 339–340
Ovarian cancer, 375–376
   hirsutism in, 245

-P-

Pain
   abdominal
     in appendicitis, 41
     and migraine in children, 343
     in pancreatitis, 379
   in back, 313–316
     in lumbar disk disorders, 315–316
     in osteoporosis, 371
   in chest (*see* Chest pain)
   in claudication, 115
   in epididymitis, 181
   in headaches, 223–228 (*see also* Headache)
   in intercourse (dyspareunia), 377–378
     in menopause, 333, 377
   in kidney stones, 297
   menstrual, 175–176
     in endometriosis, 179
   in shingles, 453
   in sickle cell crisis, 29
   in temporomandibular joint (TMJ) syndrome, 485
Painkillers (*see* specific drugs and drug types)
Palsy, Bell's, 65–66
Pancreatic disorders, 379–380
   in cystic fibrosis, 141, 379
   pernicious anemia in, 27
Pancreatitis, 379–380
   pernicious anemia in, 27
Panic disorder, 37, 39
   in motion sickness, 353
Papilloma virus, human
   and cervical dysplasia, 95, 207
   and genital warts, 207
Paralysis
   in Bell's palsy, 65–66
   infantile (poliomyelitis), immunization against, 267
   in multiple sclerosis, 355, 357
   in transient ischemic attacks and stroke, 467, 497
Parasitic infections
   lice (pediculosis), 229–230
   pinworms (Enterobius vermicularis), 391–392
   scabies (Sarcoptes scabiei) in, 441–442
   tick-borne
     Lyme disease in, 317–318
     Rocky Mountain spotted fever in, 433–434
   toxoplasmosis in, 493–496
Parkinson's disease (parkinsonism), 381–382
Paronychia (nail fungus), 361–362
Paroxetine (Paxil) in depression, 149. *see also* Antidepressant drugs
Parvovirus B19 infection, 383–384
   erythema infectiosum in, 383
Pediatric problems (*see* Children)
Pediculosis (louse infestation), 229–230
Pelvic inflammatory disease (PID), 385–386
   in chlamydial infection, 103
   in gonorrhea, 217, 385
Penbutolol (*see* Beta blockers)
Penicillamine. *see also* Antibiotics
   in kidney stones, 297
   in lead poisoning, 305
   in rheumatoid arthritis, 49
Penis
   balanitis of, 59–60
   erectile dysfunction of, 271–272
     in multiple sclerosis, 355, 357
   injection therapy in impotence, 271
Pepcid (famotidine) (*see* H2 blockers)
Peptic ulcer disease, 387–388
Pernicious anemia (vitamin B12 deficiency), 27–28
Personality disorder, 167
Pertussis vaccine, 267, 451
Pharyngitis. *see also* Common cold
   sore throat in, 463
Phendimetrazine in obesity, 365
Phenergan (*see* Antihistamines)
Phenothiazine
   in meningitis, 331
   in schizophrenia, 443
Phenytoin (Dilantin) in seizures, 449, 451. *see also* Seizures

Phobias, 37
Photosensitivity, 311–312
   in lupus erythematosus, 481
Physostigmine in glaucoma, 213
Pica (eating of non-food items), 305, 307
   lead poisoning in, 305, 307 (*see also* Lead poisoning)
Piles (hemorrhoids), 237–238
Pilocarpine in glaucoma, 213
Pindolol (*see* Beta blockers)
Pink eye (conjunctivitis), 389–390
   in chlamydial infection, 103, 389
Pinworms (Enterobius vermicularis), 391–392
Plantar warts, 527–530
Plasminogen activator, tissue, in heart attack, 231
PMS (premenstrual syndrome), 405–406
Pneumococcal vaccine, 267, 393
Pneumonia, 393–396
   bacterial, 393–394
   viral, 395–396
      adenovirus, 7
Podophyllin in genital warts, 207
Poisoning
   acetaminophen (Tylenol and others), 1–4
   carbon monoxide (CO), 89–90
   food, 195–196
      diarrhea in, 165, 195
      in Salmonella contamination, 437–440
   lead, 305–308
   snake bite, 461
   sun (light sensitivity, photosensitivity), 311–312
Poliomyelitis vaccine, 267
Posttraumatic stress disorder (PTSD), 37, 39, 397–400
   in rape (sexual assault), 417
Pravachol (*see* Cholesterol-lowering drugs)
Pravastatin (*see* Cholesterol-lowering drugs)
Prazosin in hypertension, 255
Preeclampsia, 177, 401–402
   eclampsia in, 177, 401 (*see also* Eclampsia)
Pregnancy
   in abused child, 101
   acetaminophen poisoning in, 3
   acne in, 5
   adenovirus infections in, 7
   alcohol abuse in, 11
   alopecia in, 13
   amenorrhea in, 23
   anaphylaxis in, 25
   angina pectoris in, 33
   antibiotics in
      in acne, 5
      in Rocky Mountain spotted fever, 433
      in rosacea, 435
   anxiety disorders in, 39
   asthma in, 53
   attention deficit hyperactivity disorder in, 57
   back pain in, 313, 315
   Bell's palsy in, 65
   bulimia nervosa in, 81
   carbon monoxide poisoning in, 89
   in cervical dysplasia, 95
   chickenpox (varicella) in, 99
   chlamydial infection in, 103
   cirrhosis in, 111
   common cold in, 119
   constipation in, 127
   and contraceptive practices, 129–132
   Crohn's disease in, 135
   in cystic fibrosis, 143
   depression in, 151
   dermatitis in, 153
   diabetes mellitus in, 157, 161
   diarrhea in, 165
   diverticular disease in, 171
   eclampsia in, 177–178, 401, 449
   ectopic, 515
   in endometriosis, 179
   food poisoning in, 195
   gastroesophageal reflux disease (heartburn) in, 205
   German measles (rubella) in, 209
   gonorrhea in, 217
   gout in, 219
   heart failure in, 123
   heat injury in, 235
   hemorrhoids in, 237
   hepatitis in, 239
   herpes simplex virus infection in, 241
      genital, 243
   in hirsutism, 245
   HIV infection and AIDS in, 249
   Hodgkin's disease in, 251
   hypertension in, 257
      and eclampsia, 177, 401 (*see also* Eclampsia)
      and preeclampsia, 177, 401 (*see also* Preeclampsia)
   hyperthyroidism in, 259
   immunization (vaccination) in, 267
   influenza in, 273, 275
   insomnia in, 283, 285
   iron deficiency anemia in, 287
   irritable bowel syndrome in, 289
   kidney stones in, 297, 299
   laryngitis in, 301
   lead exposure in, 307
   lupus erythematosus in, 483
   Lyme disease in, 317
   Meniere's disease in, 325
   migraine in, 343
   miscarriage (spontaneous abortion) in, 345–346, 515
   in mitral valve prolapse, 347
   mumps in, 359
   obesity in, 367
   obsessive-compulsive disorder in, 369
   osteoarthritis in, 47
   papilloma virus infection in, 207
   parvovirus B19 infection in, 383
   pelvic inflammatory disease (PID) in, 217, 385
   posttraumatic stress disorder in, 399
   preeclampsia in, 177, 401
   premature labor in, 403–404
   psoriasis in, 411
   rash in, 419, 421
   retinal detachment in, 427
   rheumatoid arthritis in, 49
   Rocky Mountain spotted fever in, 433
   rosacea in, 435
   scabies in, 441
   seizures in, 449
   in sexual assault, 415, 417
   shingles in, 453
   sickle cell anemia in, 31
   stroke in, 469
   syphilis in, 479
   toxemia of (eclampsia), 177–178, 401, 449

Pregnancy (*Continued*)
  toxic shock syndrome after, 491
  toxoplasmosis in, 493, 495
  transient ischemic attack in, 497
  ulcerative colitis in, 503
  urinary incontinence in, 507
  urinary tract infections in, 511, 513
  vaginal bleeding in, 345, 515–516
  vaginal yeast infection in, 517
  varicose veins in, 519
  vitamin deficiency in, 523
  vulvovaginitis in, estrogen deficient, 525
Premature labor, 403–404
Premenstrual syndrome (PMS), 405–406
Pressure urticaria, 419
Probenecid in gout, 219
Proctocolitis, idiopathic (ulcerative colitis), 501–504. *see also* Inflammatory bowel disease
Progesterone replacement therapy (PRT) in amenorrhea, 23
Progestogen in menopause, 333
Prolapse
  of mitral valve, 347–348
  rectal, 237
Promethazine (Phenergan). *see also* Antihistamines
  in inner ear infection, 277
  in Meniere's disease, 325
  in meningitis, viral, 331
Propranolol (*see* Beta blockers)
Prostate problems, 407–410
  benign hypertrophy (BPH), 409–410
  cancer, 407–408
  urinary incontinence in, 409, 505, 507
  urinary infections in, 407, 509
Protozoal infections
  diarrhea in, 165
  toxoplasmosis in, 493–496
Protriptyline (Vivactil) in depression, 149. *see also* Antidepressant drugs
Pruritus (*see* Itching)
Psoriasis, 411–412
Psychiatric/psychological problems
  in abused children, 101, 399
  acetaminophen poisoning in, 1
  alcohol abuse in, 9
  in Alzheimer's disease, 19, 21
  in anxiety disorders, 37–40
  in attention deficit hyperactivity disorder (ADHD), 55, 57
  in bulimia nervosa, 79, 81
  in chronic fatigue syndrome, 107
  in dementia, 147
  in depression, 149–152
  in dissociative disorders, 167–170
  insomnia in, 283, 285
  in mood disorders (*see* Mood disorders)
  obesity in, 365
  in obsessive-compulsive disorder, 37, 39, 369–370
  posttraumatic stress disorder (PTSD) in, 37, 39, 397–400, 417
  related to SIDS (crib death), 473
  in schizophrenia, 443–444
  seasonal affective disorder (SAD) in, 447–448
  in sickle cell anemia, 31
Psychoses (*see* Psychiatric/psychological problems)
PTSD (posttraumatic stress disorder), 37, 39, 397–400
  in rape (sexual assault), 417
Pubic lice ("crabs," pediculosis pubis), 229
Pulmonary disease (*see* Respiratory problems)
Pyridoxine (vitamin B6) deficiency, 521, 523

-Q-

Quinapril (*see* ACE inhibitors)

-R-

Rabies, 413–414
Radiation therapy in breast cancer, 69, 71
Radioiodine therapy in hyperthyroidism, 259
Raloxifene in breast cancer, 71
Ramipril (*see* ACE inhibitors)
Ranitidine (Zantac) (*see* H2 blockers)
Rape, 415–418
  posttraumatic stress disorder in, 417 (*see also* Posttraumatic stress disorder)
Rash, 419–422. *see also* Skin problems
  in anaphylaxis, 25
  in candidiasis, 87
  in chickenpox (varicella), 97
  in contact dermatitis, 153
  in cutaneous drug reactions, 139
  in diaper dermatitis, 163–164
  in drug allergy, 139
  in food allergy, 193, 419
  in German measles (rubella), 209
  in herpes simplex virus infections, 241
  in impetigo, 269
  in Lyme disease, 317
  in parvovirus B19 infection, 383
  in Rocky Mountain spotted fever, 433
  in shingles, 453
  in sun exposure, 419
    in photosensitivity, 311
  in toxic shock syndrome, 491
  in urticaria (hives), 419–422
Raynaud's phenomenon, 423–424
Rectal problems
  hemorrhoids (piles), 237–238
  prolapse, 237
Redux (dexfenfluramine) in obesity, 365
Reflux, gastroesophageal (heartburn), 203–206
Regional ileitis (Crohn's disease), 133–136
Renal colic (urolithiasis, kidney stones, nephrolithiasis), 297–300
Renal problems (*see* Kidney problems)
Reproductive problems
  and contraception, 129–132
  in female (*see also* Gynecologic problems)
    amenorrhea (absence of menstrual periods) in, 23–24
    miscarriage (spontaneous abortion) in, 345–346
    in pregnancy (*see* Pregnancy)
  infertility in, 189–189
  in male (*see also* Genitourinary problems, in male)
    in impotence, 271–272, 355, 357
  painful intercourse in, 377
  and sexually transmitted diseases (*see* Sexually transmitted diseases)
Respiratory problems
  in altitude illness, 15
  in anaphylaxis, 25
  in asthma, 51–54 (*see also* Asthma)
  in bronchitis
    acute, 77–78
    chronic, 109–112
  in chronic obstructive pulmonary disease (COPD), 109–112

in common cold, 117–120
in croup, 137
in cystic fibrosis, 109, 141
in emphysema, 109–112
in epiglottitis, 183
in food allergy, 193
in hay fever (allergic rhinitis), 429, 431
infections
   adenovirus, 7
   bacterial pneumonia, 393–394
   influenza (flu), 271–276
   tuberculosis, 499
   viral pneumonia, 7, 395–396
in laryngitis, 301
obstructive sleep apnea in, 457–460
in pneumonia, 7, 393–396
and sinusitis, 455 (see also Sinusitis)
Retina
  in age-related macular degeneration, 323
  detachment of, 427–428
Retin-A (tretinoin) in acne, 5
Retinoic acid in acne, 5
Retinol (vitamin A) deficiency, 521, 523
Reye's syndrome and aspirin use
  in chickenpox, 97
  in common cold, 119
  in influenza, 273, 275
  in meningitis, viral, 331
  in mononucleosis, 351
  in mumps, 359
Rheumatoid arthritis, 49–50
Rhinitis, allergic (hay fever), 429–432
  and asthma, 429 (see also Asthma)
Ribavirin
  in influenza, 273
  in pneumonia, 395
Riboflavin (vitamin B2) deficiency, 521
Rickets, 521, 523
Rickettsial infections, Rocky Mountain spotted fever in, 433–434
Rifampin. see also Antibiotics
  in tuberculosis, 499
Rimantadine
  in influenza, 273, 275
  in pneumonia, 395
Ringworm (tinea capitis), 489
Rocky Mountain spotted fever, 433–434
Rogaine (minoxidil) in alopecia, 13
Rosacea, 435–436
Rubella (German measles), 209–210
  immunization against, 209, 267, 451
Ruptured (herniated) disk, 315

-S-

SAD (seasonal affective disorder), 447–448
Salmonella infection, 437–440
Sarcoma, Kaposi's, 295–296
  in HIV infection and AIDS, 247, 295
Sarcoptes scabiei mite, 441
Scabies, 441–442
Schizophrenia, 443–444
Sciatica, back pain in, 313, 315. see also Back pain

Sclerosis, multiple, 355–358
  urinary tract problems in, 355, 357, 505
Scoliosis (spinal curvature), 445–446
Scopolamine
  in inner ear infection, 277
  in Meniere's disease, 325
  in motion sickness, 353
Seasonal affective disorder (SAD), 447–448
Sebaceous gland inflammation (acne), 5–6
Seborrheic blepharitis, 67
  with staphylococcal blepharitis, 67
Sedatives
  in insomnia, 283, 285
  in Meniere's disease, 325
Seizures, 449–452
  in eclampsia, 177, 449
  febrile, 449, 451–452
  in lead poisoning, 305, 307, 449
Seldane (see Antihistamines)
Senility, 147. see also Dementia
Serotonin re-uptake inhibitors
  in anxiety disorders, 37, 39
  in bulimia nervosa, 79
Sertraline (Zoloft) in depression, 149. see also Antidepressant drugs
Sexual abuse and assault, 415–418
  of child, 101, 415, 417
    gonorrhea in, 217
    herpes simplex virus infection in, 243
    syphilis in, 479
  posttraumatic stress disorder in, 417 (see also Posttraumatic stress disorder)
Sexual problems. see also Reproductive problems
  impotence (erectile dysfunction), 271–272
  in multiple sclerosis, 355, 357
  painful intercourse (dyspareunia) in, 377
  in menopause, 333, 377
Sexually transmitted diseases (STDs), 509, 511
  in abused child, 101
    gonorrhea in, 217
    herpes simplex virus infection in, 243
  balanitis (penile inflammation) in, 59
  candidal, 87
  cervical dysplasia in, 95
  chlamydial, 103–104
  genital warts (venereal warts, condyloma acuminata) in, 207
  gonorrhea ("clap") in, 217–218
  hepatitis in, 239, 267
  herpes simplex virus infections in, 241
    genital, 243
  HIV infection and AIDS in, 247–250
  molluscum contagiosum in, 349
  pelvic inflammatory disease (PID) in, 385
  pubic lice in, 229
  scabies in, 441
  in sexual assault, 415, 417
  syphilis in, 479
Shingles (herpes zoster), 99, 453–454
Shock
  allergic (anaphylactic), 25–26
    in food allergy, 25, 193
  hypovolemic, in cholera, 105
  toxic shock syndrome, 491–492
Sickle cell anemia, 29–32
Side effects of drugs (see Drug precautions/interactions)
SIDS (sudden infant death syndrome, crib death), 473–474
Sildenafil (Viagra) in impotence (erectile dysfunction), 271

Sinusitis (inflammation/infection of sinuses), 455–456
Situational anxiety, acute, 37
Skeletal disorders (see Bone and joint problems)
Skin (cutaneous) drug reactions, 139–140, 419
Skin problems
  in acne, 5–6
  in allergies, 153 (see also Allergy)
    to food, 193, 419
  in burns, 83
    in abused child, 83, 101
    in sun exposure, 61, 83, 475–476
  cancer
    in basal cell carcinoma, 61–62
    in Kaposi's sarcoma, 295
    in sunburn, 61, 83, 475
  in candidal infections, 87
  in chickenpox (varicella), 97
  in contact dermatitis, 153–154
  in diaper rash, 163
  in drug reactions, 139–140, 419
  in frostbite, 197
  in German measles (rubella), 209
  in hair excess (hirsutism), 245–246
  in hair loss (alopecia), 13–14
  in herpes simplex virus infections, 241, 243
  in impetigo, 269–270
  in insect bites and stings, 419
  in lupus erythematosus, 481
  in molluscum contagiosum, 349–350
  in parvovirus B19 infection, 383
  in psoriasis, 411–412
  rash in, 419–422 (see also Rash)
  in rosacea, 435–436
  in scabies (Sarcoptes scabiei), 441–442
  in shingles (herpes zoster), 453–454
  in sun exposure
    burns in, 61, 83, 475–476
    cancer risk in, 61, 83, 475
    in photosensitivity, 311
    rash in, 311, 419
  in tinea infections, 489–490
  in toxic shock syndrome, 491
  in warts, 207, 527–530
SLE (systemic lupus erythematosus), 481–484
Sleep
  apnea in, obstructive, 457–460
  in dementia, 147
    in Alzheimer's disease, 19
  in depression, 149
  enuresis in (bed wetting), 63–64, 505
  and insomnia, 283–286
  in posttraumatic stress disorder, 397
  sudden death of infant in, 473
Sleep-walking in dissociative disorders, 167
Snake bites, 461–462
Solar rash, 419. see also Photosensitivity
Sore throat, 463–464
  in common cold, 117 (see also Common cold)
  in influenza, 273
  in laryngitis, 301–302 (see also Laryngitis)
  in pharyngitis, 463
Spastic colon (irritable bowel syndrome), 389–390
Spermicides, 129
Spider bites, 279, 281
Spinal cord inflammation in meningitis, 329–332
Spinal curvature (scoliosis), 445–446

Spinal problems
  back pain in, 315–316
  in osteoporosis, 371, 373
  scoliosis in, 445–446
Spontaneous abortion (miscarriage), 345–346
Sprains and strains, 465–466
"Staph" infections, 67, 471, 491–492
Staphylococcal infections
  blepharitis in, 67
  stye in, 471
  toxic shock syndrome in, 491–492
STDs (see Sexually transmitted diseases)
Sterilization, tubal, 129
Steroids
  in allergic rhinitis (hay fever), 429
  in alopecia, 13
  in anaphylaxis, 25
  in asthma, 51, 53
  in Bell's palsy, 65
  in bursitis, 85
  in carpal tunnel syndrome, 91
  in chronic obstructive pulmonary disease, 109
  in contact dermatitis, 153
  in Crohn's disease, 133
  in diaper rash, 163
  in gingivitis, 211
  in hepatitis, 239
  in insect bites and stings, 281
  precautions/interactions, 13
  in rash, 421
  in rheumatoid arthritis, 49
Stings, insect, 279–282
  anaphylaxis in, 25
Stomach problems. see also Gastrointestinal problems
  cancer in pernicious anemia, 27
  inflammation of lining (gastritis), 201–202
  peptic ulcer disease, 387–388
Stones
  gallstones (cholelithiasis), 199–200
    pancreatitis in, 379
  kidney (nephrolithiasis, renal colic, urolithiasis), 297–300
Stool
  impaction of, 187
  incontinence of (encopresis), 187–188
  softening agents
    in constipation, 125
    in heart attack, 231
    in hemorrhoids, 237
Strains and sprains, 465–466
Stress
  anxiety disorders in, 37–40
  and posttraumatic stress disorder, 37, 39, 397–400
    in rape (sexual assault), 417
  temporomandibular joint syndrome in, 485
  tension headache in, 225
Stress incontinence, 505, 507
Stroke (cerebrovascular accident, brain attack), 467–470
  dementia in, multi-infarct, 147
  in hypertension, 467, 469, 497 (see also Hypertension)
  mini-stroke or transient ischemic attack, 147, 497–498
Stroke in heat exposure (hyperthermia), 235–236
Stye (hordeolum), 471–472
Substance abuse
  of alcohol, 9–12 (see also Alcohol use and alcoholism)
  hepatitis in, 239, 267
  HIV infection and AIDS in, 247

Sudden infant death syndrome (SIDS, crib death), 473–474
Suicidal behavior
   acetaminophen poisoning in, 1
   in Alzheimer's disease, 21
   in bulimia nervosa, 79, 81
   carbon monoxide poisoning in, 89
   in depression, 149, 151
Sulfasalazine
   in Crohn's disease, 133, 135
   in ulcerative colitis, 501, 503
Sun exposure
   rash in, 311, 419
   risk for skin cancer in, 61, 83, 475
   and seasonal affective disorder, 447
   sensitivity to (sun poisoning, photosensitivity), 311–312
      in lupus erythematosus, 481
   sunburn in, 61, 83, 475–476
   in vitamin D deficiency, 521, 523
Sunburn, 83, 475–476
   risk for skin cancer in, 61, 83, 475
Suppositories, rectal, in constipation, 125
Swelling (see Edema)
Swimmer's ear (otitis externa), 477–478
Synthetic salmon calcitonin drugs (Miacalcin, Calcimar, Osteocalcin)
      in osteoporosis, 371
Synthroid (levothyroxine)
   in hypothermia, 261
   in hypothyroidism, 265
Syphilis, 479–480
Systemic lupus erythematosus (SLE), 481–484

-T-

Tagamet (cimetidine) (see H2 blockers)
Tamoxifen. see also Chemotherapy
   in breast cancer, 69, 71
Tampon-related toxic shock syndrome, 491
Tavist (see Antihistamines)
Teeth (see Dental problems)
Temperature-related problems
   in cold exposure
      frostbite in, 197–198
      hypothermia in, 261–264
      rash in, 419
      Raynaud's phenomenon in, 423–424
      febrile seizures in, 449, 451–452
   in heat exposure
      exhaustion and heat stroke in (hyperthermia), 235–236
      rash in, 419
      sunburn in, 61, 83, 475–476
Temporomandibular joint (TMJ) syndrome, 485–486
Tendinitis (inflammation of tendon), 487–488
Tension headaches, 225–228
   chronic, 225
   episodic, 225
Terazosin in hypertension, 255
Terfenadine (Seldane) (see Antihistamines)
Testicular effects of mumps (orchitis), 359
Tetanus immunization, 267, 451. see also Animal bites
Tetracycline. see also Antibiotics
   in acne, 5
   in cholera, 105
   in Rocky Mountain spotted fever, 433
   in rosacea, 435
Theophylline
   in asthma, 51 (see also Anti-asthma drugs)
   in chronic obstructive pulmonary disease, 109
Thiamine (vitamin B1)
   deficiency of, 521, 523
   in dysmenorrhea, 175
Thioridazine (Mellaril)
   in dementia, 147
   in dissociative disorders, 167
Throat, sore (see Sore throat)
Thrombolytic (clot-busting) drugs
   in heart attack, 231
   in stroke, 467
Thyroid problems
   excess (hyperthyroidism), 259–260
   insufficiency (hypothyroidism, myxedema), 265–266
Tick-borne infections, 279, 281
   Lyme disease in, 317–318
   Rocky Mountain spotted fever in, 433–434
Ticlopidine
   in arteriosclerotic heart disease, 43
   in claudication, 115
   in transient ischemic attack and stroke, 467, 497
Timolol (see Beta blockers)
Tinea infections (ring worm, jock itch, athlete's foot), 489–490
   alopecia in, 13
Tinnitus (ringing in ear)
   in inner ear infection, 277
   in Meniere's disease, 325
   in pernicious anemia, 27
Tissue plasminogen activator (alteplase, TPA) in heart attack, 231
TMJ (temporomandibular joint) syndrome, 485–486
alpha-Tocopherol deficiency, 521, 523
Toxemia of pregnancy (eclampsia), 177–178, 401, 449
Toxic conditions (see Poisoning)
Toxic shock syndrome (Staphylococcus aureus), 491–492
Toxoplasma gondii, 493
Toxoplasmosis, 493–496
TPA (tissue plasminogen activator) in heart attack, 231
Transient ischemic attacks (mini-strokes, TIAs), 497–498. see also Stroke
   dementia in, 147
   in hypertension, 497 (see also Hypertension)
Trauma
   in animal bites, 35–36
      rabies in, 413–414
      from snakes, 461–462
   in burns, 83–84
      in abused child, 83, 101
      in sun exposure, 61, 83, 475–476
   bursitis in, 85
   in child abuse, 101 (see also Child abuse)
   in cold exposure, frostbite in, 197
   dissociative disorders in, 167, 169
   in heat exposure, 235
   in insect bites and stings, 279–282
   and posttraumatic stress disorder, 37, 39, 397–400
      in rape (sexual assault), 417
   in sexual abuse and assault, 415–418 (see also Sexual abuse and assault)
   sprains and strains in, 465
   tendinitis in, 487
Travel
   altitude illness in, 15–18
   cholera in, 105

Travel (*Continued*)
  diarrhea in, 165
  jet lag (circadian dysrhythmia) in, 293–294
    and insomnia, 283
  motion sickness in, 353–354
  rabies exposure in, 413
  vaccinations in, 267
Tretinoin (Retin-A) in acne, 5
Tri-cyclic antidepressants. *see also* Antidepressant drugs
  in anxiety disorders, 37, 39
  in insomnia, 283
  in nocturnal enuresis, 63
Trimethoprim-sulfamethoxazole (*see* Antibiotics)
L-Tryptophan in insomnia, 285
Tuberculosis, 499–500
Tumors (*see* Cancer)
Tylenol (*see* Acetaminophen)

-U-

Ulcerative colitis (idiopathic proctocolitis), 501–504. *see also*
    Inflammatory bowel disease
Ulcers
  in blepharitis, staphylococcal, 67
  peptic, 387–388
Urinary incontinence, 505–508
  infections of urinary tract in, 507, 509, 513
  nocturnal, bed wetting in, 63–64, 505
  in prostate problems, 409, 505, 507
  stress, 505, 507
  and vulvovaginitis, estrogen deficient, 525
Urinary tract problems, 505–514. *see also* Genitourinary problems
Urolithiasis (kidney stones, nephrolithiasis, renal colic),
    297–300
Ursodiol in gallstones, 199
Urticaria (hives), 419–422. *see also* Rash; Skin problems
Uterus
  cervical dysplasia of, 95–96
    in papilloma virus infections, 95, 207
  dysfunctional bleeding from, 173–174
  endometriosis of, 179–180
    fertility problems in, 179, 189
UTIs (urinary tract infections), 509–514
  in men, 59, 407, 509–510
  in urinary incontinence, 507, 509, 513
  in women, 511–514
UV light exposure (*see* Sun exposure)

-V-

Vaccination (immunization), 267–268
  cholera, 105
  febrile seizures after, 451
  hepatitis, 239, 267
  influenza, 267, 275, 395
  mumps, 267, 359, 451
  pneumococcal, 267, 393
  in pregnancy, 267
  rabies, 413

  recommendations on, 267–268
  rubella (German measles), 209, 267, 451
  varicella zoster virus, 97, 267
Vaginal problems
  bleeding in pregnancy, 515–516
    miscarriage in, 345, 515 (*see also* Miscarriage)
  in estrogen deficiency, 525–526
  infections, 517–518
    candidal, 87, 517–518
    and tampon-related toxic shock syndrome, 491
Valacyclovir
  in herpes simplex virus infections, 241, 243
  in shingles, 453
Valium (*see* Benzodiazepines)
Varicella (chickenpox), 97–100
  immunization, 97, 267
  shingles after, 99, 453
Varicose veins, 519–520
Vasectomy, 129
Vasodilators
  in claudication, 115
  in heart failure, 121
  in hypertension, 255
Venereal warts (genital warts, condyloma acuminata),
    207–208
Venlafaxine (Effexor) in depression, 149. *see also*
    Antidepressant drugs
Verapamil. *see also* Calcium channel blockers
  in cluster headache, 223
Vertigo (dizziness)
  in inner ear infection, 277
  in Meniere's disease, 325
Viagra (sildenafil) in impotence (erectile dysfunction),
    271
Vibratory urticaria, 419
Vibrio cholerae infection, 105–106
Viral infections
  adenovirus, 7–8
  bronchitis in, acute, 77
  chickenpox (varicella) in, 97–100, 267
  common cold in, 117–120
  croup in, 137–138
  diarrhea in, 165
  German measles (rubella) in, 209, 267
  glomerulonephritis, 216
  hepatitis in, 239–240, 267
  herpes simplex, 241–244
    genital, 241, 243–244
  herpes zoster (shingles), 99, 453–454
  HIV/AIDS, 247–250, 295, 493
  influenza, 267, 273–276
  of liver, 239–240, 267
  meningitis (brain/spinal cord inflammation) in,
      331–332
  molluscum contagiosum in, 349
  mononucleosis in, 351–352
  mumps in, 267, 359
  papilloma virus
    and cervical dysplasia, 95, 207
    and genital warts, 207
  parvovirus B19, 383–384
  pneumonia in, 7, 395–396
  rabies in, 413–414
  sore throat in, 463
  warts in, 207, 527–530

Virilization, 245
Vision problems
   in cataracts, 93
   in glaucoma, 213
   in lazy eye (amblyopia), 303
   in macular degeneration, age-related, 323
   in retinal detachment, 427
Vitamin A deficiency, 521, 523
Vitamin B1
   deficiency of, 521, 523
   in dysmenorrhea, 175
Vitamin B2 deficiency, 521
Vitamin B3 deficiency, 521
Vitamin B6 deficiency, 521, 523
Vitamin B12 deficiency, 27–28, 521
Vitamin C
   in common cold, 117
   deficiency of, 521
Vitamin D
   deficiency of, 521, 523
   in osteoporosis, 371, 373
Vitamin E deficiency, 521, 523
Vitamin K deficiency, 521, 523
Vitamins, 521–524
   deficiency of, 521–524
      anemia in, 27–28, 521
   in macular degeneration, age-related, 323
Vulvovaginitis
   candidal (vaginal yeast infection), 87, 517–518
   in estrogen deficiency, 525–526

-W-

Wakefulness (insomnia), 283–286
Warts, 527–530
   genital (venereal warts, condyloma acuminata), 207–208
   plantar and other nonvenereal, 527–530
"Water pills" (*see* Diuretics)
Water rash, 419
Worms
   pinworms (Enterobius vermicularis), 391–392
   ringworm (tinea capitis), 489
Wounds (*see* Trauma)

-Y-

Yeast infections (candidal), 87–88
   of nails, 87, 361
   vaginal, 87, 517–518

-Z-

Zantac (ranitidine) (*see* H2 blockers)
Zolpidem in insomnia, 283
Zovirax (*see* Acyclovir)

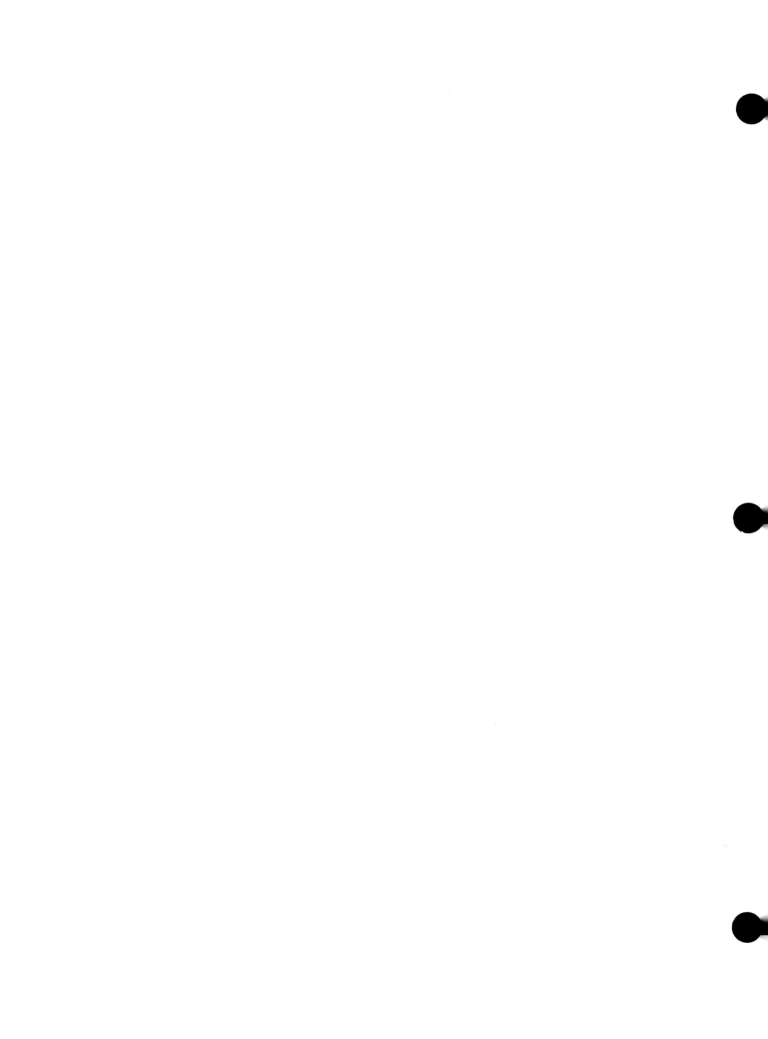

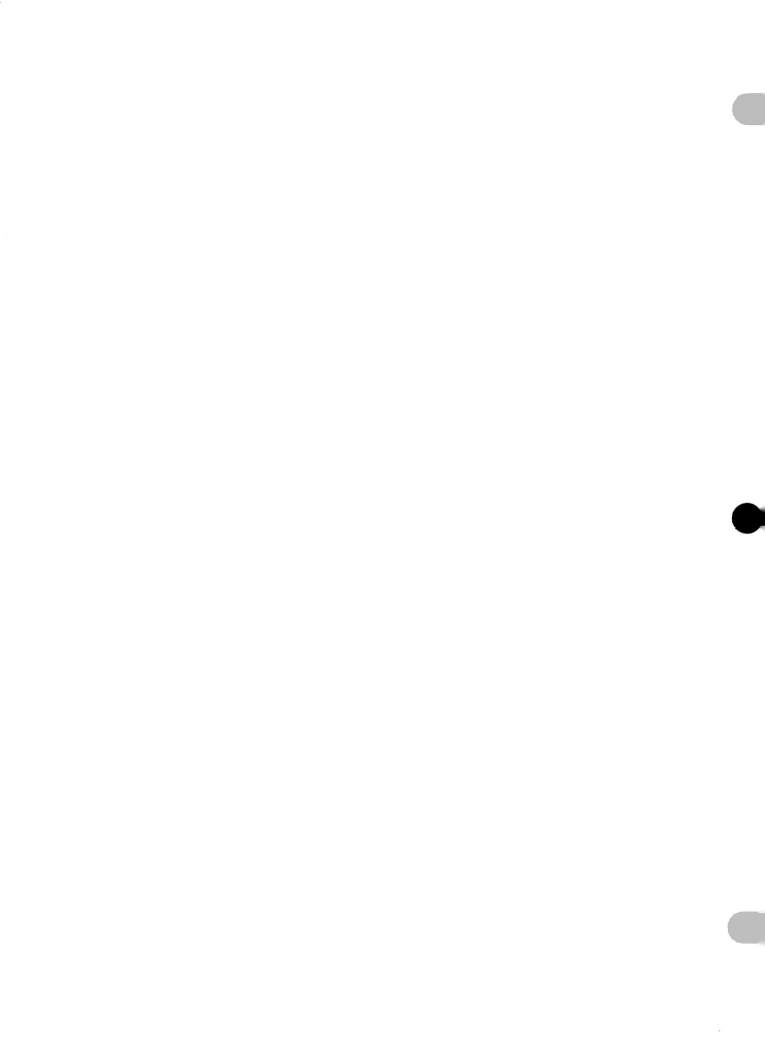

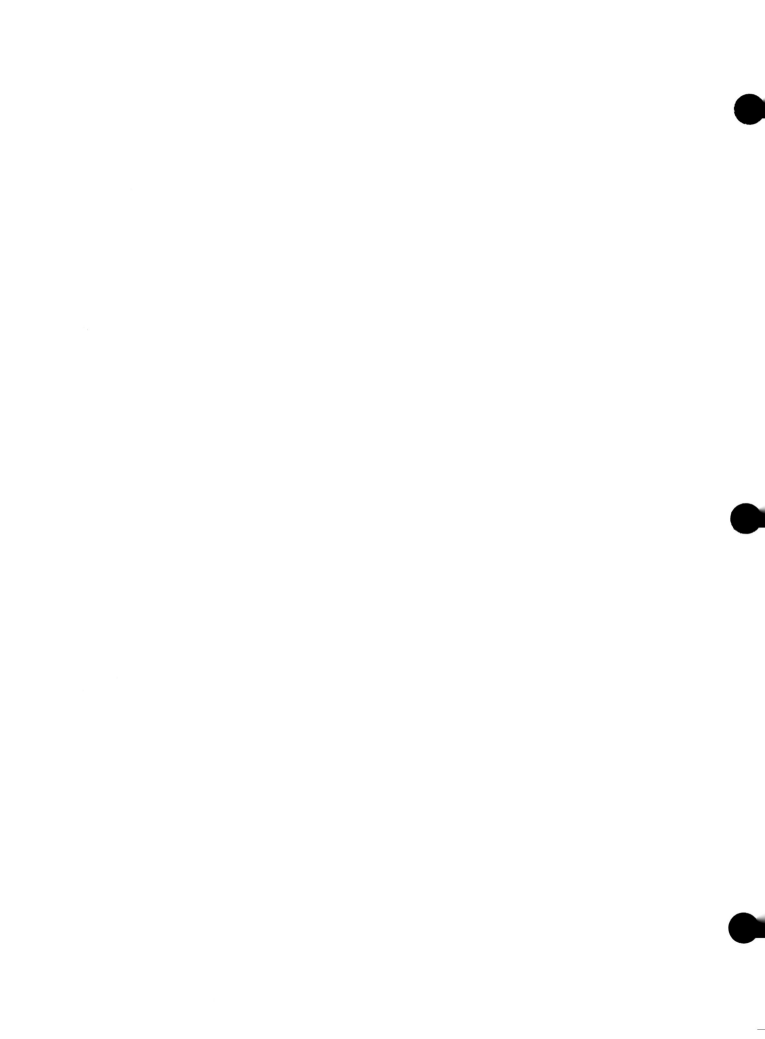